PSYCHOLOGICAL, NEUROPSYCHIATRIC, AND SUBSTANCE ABUSE ASPECTS OF AIDS

Advances in Biochemical Psychopharmacology
Volume 44

Advances in Biochemical Psychopharmacology

Series Editors

E. Costa, M.D.
Director
Fidia Georgetown Institute for the Neurosciences
Georgetown Medical Center
Washington, D.C. 20007

Paul Greengard, Ph.D.
Professor of Molecular and Cellular Neuroscience
The Rockefeller University
1230 York Avenue
New York, New York 10021

Psychological, Neuropyschiatric, and Substance Abuse Aspects of AIDS

Advances in Biochemical Psychopharmacology
Volume 44

Volume Editors

T. Peter Bridge, M.D.

Alcohol, Drug Abuse, and Mental
Health Administration
Intramural Research Program
National Institute of Mental Health
National Institutes of Health
Bethesda, Maryland

Allan F. Mirsky, Ph.D.

Laboratory of Psychology
and Psychopathology
Intramural Research Program
National Institute of Mental Health
National Institutes of Health
Bethesda, Maryland

Frederick K. Goodwin, M.D.

National Institute of Mental Health
National Institutes of Health
Bethesda, Maryland

Raven Press *New York*

Raven Press, 1185 Avenue of the Americas, New York, New York 10036

Made in the United States of America

Library of Congress Cataloging-in-Publication Data

Psychological, neuropsychiatric, and substance abuse
   aspects of AIDS.

   (Advances in biochemical psychopharmacology ; v. 44)
   Includes bibliographies and index.
   1. AIDS (Disease)—Immunological aspects. 2. AIDS (Disease)—
Complications and sequelae. 3. Substance abuse—Complications and
sequelae. 4. Immune system—Effect of chemicals on. I. Bridge,
T. Peter. II. Mirsky, Allan F. III. Goodwin, Frederick K., 1936–
IV. Series. [DNLM: 1. Acquired Immunodeficiency Syndrome—
complications. 2. Acquired Immunodeficiency Syndrome—etiology.
3. Acquired Immunodeficiency Syndrome—psychology. 4. Substance
Abuse—complications. W1 AD437 v.44 / WD 308 P9745]
RM315.A4 vol. 44 [RC607.A26]   615'.78s   87-42723
ISBN 0-88167-396-X   [616.9'792]

9 8 7 6 5 4 3 2 1

Preface

Responding to the changing perception of the relationship of human immunodeficiency virus (HIV) infection to the CNS manifestations of AIDS, the fields of neuroscience, neuropsychology, and substance abuse research are now critical components to the fight against AIDS. HIV is transferred early in the course of the infection to the brain, probably by a macrophage-mediated mechanism. Once present in the CNS, HIV renders the brain a reservoir for constant reinfection of cells susceptible to HIV. Put simply, any treatment for HIV infection must be effective in the brain. Compelling evidence also documents the immensely disabling symptomatology associated with the direct infection of the brain by HIV. Hence the research areas represented in these chapters offer the hope of perhaps the most important treatment for AIDS, that is, in the brain.

The chapters in this volume span relevant research areas from the molecular to the psychosocial, emphasizing traditional and recently developed research approaches to the most important public health challenge of the last half of the 20th century. These articles are of vital interest to those researchers studying the immune, virologic, and CNS-mediated mechanisms of HIV infection. It is exactly these areas that will contribute to the identification, development, and integration of CNS specific treatments for AIDS and mechanisms for the behaviorally oriented prevention of HIV transmission.

Introduction

If there is one overarching characteristic of the field of AIDS research, it is the extraordinarily dynamic pace at which new concepts emerge and are assimilated. This is in large measure due to the considerable productivity of this research area and the availability of resources for this research.

The field of AIDS research underwent several important changes approximately 2 years ago. Prior to that point, it was believed that any central nervous system (CNS) disability seen in AIDS patients was most likely the result of opportunistic infections or lymphomas previously observed in AIDS patients. At that time, there was a growing perception that much of the CNS disability associated with AIDS could not be accounted for by the presence of these opportunistic conditions. The operant assumption was that a direct infection of the brain by the etiologic agent for AIDS, the human immunodeficiency virus (HIV), was causing the clinical triad of what has come to be known as AIDS dementia complex. This triad, composed of cognitive, behavioral, and motoric deficits most closely related to subcortical dementias, has stimulated numerous research strategies, both basic and clinical, described within the chapters presented here. Central to the progress documented in these collected articles in the area of AIDS neuroscience research is the interdigitation of disciplines spanning the molecular to the clinical. Unique to this area of research has been the focus on behavioral impact on disease outcome and behavioral expression as a consequence of disease manifestation.

At about the same time, the central importance of drug abuse in the fight against AIDS became clearly apparent. Not only are intravenous drug abusers (IVDAs) the second most common group at risk for HIV infection after gay and bisexual males, but they represent the most likely conduit of the infection to the heterosexual community. The vast majority of female IVDAs acknowledge relying at least occasionally on prostitution to support their drug addiction. Further, IVDAs are the group most associated with the birth of HIV-infected children. As detailed in the chapters in this volume, exposure to psychoactive agents may well represent yet another risk factor independent of the needle sharing demonstrated to be the primary drug-associated, high-risk behavior involved in the transmission of HIV infection.

Given the similarities of HIV to other lentiviruses, which are neurotropic, the acceptance that HIV would directly produce CNS pathology proceeded quickly. Persuasive data then emerged, documenting the clinical pathologic correlates of a subcortical dementia in AIDS patients in which no space-occupying or tissue-destructive lesion was identified. In the short period of 2 years, therefore, the relevance of neuroscience to the fight against AIDS has gone from the occasional consult for choice of CNS antifungals or for treatment of secondary depression to potentially providing the final, and we think most important, treatment for AIDS— that is, in the CNS.

HIV not only infects the brain, but crosses the blood brain barrier early in the course of the infection. The brain remains a reservoir for continual reinfection of susceptible cells, i.e., those with the CD4 or OKT4 receptor. Hence any ultimately successful treatment for HIV infection must penetrate the CNS, and do so in effective concentrations that can kill the virus or render it nontoxic. Absent such therapies, we face institution of continuous antiviral treatments to arrest immune dysfunction in the 1 to 1½ million HIV-infected persons in the United States. Worse than this would be the potential scenario that only peripherally effective anti-HIV treatments would be available. Such an outcome would lead us to envision growing numbers of immunologically intact HIV-infected persons exposed for ever-increasing periods of time to the toxic presence of HIV and HIV products in the CNS.

Propelled principally by the work of Navia and Price (1,2), acceptance of the concept of an HIV-mediated CNS disorder resulted in the codification of a diagnostic schema for ADC within the last 2 years. Most recently, the Centers for Disease Control modified the criteria by which patients are diagnosed as having AIDS. The diagnosis of AIDS can now be made by the presence of dementia in a seropositive individual without the requisite opportunistic infection or Kaposi's sarcoma. This action was based on the relatively common observation that dementia can be the initial clinical presentation of AIDS in as many as one-fourth of patients.

Although the vast majority of cases of AIDS have been seen in adults, the disease also appears in infants born to seropositive parents, primarily IVDAs. It is clear that HIV infection in children is as neurotropic, if not more so, than in adults.

Important data are now emerging from several studies that HIV antibodies can be identified in the cerebrospinal fluid (CSF) of patients in the early stages of HIV infection. Further data from these asymptomatic and lymphadenopathy patients indicate that HIV can be recovered by culture techniques from the CSF as well. Given what are persuasive data that HIV enters the CNS early in the course of the infection, it would likely follow that neuropsychiatric abnormalities would also appear early in the natural history of the disease. This is an area of considerable research activity and importance emerging from a rapidly changing view of the importance of neuroscience research to the understanding and treatment for AIDS.

The prospects for the treatment of HIV infection in the CNS are not relentlessly dismal. Several antiviral studies have focused on the CNS manifestations of HIV infection as outcome measures. These studies, although quite preliminary in their nature, indicate that relatively brief treatment periods by drugs such as AZT or Peptide T can lead to reversal to normative values in such neuropsychiatric measures as cognitive assessment and brain imaging including PET and MRI scans. Although far from providing definitive evidence that such drugs are efficacious at present, these studies make the point that research for medical treatment and prevention must utilize the methods of neuroscience research to provide effective treatment for AIDS and HIV infection. Such research will span the cellular modes of transmission of the virus into the brain; the attachment and entrance mechanisms of HIV, or its products, into cells of the CNS; behavioral correlates of HIV infection including risk factors, cofactors, and symptomatic expression secondary to the presence of HIV in the CNS; and treatment modalities specific to the CNS including cognitive impairment, drug abuse, affective disorder, and motor dysfunction.

T. Peter Bridge, M.D.

REFERENCES

1. Navia, B. A., Jordan, B. D., and Price, R. W. (1986): The AIDS dementia complex I. Clinical features. *Ann. Neurol.*, 19:517–524.
2. Navia, B., and Price, R. W. (1987): AIDS dementia complex as the presenting sole manifestation of HIV infection. *Ann. Neurol.*, 44:65–69.

Contents

Contributors

Robert Ader
Department of Psychiatry
University of Rochester
*   School of Medicine and Dentistry*
Rochester, New York 14642

Rob Berman
Section on Brain Biochemistry
Clinical Neuroscience Branch
Intramural Research Program
National Institute of Mental Health
Alcohol, Drug Abuse,
*   and Mental Health Administration*
National Institutes of Health
Bethesda, Maryland 20892

J. Edwin Blalock
Department of Physiology and Biophysics
University of Alabama at Birmingham
Birmingham, Alabama 35294

D. K. Blanchard
Department of Medical Microbiology
*   and Immunology*
University of South Florida
*   College of Medicine*
Tampa, Florida 33612

George Bone
Laboratory of Clinical Studies
National Institute on Alcohol Abuse
*   and Alcoholism*
Bethesda, Maryland 20892

T. Peter Bridge
Alcohol, Drug Abuse,
*   and Mental Health Administration*
Intramural Research Program
National Institute of Mental Health
National Institutes of Health
Bethesda, Maryland 20892

Pim Brouwers
Laboratory of Psychology and
*   Psychopathology*
Intramural Research Program
National Institute of Mental Health
National Institutes of Health
Bethesda, Maryland 20892

Nicholas Cohen
Department of Microbiology
*   and Immunology*
University of Rochester
*   School of Medicine and Dentistry*
Rochester, New York 14642

Samuel I. Cohen
Department of Psychiatry
Boston University School of Medicine
Boston, Massachusetts 02118, and
Health and Behavior Branch
Division of Basic Science
National Institute of Mental Health
National Institutes of Health
Rockville, Maryland 20857

Don C. Des Jarlais
New York State Division
*   of Substance Abuse Services*
New York, New York 10047

L. David Dion
Department of Physiology and Biophysics
University of Alabama at Birmingham
Birmingham, Alabama 35294

R. M. Donahoe
Laboratory of Psychoimmunology
Department of Psychiatry
Emory University School of Medicine
Georgia Mental Health Institute
Atlanta, Georgia 30306

Diana Donnelly-Roberts
Departments of Cell Biology
  and Pharmacology
Yale University School of Medicine
New Haven, Connecticut 06510

Michael J. Eckardt
Laboratory of Clinical Studies
National Institute on Alcohol Abuse
  and Alcoholism
Bethesda, Maryland 20892

A. Falek
Human and Behavioral Genetics
  Laboratory
Department of Psychiatry
Emory University School of Medicine
Georgia Mental Health Institute
Atlanta, Georgia 30306

William L. Farrar
Laboratory of Molecular
  Immunoregulation
Biological Response Modifiers Program
Division of Cancer Treatment
National Cancer Institute
Frederick Cancer Research Facility
Frederick, Maryland 21701

Herman Friedman
Department of Medical Microbiology
  and Immunology
University of South Florida
  College of Medicine
Tampa, Florida 33612

Samuel R. Friedman
Narcotic and Drug Research, Inc.
New York, New York 10027

Ronald Glaser
Department of Medical Microbiology
  and Immunology
Comprehensive Cancer Center
The Ohio State University
  College of Medicine
Columbus, Ohio 43210

Curtis C. Harris
Laboratory of Human Carcinogenesis
National Cancer Institute
National Institutes of Health
Bethesda, Maryland 20892

Harry W. Haverkos
Clinical Medicine Branch
Division of Clinical Research
National Institute on Drug Abuse
Alcohol, Drug Abuse,
  and Mental Health Administration
Rockville, Maryland 20857

Edward Hawrot
Departments of Cell Biology
  and Pharmacology
Yale University School of Medicine
New Haven, Connecticut 06510

Joanna M. Hill
Section on Brain Biochemistry
Clinical Neuroscience Branch
Intramural Research Program
National Institute of Mental Health
Alcohol, Drug Abuse,
  and Mental Health Administration
National Institutes of Health
Bethesda, Maryland 20892

Thomas R. Jerrells
Department of Pathology
University of Texas Medical Branch
Galveston, Texas 77550

Russell T. Joffe
Biological Psychiatry Branch
Intramural Research Program
National Institute of Mental Health
National Institutes of Health
Bethesda, Maryland 20892

Janice Kiecolt-Glaser
Department of Psychiatry
The Ohio State University
  College of Medicine
Columbus, Ohio 43210

Patricia L. Kilian
Department of Immunopharmacology
Hoffman-LaRoche
Nutley, New Jersey 07110

Thomas W. Klein
Department of Medical Microbiology
  and Immunology
University of South Florida
  College of Medicine
Tampa, Florida 33612

H. Clifford Lane
Laboratory of Immunoregulation
National Institute of Allergy and
 Infectious Disease
National Institutes of Health
Bethesda, Maryland 20892

Thomas L. Lentz
Departments of Cell Biology
 and Pharmacology
Yale University School of Medicine
New Haven, Connecticut 06510

Maxine A. Lesniak
Diabetes Branch
National Institute of Diabetes, Digestive
 and Kidney Diseases
National Institutes of Health
Bethesda, Maryland 20892

Sandra M. Levy
Pittsburgh Cancer Institute
University of Pittsburgh
 School of Medicine
Pittsburgh, Pennsylvania 15213

Dean L. Mann
Laboratory of Human Carcinogenesis
National Cancer Institute
National Institutes of Health
Bethesda, Maryland 20892

Cheryl A. Marietta
Laboratory of Physiologic
 and Pharmacologic Studies
National Insitute on Alcohol Abuse
 and Alcoholism
Rockville, Maryland 20852

George E. Mark
Laboratory of Human Carcinogenesis
National Cancer Institute
National Insitutes of Health
Bethesda, Maryland 20892

Allan F. Mirsky
Laboratory of Psychology
 and Psychopathology
Intramural Research Program
National Institute of Mental Health
National Institutes of Health
Bethesda, Maryland 20892

Catherine A. Newton
Department of Medical Microbiology
 and Immunology
University of South Florida
 College of Medicine
Tampa, Florida 33612

David G. Ostrow
Department of Psychiatry
University of Michigan
 School of Medicine, and
Ann Arbor Veterans Administration
 Medical Center
Ann Arbor, Michigan 48105

Candace B. Pert
Section of Brain Biochemistry
Clinical Neuroscience Branch
Intramural Research Program
National Institute of Mental Health
National Institutes of Health
Bethesda, Maryland 20892

Andrea Pfeifer
Laboratory of Human Carcinogenesis
National Cancer Institute
National Institutes of Health
Bethesda, Maryland 20892

Susan Pross
Department of Medical Microbiology
 and Immunology
University of South Florida
 College of Medicine
Tampa, Florida 33612

Jesse Roth
Diabetes Branch
National Institute of Diabetes,
 Digestive and Kidney Disease
National Institutes of Health
Bethesda, Maryland 20892

David R. Rubinow
Biological Psychiatry Branch
Intramural Research Program
National Institute of Mental Health
National Institutes of Health
Bethesda, Maryland 20892

Michael R. Ruff
Cellular Immunology Section
Laboratory of Microbiology
and Immunology
National Institute of Dental Research
National Institutes of Health
Bethesda, Maryland 20892

Frank Ruscetti
Laboratory of Molecular
Immunoregulation
Biological Response Modifiers Program
National Cancer Institute
Frederick, Maryland 21701

Steven Specter
Department of Medical Microbiology
and Immunology
University of South Florida
College of Medicine
Tampa, Florida 33612

Kathleen Squillace
Laboratory of Psychology and
Psychopathology
Intramural Research Program
National Institute of Mental Health
National Institutes of Health
Bethesda, Maryland 20892

Lydia Temoshok
Department of Psychiatry
Langley Porter Psychiatric Institute
University of California at San Francisco
School of Medicine
San Francisco, California 94143

Forrest F. Weight
Laboratory of Physiologic
and Pharmacologic Studies
National Institute on Alcohol Abuse
and Alcoholism
Rockville, Maryland 20852

Raymond Widen
Department of Medical Microbiology
and Immunology
University of South Florida
College of Medicine
Tampa, Florida 33612

Paul T. Wilson
Departments of Cell Biology
and Pharmacology
Yale University School of Medicine
New Haven, Connecticut 06510

PSYCHOLOGICAL, NEUROPSYCHIATRIC, AND SUBSTANCE ABUSE ASPECTS OF AIDS

Advances in Biochemical Psychopharmacology
Volume 44

Psychological, Neuropsychiatric, and
Substance Abuse Aspects of AIDS,
edited by T. Peter Bridge et al.
Raven Press, New York © 1988.

AIDS and HIV CNS Disease: A Neuropsychiatric Disorder

T. Peter Bridge

Alcohol, Drug Abuse, and Mental Health Administration, Intramural Research Program, National Institute of Mental Health, National Institutes of Health, Bethesda, Maryland 20892

Identified as the number-one health priority of the United States Department of Health and Human Services, the acquired immunodeficiency syndrome (AIDS) has become the object of intensive medical research in the United States as well as internationally, and massive prevention and education efforts to modify high risk behaviors are under way.

The infection is not known to have existed in this country prior to 1977 and presumably entered the United States with infected individuals from Africa, through Haiti. AIDS was first observed to occur in the United States in gay males in 1981 (14,15). Transmission of the illness occurred so rapidly that it is estimated there are between one and two million persons in the United States who have been exposed to the virus (14,15).

Compared to earlier epidemics, we know a great deal about AIDS. Gathered over a relatively short period of time, our knowledge about AIDS results in large measure from a decade of retrovirology research that preceded the appearance of the virus-caused illness. Because we were able to assemble currently available medical technology, medical research has (a) identified the etiologic agent, human immunodeficiency virus (HIV), for the illness (5,30,45), (b) developed a diagnostic test to screen blood supplies for the presence of antibody to the virus (68), and (c) begun identification and evaluation of antiviral agents and development of vaccines against HIV (25).

HIV CNS DISEASE

Although much remains to be accomplished in the fight against AIDS, current knowledge of the illness spans medical research fields such as epidemiology, immunology, and virology and has recently expanded to include neuroscience and addiction research. AIDS is not only a viral immune disorder, it is also a neuropsychiatric disorder (11,38,52). AIDS and HIV patients develop neuropsychiatric symptoms believed secondary to a direct infection of the brain by HIV (31,37,44,52,56,64). Characteristic of this infection, AIDS patients demonstrate cognitive, motor, and affective symptoms, sometimes antecedent to the diagnosis of AIDS (52). Nearly 25% of all AIDS patients are intravenous drug abusers capable of transmitting their infection sexually and by needle sharing (33). Although the central nervous system (CNS) aspects of AIDS were not an immediate focus in the research on AIDS, the knowledge base in retrovirology predicted the neurotrophic nature of HIV. In addition, the evolving field of psychoneuroimmunology, which is defining the extensive interdigitations of the immune, endocrine, and central nervous systems, also predicts that any disorder of the immune system will have interacting ramifications in neuropsychiatric function (1,6,7,10,57).

AIDS research is entering a second phase in which both neuroscience and addiction research must be involved as well as the continuing contributions of epidemiology, immunology, and virology. Furthermore, these research fields are most likely to be maximally productive when their efforts are as interdigitated as the physiologic systems on which their research is based.

Although the characteristics of the retroviruses predict CNS involvement in AIDS (34), it nonetheless came as something of a clinical "surprise" that AIDS patients were manifesting early CNS symptomatology. It is now generally conceded that cognitive impairment is nearly ubiquitous in AIDS patients (67). In fact, some patients demonstrate signs of cognitive decline in advance of the diagnosis of AIDS (52). These observations are independent of the presence of opportunistic CNS disease in AIDS patients and have fostered considerable research interest in the neuropsychiatric manifestations of HIV infection, in the pathologic evidence for HIV infection of the brain, and in the utilization of CNS diagnostic methods to detect the presence of HIV infectious processes in AIDS patients.

The manifestations associated with CNS HIV disease include early cognitive (forgetfulness, poor concentration, confusion, slowed thinking) and motor symptoms (loss of balance, poor handwriting, leg weakness) as well as depression, fatigue, paranoia, hallucinations, and anergy. Early signs include impaired cognition, moderate to severe psychomotor retardation, ataxia, tremor, paresis, pyramidal tract signs, as well as behavioral signs (apathy, dysphoria, psychosis, regression) (52).

In the later course of the illness, frank dementia is apparent with mutism, ataxia, hypertonia, moderate to severe paresis, incontinence, tremor, facial release signs, myoclonus, seizures, and psychosis (52).

NEUROPATHOLOGIC FINDINGS IN HIV DISEASE

Based on these clinical findings, researchers set out to assess the evidence for the presence of HIV in the brain in association with cognitive and behavioral symptoms in AIDS patients. These workers demonstrated HIV in the brains and CSF of AIDS patients with various neuropsychiatric symptoms thought attributable to HIV infection of the brain. Less clear, however, was the likelihood of finding HIV within brain cells. Epstein and co-workers identified retrovirus-like particles in both CSF and brain tissue at autopsy from AIDS patients, including children with AIDS (23,24). In a study of two patients with HIV dementia, Koenig (44) demonstrated the presence of HIV in giant mononuclear and multinucleated cells in their brains. Immunohistochemical and *in situ* hybridization techniques showed multinucleated giant cells with HIV RNA near blood vessels in brain and clustered in brain parenchyma. Electron microscopy demonstrated giant multinucleated cells in brain parenchyma with budding HIV virions. Retrovirus particles were not observed in lymphocytes or endothelial or glial cells. In another study, Stoler and colleagues (64) also used *in situ* hybridization techniques to detect HIV RNA and observed the presence of HIV RNA in macrophages, as had Koenig and colleagues, but also found evidence for HIV in astrocytes, oligodendroglia, and occasional neurons. Levy and colleagues (46) also isolated HIV in both CSF and brain tissue of patients with AIDS. Gabuzda and co-workers (29) used immunoperoxidase methods to study the brains of 13 AIDS patients post-mortem. Whereas 11 of the 13 demonstrated positive HIV viral cultures, only five of the 13 demonstrated the presence of HIV antigen observed by the immunoperoxidase method. In those HIV antigen-positive brains, the rare positive cells, resembling monocytes/macrophages, were observed associated with capillaries and near microglial nodules.

Having established that HIV is present in brain specimens of AIDS patients with neuropsychiatric impairment, scientists next endeavored to determine the means by which HIV entered the brain. The OKT4 or CD4 receptor had been established as the entry route for HIV into the lymphocyte (21,43). Pert and colleagues demonstrated the presence of the OKT4 receptor in brain, thus arriving at the shared route of entry for the CNS and the immune system (56). In addition, Ho and colleagues (37) also demonstrated that macrophages can be infected by HIV, thus establishing a mode of transfer of HIV from the periphery to the CNS. With these data, then, it can be concluded that HIV has a specific affinity not only for the OKT4 lymphocyte but also for cells in the CNS.

If HIV can be identified in brain and cultured from it, the next question of paramount concern is whether or not the virus can transfer from brain to other cells susceptible to HIV infection. This is of particular concern for the uninfected hematopoietic cells. Gartner and colleagues demonstrated that a brain specimen from an AIDS patient with dementia produced HIV in culture and was capable of transferring the infection to peripheral monocytes (31). The source of the infection in brain was presumably monocyte/macrophage cells present in the patient's brain tissue. Ominously, Chiodi and colleagues (16) report recovering HIV from the CSF of a seropositive person without active HIV neuropsychiatric symptomatology. Furthermore, production of HIV in culture was stimulated by contact with PHA-stimulated blast cells, suggesting evidence that the CNS can function as a reservoir for HIV infection in the face of adequate immunologic challenge.

To specify the histopathological substrate of the AIDS dementia complex, Navia and colleagues (51) conducted neuropathological examinations of the brains and spinal cords of all the AIDS patients. The findings indicated mild to moderate–mild atrophy. The principal microscopic abnormalities were reactive cellular changes in the white matter and subcortical gray structures. Inflammation was present and included perivascular and parenchymal infiltrates of lymphocytes and macrophages. White matter abnormalities consisted of three types: ill-defined large areas of pallor, focal rarefaction containing infiltrates, and vacuolation. A generally diffuse appearance was the most prominent feature in the centrum semiovale region. Vacuolation was most commonly noted in the centrum semiovale and less often in the internal capsule, brainstem, and cerebellum. In some instances the areas of vacuolation contained multinucleated cells and macrophages.

Subcortical gray matter involvement was characterized by macrophages, multinucleated cells, and lymphocytes with reactive astrocytosis and generally involved the putamen, caudate, and claustrum and less frequently the globus pallidus. Similar lesions were found in the brainstem, particularly in the pons. Several patients had severe subcortical gray matter involvement that ran parallel to the white matter changes or occasionally was the most conspicuous disorder. In contrast, the cerebral cortex was relatively spared, with astrocytosis being restricted to the lowest layers. Marked cortical neuronal loss and gross architectural changes were detected only in the brains of those with the most advanced disease. White matter pallor and vacuolation were primarily seen in demented patients but were also observed in nondemented patients. On the other hand, subcortical gray matter changes were discovered in the basal ganglia and brainstem of more than 80% of patients with dementia, whereas the same abnormalities were present in fewer than a third of those without dementia. Vacuolar myelopathy occurred in almost 30% of all AIDS patients, and over 90% of persons with this neuropathological finding were demented.

Based on their findings, Navia and co-workers (51) proposed the following summary of the pathological progression of AIDS. The earliest features include diffuse pallor and mild vacuolation of the white matter accompanied by mild perivascular lymphocytic reaction. These changes, frequently seen in the nondemented group of patients, are consistent with their subclinical state and suggest that these conditions occur in the great majority of AIDS patients. As the disease progresses past the asymptomatic stage, demyelination and cell reactions become more prominent. In patients with the most severe symptoms, the presence of macrophages and multinucleated cells and widespread loss of white matter substance are conspicuous and are clinically associated with profound cognitive impairment. In contrast, patients in the demented group without multinucleated cells were distinguished by the remarkably bland nature of the CNS changes despite severe dementia.

Although autopsy studies find fewer than 5% of the brains of AIDS patients without any demonstrable defect (51,52), it is nonetheless troubling that there is a relative absence of CNS pathology detectable either pre- or postmortem that is associated with dramatic HIV CNS symptomatology. Without question, the potential for devastating cognitive change with AIDS and HIV infection has been demonstrated, but the underlying neuropathologic processes are far from clear. Because these changes occur in the absence of other opportunistic CNS infections or neoplasms, the presumption remains that the neuropsychiatric pathology demonstrated is a consequence of a direct HIV infection of the brain. The data are not yet sufficient to provide an explanation of the mechanisms by which HIV is capable of producing the degree of clinical pathology observed when autopsy studies demonstrate relatively minimal presence of the virus in brain cells. Although the approaches to this research challenge may be multiple, one of those approaches must be the continued postmortem examination of patients with HIV CNS disease.

BRAIN IMAGING IN HIV CNS DISEASE

Brain imaging has proved to be essential in the evaluation of focal and diffuse disease. Several neurodiagnostic studies were performed on AIDS patients with dementia by Navia and colleagues (52). Computed tomographic (CT) scans, with or without contrast enhancement, demonstrated varying degrees of cortical atrophy in 32 patients. The cortical atrophy was accompanied by ventricular dilatation. Magnetic resonance imaging (MRI) studies in three subjects also found discrete focal areas of increased signal on T2 imaging in the white matter. Lumbar puncture studies revealed a series of elevated protein levels that progressively increased during the clinical course of the illness. The cortical atrophy was detected by CT scans and MRI 1 to 4 months before the onset of clinical dementia, suggesting that these imaging techniques may provide evidence of CNS pathology prior to the appearance of any clinical symptoms (51,53).

MRI is a sensitive tool for detecting CNS lesions. Recent studies have shown that patchy white matter lesions (focal areas of increased signal intensity on T2-weighted images) seen on MRI scans often reflect areas of focal rarefaction and perivascular atrophy, pathological changes similar to those seen in early stages of the AIDS dementia complex even prior to the onset of the symptoms of dementia. De La Paz (22) observed brain abnormalities in 18 of 24 patients with AIDS. The most common abnormality was toxoplasmosis. Significantly more patients and lesions were identified by MRI than by CT scans. Other brain lesions observed include lymphoma, progressive multifocal leukoencephalopathy, candidiasis, and diffuse bilateral white matter abnormalities. These diffuse white matter abnormalities were considered likely to be reflective of AIDS dementia complex. De La Paz reported that MRI screening of AIDS patients may influence treatment and monitoring of therapy by detecting lesions at an earlier stage than is possible with CT scans and demonstrating any change in their appearance and number during treatment. In conclusion, De La Paz reports that it is appropriate to screen all AIDS patients for neurological disease with MRI.

Post and colleagues (58), in a prospective study comparing the abilities of high-resolution CT and MRI in the detection and evaluation of CNS disease in neurologically symptomatic patients with AIDS, showed that MRI imaging was superior to CT scanning in the evaluation of white matter lesions and detection of small lesions surrounded by an edema that is probably related to the AIDS dementia complex. Levy and colleagues (47) reported radiologic studies of 200 AIDS patients with neurological symptoms. They showed that of 81 patients with initially normal CT scans, four developed progressive neurological illness. In addition, 75 patients had CT evidence of diffuse cerebral atrophy, and 12 of these later developed other CT abnormalities or postmortem CNS disease. The CT scans showed mass lesions in 44 patients and later in an additional seven patients. The authors also report that MRI seems to be more sensitive than CT in detecting intercranial disease related to AIDS.

HIV DEMENTIA: NEUROPSYCHOLOGIC MANIFESTATIONS

Several researchers have pointed out the similarities between the clinical profiles of the AIDS dementia complex and other subcortical dementias (51,52). Although the validity of the concept of subcortical dementias is still controversial, these authors argue that the clinical manifestations of AIDS correspond more closely to those of the subcortical dementias. Because of the lack of well-designed studies on the behavioral and clinical symptoms of AIDS dementia, however, the exact nature of this illness still needs to be detailed and verified.

Because a variety of diseases can cause dementia, there is a definite need to describe the distinctive characteristics of each syndrome. In the early 1970s, the term subcortical dementia was introduced to describe the intellectual deterioration secondary to diseases that are primarily distinguished by pathologic alterations in subcortical (i.e., striatum, thalamus, and brainstem) rather than cortical structures (2,50). Thus, the subcortical dementias have included progressive supranuclear palsy, Huntington's disease (HD), Parkinson's disease (PD), and other extrapyramidal disorders (19), whereas the classic cortical dementia is Alzheimer's disease (AD).

The current clinical picture of these two types of dementia is based on numerous investigations (2,19,39). The cardinal features of subcortical dementias include slowing of mental processes, progressive impairment of memory (i.e., difficulty in retrieving already stored material), and deficits in manipulating or using spontaneously acquired information (i.e., poor problem solving). However, unlike the cortical dementias, higher-order associative function is preserved, and intellectual impairment is milder in the subcortical dementias. Other clinical signs are personality and affective changes and dysfunctions of the motor system, including speech, posture, gait, motor speed, and movement disorder.

In contrast, the prominent characteristics of cortical dementias usually involve progressive deterioration of memory (i.e., difficulty in learning new material) and higher-order associative functions. The latter include increasing impairment of expressive and comprehensive language (aphasia), misnaming of objects, failure to recall names of acquaintances (anomia), word intrusion, perceptual misinterpretations (agnosia), and deficiencies in perceptual–motor activity (apraxia). Personality tends to be unconcerned or euphoric, and mood is normal. The motor system is also generally unaffected.

This distinction between cortical and subcortical dementias on the basis of strict anatomical criteria, however, has been strongly criticized because of the lack of clinical and neuropsychological evidence to validate the hypothetical framework (70). Few systematic controlled studies have been conducted. More importantly, pathological studies have indicated that both cortical and subcortical structures are involved in most dementias. On the one hand, subcortical changes have been found in AD patients in the nucleus basalis of Meynert (4,65,72), locus coeruleus (9,26,36,55), and raphe nucleus (20). Similar neuronal loss has been observed in the nucleus basalis and locus coeruleus for some, but not all, subcortical dementias (13,17,71). At the same time, there have been reports of cortical alterations in PD (3,8,32,35,40) and HD (12,27,49) that are indistinguishable from those in patients with AD (8,35). Therefore, there may actually exist varying degrees of independence and interdependence between the involvement of subcortical and cortical regions of the brain, and the saliency of the specific CNS area may change over the course of the dementing condition.

Although the anatomical data raise serious questions regarding the accuracy of the cortical/subcortical distinction, the evidence does not necessarily invalidate the use of a cortical/subcortical classification system to differentiate dementias on a clinical basis. Based on current knowledge of various dementias, research efforts must be directed toward the development of reliable, objective, and descriptive cognitive and motor instruments for the diagnosis and continued monitoring of the AIDS dementia complex.

Prospective studies of AIDS patients should prove to be very important in the development of AIDS-relevant neuropsychological assessment instruments, allowing for the collection of longitudinal data on the systematic specification of mental and motor deficits observed during different sequential stages of HIV illness. As mentioned earlier, neuroimaging techniques may also detect CNS pathology before the onset of any clinical symptoms. Consequently, the combined used of neuropsychological and MRI evaluations may provide a very sophisticated approach for the early diagnosis of neurological changes in AIDS patients. Systematic comparisons of the AIDS and other subcortical dementias may further generate invaluable insights into the anatomical and histopathologic correlates of the cognitive, motor, and behavioral disturbances of this type of illness and provide evidence for the validation of the concept of subcortical dementias.

HIV NEUROPSYCHIATRIC DISEASE

Given the extent of CNS disease associated with HIV infection, it comes as no surprise that there are neuropsychiatric symptoms specific to this infection. Although some of the boundaries between neuropathology, neuropsychology, and neuropsychiatry can blur in a disease such as HIV CNS infection, there are nonetheless

HIV-related neuropsychiatric syndromes that have emerged. The cognitive changes presumed secondary to a direct HIV infection of the brain have been discussed above, but behavioral and affective components of this infection exist as well. Additionally, motor changes discussed previously complete the spectrum of HIV CNS disease identified at present.

In the current social environment that surrounds the AIDS epidemic, it is not facetious to observe that there is considerable psychological distress among those who perceive themselves to be at risk for AIDS, informally referred to as "AIDS phobia." Further, massive public anxiety regarding the spread of the epidemic from the currently identified risk groups to the general population exists as well. Although supportive psychosocial and information dissemination techniques have been employed on an individual basis in addressing the needs of seronegative risk group members, information and education techniques are also being employed to assuage the unrealistic fears of the general public regarding the spread of HIV infection. In both instances, however, the consistent delivery of data-based recommendations regarding behavioral change and/or precautions necessary to prevent the spread of HIV infection is needed. For those whose behavioral change requirements are the greatest or are perceived as being accomplished with difficulty, supportive interventions already employed in substance abuse or medical care settings are appropriate (e.g., Alcoholics Anonymous, colostomy groups, etc.).

Among seropositive individuals, there are persuasive data that considerable affective response is present. Both anxiety and depression are present, as might be expected in the face of a life-threatening illness with no known effective treatment. Although apparently counterintuitive, it is those individuals with ARC, rather than AIDS, who demonstrate the greatest affective response to the illness (38). Experientially, patients perceive their reduced psychological distress to be associated with the resolution of their fate: AIDS is fatal; ARC may not be. The relationship of this distress, which is common but not universal among ARC patients, to the progression of the illness is speculative but an intriguing research lead.

The association of antecedent psychiatric illness, particularly affective, with disease trajectory in HIV infection may prove to be another research lead worthy of pursuit. The presence of depression, in one study of AIDS patients, was associated with a history of prior depression (41). Immunodysregulation associated with depression has been shown in various studies (60–63). Further, psychoactive agents used to treat these disorders have demonstrated immunomodulatory effects as well (48,66). As before, the effective impact of all of these factors remains to be demonstrated in HIV illness but cannot be dismissed. Thought disorders and mania have as well been observed in association with HIV infection (28,42,54), and retroviral infection has been the subject of hypothetical proposals in psychotic disorders (18).

Early reports of treatment for HIV infection indicate that relatively short periods of treatment demonstrate changes in neuropsychological and brain-imaging studies (69,73). As encouraging as these pilot studies may ultimately prove to be, these results underscore the considerable dearth of knowledge of the mechanism by which HIV exacts its effects in the CNS. Such responsiveness of the CNS to treatment is suggestive of a biologic response-mediated mechanism for HIV dementia rather than cell death. Further, the identification of the CD4 receptor in brain and of potential synthetic and endogenous ligands for that receptor points to research directions in HIV pathophysiology and intervention (56,59).

CONCLUSION

Both the evidence presented to date and summarized above and the data contained in the other chapters in this volume persuasively argue that HIV infection is a neuropsychiatric disorder as well as an immunologic disorder. Although the data point unquestionably to an infectious process that initiates the physiologic sequelae comprising AIDS and HIV disease, many questions about the pathophysiology remain unanswered. First and foremost, of course, is the absence of effective treatment for the infection and of available vaccines. The data presented here argue, however, that success in achieving the goals of developing treatment and prevention measures must involve the fields of neuroscience, behavior, and substance abuse research.

The interdigitations of the immune and central nervous systems already described in non-AIDS research make the point that these two biological systems are interconnected, forming a homeostatic network in the body. They contain and produce peptide compounds capable of eliciting responses in both the system of origin and the other system. Neurotransmitters and immunotransmitters are often identical. When they are not, they nonetheless elicit responses in the other system (e.g., interferon effects in the CNS). Knowledge of this interrelatedness of the immune system and CNS still leaves a great deal unknown about the pathophysiology of HIV infection. Direct measures of immuno- and neurotransmitter changes secondary to HIV infection and treatment have generally not been undertaken. Given the paucity of cellular damage in the CNS associated with HIV infection, it is probable that a neurochemical-mediated process will be found to play an important role in HIV CNS disease.

Efforts to encourage behavioral change, the only available prevention technique at present, are under way but are of uncertain efficacy. Preliminary data on this question are incomplete and contradictory. Considerable research is needed both to demonstrate the effectiveness of these techniques in this epidemic as well as to identify and evaluate novel approaches to modify high-risk sexual and drug abuse behaviors.

Compelling evidence exists of the extent and severity of the CNS compromise secondary to HIV infection and AIDS. Less clear, however, is the means by which what appears to be a relatively limited direct infection of the CNS by HIV produces this result. Although direct penetration of cells of the CNS appears quite limited, it is not different in kind from the estimates of one in 100 T4 cells infected by HIV in AIDS patients. Similarly, the early findings of reversal of HIV CNS symptoms and signs in four patients treated with AZT, including PET scan results, suggest mechanisms other than cell death as responsible for the HIV dementia. Much more needs to be known about the neurophysiology of HIV dementia in order to provide adequate treatment for this disorder.

Suggestive evidence, discussed elsewhere in this volume, implicates a potential role for psychoactive drugs in the pathophysiology of AIDS. Whether through their impact on receptor-mediated events or through their effect on immune-mediated mechanisms, psychoactive agents will likely exert some effect, of unknown significance presently, on the cascade of events leading to AIDS. Similarly, the presence of affective disease, with its close links to neurohumoral perturbations, is likely to be consequential in the natural history of AIDS. Finally, through the interconnections of the immune and central nervous systems, the panoply of psychosocial variables already known to be associated with AIDS will potentially impact on the pathophysiology of AIDS.

The chapters in this volume address many of these questions and in concert make the point that the fields of neuroscience, behavior, and substance abuse research have research and clinical methods of high relevance to the understanding of the natural history of HIV infection. As well, they are most likely to contribute to the discovery and/or implementation of effective treatments and preventive approaches for HIV infection. Clearly, any treatment or prevention for HIV infection that is not effective in the brain will only prove of limited value for the AIDS patient.

REFERENCES

1. Ader, R. (1980): Presidential address, 1980: Psychosomatic and psychoimmunologic research. *Psychosom. Med.*, 42:307–321.
2. Albert, M. L., Feldman, R. G., and Willis, A. L. (1974): The 'subcortical dementia' of progressive supranuclear palsy. *J. Neurol. Neurosurg. Psychiatry*, 37:121–130.
3. Alvord, E. C., Jr. (1968): The pathology of parkinsonism. In: *Pathology of the Nervous System, Vol. 1,* edited by J. Minckler, pp. 1152–1161. McGraw-Hill, New York.
4. Arendt, T., Bigl, V., Arendt, A., and Tennstedt, A. (1983): Loss of neurons in the nucleus basalis of Meynert in Alzheimer's disease, paralysis agitans, and Korsakoff's disease. *Acta Neuropathol. (Berl.),* 61:101–108.
5. Barre-Sinoussi, F. J. C., Chermann, F. R., and Nugeyre, M. T. (1983): Isolation of a T-lymphotropic retrovirus from patients at risk for AIDS. *Science,* 220:868–871.
6. Blalock, J. E. (1984) Relationships between neuroendocrine hormones and lymphokines. *Lymphokines,* 9:1–13.
7. Blalock, J. E., McMenamin, D. H., and Smith, E. M. (1985): Peptide hormones shared by the neuroendocrine and immunologic systems. *J. Immunol.,* 135:858s–861s.
8. Boller, F., Mizutani, T., Roessmann, U., and Gambetti, P. (1980): Parkinson disease, dementia, and Alzheimer disease: Clinicopathological correlations. *Ann. Neurol.,* 7:329–335.
9. Bondareff, W. (1984); Effect of aging on loss of neurons in dementia of the Alzheimer type (DAT). In: *Alzheimer's Disease: Advances in Basic Research and Therapies,* edited by R. J. Wurtman, S. H. Corkin, and J. H. Growdon. International Study Group on the Treatment of Memory Disorders Associated with Aging, Zurich.
10. Bridge, T. P. (1987): AIDS and future psychoimmunologic research. In: *Behavior and STD,* edited by D. Ostrow. Raven Press, New York (*in press*).
11. Bridge, T. P., and Macdonald, D. I. (1986): AIDS and the brain. *Psychopharmacol. Bull.,* 22:675–677.
12. Bruyn, G. W., Botts, G. T. A. M., and Dom, R. (1979): Huntington's chorea: Current neuropathological status. In: *Advances in Neurology, Vol. 23: Huntington's Disease,* edited by T. N. Chase, N. X. Wexler, and A. Barbeau, pp. 83–93. Raven Press, New York.

13. Candy, J. M., Perry, R. H., and Perry, E. K. (1983): Pathological changes in the nucleus of Meynert in Alzheimer's and Parkinson's diseases. *J. Neurol. Sci.*, 59:277–289.
14. Centers for Disease Control (1985): Revision of the case definition of acquired immunodeficiency syndrome for national reporting—United States. *Morbid. Mortal. Week. Rep.*, 34:373–375.
15. Centers for Disease Control (1986): Update: Acquired immunodeficiency syndrome. *Morbid. Mortal. Week. Rep.*, 35:222–223.
16. Chiodi, F., Asjo, B., and Fenyo, E. M. (1986): Isolation of human immunodeficiency virus from cerebrospinal fluid of antibody-positive virus carrier without neurological symptoms. *Lancet*, 2:1276–1277.
17. Clark, A. W., Parhad, I. M., and Folstein, S. E. (1983): The nucleus basalis in Huntington's disease. *Neurology (N.Y.)*, 33:1262–1267.
18. Crow, T. J. (1984): A re-evaluation of the viral hypothesis: Is psychosis the result of retroviral integration at a site close to the cerebral dominance gene? *Br. J. Psychiatry*, 145:243–253.
19. Cummings, J. L., and Benson, D. F. (1984): Subcortical dementia: Review of an emerging concept. *Arch. Neurol.*, 41:874–879.
20. Curcio, C. A., and Kemper, T. (1984): Nucleus raphe dorsalis in dementia of the Alzheimer type: Neurofibrillary change and neuronal packing density. *J. Neuropathol. Exp. Neurol.*, 43:359–368.
21. Dalgleish, A. G., Beverley, P. C. L., and Clapham, P. R. (1984): The CD4 (T4) antigen is an essential component of the receptors for the AIDS retrovirus. *Nature*, 312:763–767.
22. De La Paz, R. (1986): MRI may influence treatment of AIDS. *Radiography*, 52:10.
23. Epstein, L. G., Sharer, L. R., and Cho, E. S. (1984): HTLV-III/LAV-like retrovirus particles in the brains of patients with AIDS encephalopathy. *AIDS Res.*, 1:447–454.
24. Epstein, L. G., Sharer, L. R., and Joshi, V. V. (1985): Progressive encephalopathy in children with acquired immune deficiency syndrome. *Ann. Neurol.*, 17:488–496.
25. Fauci, A. S., Masur, H., and Gelmann, E. P. (1985): The acquired immunodeficiency syndrome: An update. *Ann. Intern. Med.*, 102:800–813.
26. Forno, L. S., Barbour, P. J., and Norville, R. L. (1978): Presenile dementia with Lewy bodies and neurofibrillary tangles. *Arch. Neurol.*, 35:818–822.
27. Forno, L. S., and Jose, C. (1973): Huntington's chorea: A pathological study. In: *Advances in Neurology, Vol. 1: Huntington's Chorea 1872–1972*, edited by A. Barbeau, T. N. Chase, and G. W. Paulson, pp. 453–470. Raven Press, New York.
28. Gabel, R. H., Baranar, N., and Norko, M. (1986): AIDS presenting as mania. *Compr. Psychiatry*, 27:251–254.
29. Gabuzda, D. H., Ho, D. D., and Monte, S. M. (1986): Immunohistochemical identification of HTLV-III antigen in brains of patients with AIDS. *Ann. Neurol.*, 20:289–295.
30. Gallo, R. C., Salahuddin, S. Z., and Popovic, M. (1984) Frequent detection and isolation of cytopathic retroviruses (HTLV-III) from patients with AIDS. *Science*, 224:500–502.
31. Gartner, S., Markovits, P., and Markovitz, D. M. (1986): Virus isolation from and identification of HTLV-III/LAV-producing cells in brain tissue from a patient with AIDS. *J.A.M.A.*, 256:2365–2371.
32. Gaspar, P., and Gray, F. (1984): Dementia in idiopathic Parkinson's disease: A neuropathological study of 32 cases. *Acta Neuropathol. (Berl.)*, 64:43–52.
33. Ginzburg, H. M., and Weiss, S. H. (1986): *HTLV-III and Drug Abusers*. Committee on a National Strategy for AIDS, Washington.
34. Gonda, M. A., Wong-Stall, F., and Gallo, R. C. (1985): Sequence homology and morphologic similarity of HTLV-III and visna virus, a pathologic lentivirus. *Science*, 227:173–177.
35. Hakim, A. M., and Mathieson, G. (1979): Dementia in Parkinson disease: A neuropathologic study. *Neurology (N.Y.)*, 29:1209–1214.
36. Hirano, A., and Zimmerman, H. M. (1962): Alzheimer's neurofibrillary changes: A topographic study. *Arch. Neurol.*, 7:227–242.
37. Ho, D. D., Rota, T. R., and Schooley, R. T. (1985): Isolation of HTLV-III from cerebrospinal fluid and neural tissues of patients with neurological syndromes related to the acquired immunodeficiency syndrome. *N. Engl. J. Med.*, 313:1493–1497.
38. Holland, J. C., and Tross, S. (1985): The psychosocial and neuropsychiatric sequelae of the immunodeficiency syndrome and related disorders. *Ann. Intern. Med.*, 103:760–764.
39. Huber, S. J., and Paulson, G. W. (1985): The concept of subcortical dementia. *Am. J. Psychiatry*, 142:1312–1317.

40. Jellinger, K., and Grisold, W. (1982): Cerebral atrophy in Parkinson syndrome. *Exp. Brain Res. [Suppl.]*, 5:26–35.
41. Joffe, R. T., Rubinow, D. R., and Squillace, K. (1986): Neuropsychiatric aspects of AIDS. *Psychopharmacol. Bull.*, 22:684–688.
42. Jones, G. H., Kelly, C. L., and Davies, J. A. (1987): HIV and onset of schizophrenia. *Lancet*, 1:982.
43. Klatzmann, D. E., Champagne, E., and Chamaret, S. (1984): T-lymphocyte T4 molecule behaves as the receptors for human retrovirus LAV. *Nature*, 312:767–768.
44. Koenig, S., Gendelman, H. E., and Orenstein, J. M. (1986): Detection of AIDS virus in macrophages in brain tissue from AIDS patients with encephalopathy. *Science*, 213:1089–1093.
45. Levy, J. A., Hoffman, A. D., and Kramer, S. M. (1984): Isolation of lymphocytotrophic retroviruses from San Francisco patients with AIDS. *Science*, 225:840–842.
46. Levy, J. A., Shimabukuro, J., and Hollander, H. (1985): Isolation of AIDS-associated retroviruses from cerebrospinal fluid and brain of patients with neurological symptoms. *Lancet*, 2:586–588.
47. Levy, R. M., and Rosenblum, M. L. (1986): Neuroradiologic findings in AIDS. *Am. J. Radiol.*, 147:977–983.
48. Lieb, J. (1983): Remission of rheumatoid arthritis and other disorders of immunity in patients taking monoamine oxidase inhibitors. *Int. J. Immunopharmacol.*, 5:353–357.
49. McCaughey, W. T. E. (1961): The pathologic spectrum of Huntington's chorea. *J. Nerv. Ment. Dis.*, 133:91–103.
50. McHugh, P. R., and Folstein, M. F. (1975): Psychiatric syndromes of Huntington's chorea: A clinical and phenomenologic study. In: *Psychiatric Aspects of Neurologic Disease*, edited by D. F. Benson and D. Blumer, pp. 267–286. Grune & Stratton, New York.
51. Navia, B., Cho, E., and Petito, C. K. (1986): AIDS dementia complex II. Neuropathology. *Ann. Neurol.*, 19:525–535.
52. Navia, B. A., Jordan, B. D., and Price, R. W. (1986): The AIDS dementia complex I. Clinical features. *Ann. Neurol.*, 19:517–524.
53. Navia, B., and Price, R. W. (1987): AIDS dementia complex as the presenting sole manifestation of HIV infection. *Ann. Neurol.*, 44:65–69.
54. Nurnberg, H. G., Prudic, J., and Fiori, M. (1984): Psychopathology complicating AIDS. *Am. J. Psychiatry*, 141:95–96.
55. Perry, E. K., Tomlinson, B. E., and Blessed, G. (1981): Neuropathological and biochemical observations on the noradrenergic system in Alzheimer's disease. *J. Neurol. Sci.*, 51:279–287.
56. Pert, C. B., Hill, J. M., and Ruff, M. R. (1986): Octapeptide deduced from the neuropeptide receptor-like pattern of antigen T4 in brain potently inhibit human immunodeficiency virus receptor binding and T cell infectivity. *Proc. Natl. Acad. Sci. U.S.A.*, 23:9254–9258.
57. Pert, C. B., Ruff, M. R., and Weber, R. J. (1985): Neuropeptides and their receptors: A psychosomatic network. *J. Immunol.*, 135:820s–826s.
58. Post, M. J. D., Sheldon, J. J., and Hensley, G. T. (1986): CNS disease in AIDS: Prospective correlation using CT, MRI and pathologic studies. *Neuroradiology*, 158:141–148.
59. Ruff, M. R., Martin, B. R., and Ginns, E. D. (1987): CD4 receptor binding peptides that block HIV infectivity cause human monocyte chemotaxis: Relationship to VIP. *FEBS Lett.*, 211:17–22.
60. Schleifer, S. J., Keller, S. E., and Camerino, M. (1983): Suppression of lymphocyte stimulation following bereavement. *J.A.M.A.*, 250:374–377.
61. Schleifer, S. J., Keller, S. E., and Meyerson, A. T. (1984) Lymphocyte function in major depressive disorders. *Arch. Gen. Psychiatry*, 41:484–486.
62. Schleifer, S. J., Keller, S. E., and Siris, S. G. (1985): Depression and immunity. *Arch. Gen. Psychiatry*, 42:129–133.
63. Stein, M., Keller, S. E., and Schleifer, S. J. (1985): Stress and immunomodulation. *J. Immunol.*, 135:827s–830s.
64. Stoler, M. H., Eskin, T. A., and Benn, S. (1986): HTLV-III infection of the central nervous system. *J.A.M.A.*, 256:2360–2364.
65. Tagliavini, F., and Pilleri, G. (1983): Neuronal counts in basal nucleus of Meynert in Alzheimer disease and in simple senile dementia. *Lancet*, 1:469–470.
66. Verma, D. S., Spitzer, G., and Gutterman, J. U. (1982): Human leukocyte interferon mediated granulopoietic differentiation arrest and its abrogation by lithium carbonate. *Am. J. Hematol.*, 12:39–46.

67. Volberding, P. A. (1986): Variation in AIDS related illnesses: Impact on clinical research. In: *Abstracts of the Second International Conference on AIDS, Paris.* Elsevier, Amsterdam/New York.
68. Weiss, S. H., Goedert, J. J., and Sarngadharan, M. (1985): Screening test for HTLV-III antibodies. *J.A.M.A.,* 253:221–225.
69. Wetterberg, L., Alexius, B., and Sass, J. (1987): Peptide T in the treatment of AIDS. *Lancet,* 1:159.
70. Whitehouse, P. J. (1986): The concept of subcortical and cortical dementia: Another look. *Ann. Neurol.,* 19:1–6.
71. Whitehouse, P. J., Hedreen, J. C., White, C. L. III, and Price, D. L. (1983): Basal forebrain neurons in the dementia of Parkinson disease. *Ann. Neurol.,* 13:243–248.
72. Whitehouse, P. J., Price, D. L., and Clark, A. W. (1981): Alzheimer disease: Evidence for selective loss of cholinergic neurons in the nucleus basalis. *Ann. Neurol.,* 10:122–126.
73. Yarchoan, R., Brouwers, P., and Spitzer, A. R. (1987): Response of human-immunodeficiency-virus-associated neurological disease to 3'-azido-3'deoxythymidine. *Lancet,* 1:132–135.

Psychological, Neuropsychiatric, and
Substance Abuse Aspects of AIDS,
edited by T. Peter Bridge et al.
Raven Press, New York © 1988.

Neuroendocrine Properties
of the Immune System

L. David Dion and J. Edwin Blalock

*Department of Physiology and Biophysics, University of Alabama at Birmingham,
Birmingham, Alabama 35294*

Control of the immune response by the neuroendocrine system is an expanding subdiscipline of both immunology and neuroendocrinology. This field of work is often referred to by such titles as neuroimmunoendocrinology, neuroimmunomodulation, psychoimmunology, and psychoneuroimmunology, without any one of these terms being predominant. The classic examples of this interaction are the steroid-mediated immunosuppressive effects of stress; however, that other, nonsteroidal mechanisms such as direct innervation of lymphoid tissues and peptide-mediated responses exist is also now widely accepted. Currently, the field is emerging from its phenomenologic beginnings with the identification of the molecular basis of these mechanisms. Recently, a new and intriguing twist has been added that offers to expand further and explain the scope of the interaction between these two systems. It is now apparent that cells of the immune system can produce neuroendocrine hormones at physiologically significant levels. The central theme of this chapter is that the neuroendocrine and immune systems are bidirectionally interconnected as a result of shared expression of the same messenger molecules as well as receptors for those molecules. Given this interconnection, it might be anticipated that a disease such as AIDS could have neuroendocrine manifestations as a direct result of its immunosuppressive effects.

The immune system is modulated by the neuroendocrine system through a number of different mechanisms. For example, the immunosuppressive effect of stress-induced steroids has been extensively investigated (25). In addition, all of the major lymphoid organs are now known to be innervated directly, suggesting possible control by neurotransmitters (9). More recently, it has become apparent that various components of the immune system are responsive to neuroendocrine peptide hormones (6). For example, the enkephalins have been shown to enhance lymphocyte responsiveness to mitogens, increase survival time of transplanted tumors, and increase lymphoid organ size (13,24). Alternatively, adrenocorticotropin (ACTH) has been shown to suppress the *in vitro* antibody response as well as the γ interferon response of murine lymphocytes (17,18).

Since cells of the immune system demonstrate specific responses to neuroendocrine peptides, it is not surprising that there has been a steady accumulation of evidence demonstrating the presence of high-affinity receptors for neurotransmitters and neuropeptides on cells of the immune system (17,23,32,35). For example, Bost and Blalock (7) have isolated ACTH receptors from mouse adrenal Y-1 cells as well as mouse and human lymphocytes. Physically, the ACTH receptor seems to be highly conserved across both tissue and species boundaries, having in this case identical intact and subunit structures from these different sources, including lymphocytes. With this peripheral source of ACTH receptors, it should now be possible to study altered structure and function of receptors that were traditionally thought to be present only at inaccessible sites such as the adrenal gland. Smith et al. (30) have, in fact, reported on the use of peripheral human lymphocytes to demonstrate that a patient with adrenal insufficiency was the victim of an ACTH receptor defect.

Lymphocyte-derived β-adrenergic receptors are also apparently functionally identical to those on neural tissue. This identity has been exploited to correlate altered receptor activities with depression and psychomotor agitation (23). Most of the other lymphocyte-derived receptors still need to be characterized structurally and functionally to compare their relatedness to the *bona fide* receptors of the neuroendocrine system. If other neurotransmitter and neuropeptide hormone receptors also prove to be identical across tissue boundaries, this approach to understanding neuroendocrine disorders may find wider application.

In contrast to responding to and expressing receptors for neuroendocrine hormones, it is becoming clear that components of the immune system can in turn directly affect the neuroendocrine system. Induction of fever during an infection is an example of such interaction. It is generally thought that the induction of fever is through macrophage-produced IL-1 affecting thermoregulatory centers in the hypothalamus. Recently, the structural and functional similarities between IL-1 and endogenous pyrogen have been noted, and synthesis of an IL-1-like peptide in the brain has been described (10). Regardless of the source of the physiologically active pyrogen, this is an example of the immune system being integrated with the neuroendocrine system by the shared synthesis and response to a common messenger. Another example has been provided by Besedovsky et al. (3), who have shown that during the immune response there is an increase in the firing rate of neurons in the hypothalamus and an accompanying increase in glucocorticoid levels. They have also shown that concanavalin-A- (ConA) and phytohemagglutinin (PHA)-stimulated leukocyte cultures secrete a factor(s) into culture medium that can raise corticosterone levels in rats (4). They have shown that the lymphocyte-derived mediator of this increase is probably not ACTH, since the effect is dependent on an intact pituitary gland. The molecular agent involved has recently been identified as IL-1 by neutralization with antisera to IL-1. Therefore, in this system, the IL-1 seems to act as a corticotropin-releasing factor (5). That IL-1 can have *in vitro* corticotropin-releasing factor activity has also been reported by others (1,19,34).

Other studies have identified lymphocyte-synthesized peptides that are similar or identical to known neuropeptides. Smith and Blalock have shown that both human peripheral leukocytes and mouse spleen cells produce ACTH and endorphins in response to virus infection or a B-cell mitogen, bacterial lipopolysaccharide (LPS) (15,27). The induction of ACTH was specific in that other hormones (TSH, CG, FSH, and LH) were not detectable. Initially, this lymphocyte-derived ACTH was detected by monospecific antisera and thus was referred to as immunoreactive ACTH (irACTH). It has since been characterized by molecular weight, reverse-phase HPLC, and biological activity as being identical to ACTH. Using immuno-fluorescent staining, Lolait et al. (21) also found that resting splenic macrophages synthesize both ACTH and β-endorphin-related peptides. Siegel et al. (26) have similarly shown that chickens injected with *Salmonella* antigen also have increased corticosteroid levels, which may be a result of splenic leukocyte production of ACTH.

Not only can lymphocytes produce ACTH, but control of such ACTH synthesis appears to be similar to the mechanisms of control that operate in the pituitary gland. Smith et al. (31) have shown that lymphocytes can be induced by corticotropin-releasing factor (CRF) to synthesize ACTH and that such synthesis is under negative control by dexamethasone. In the pituitary, ACTH is one of several peptides that are processed from a common precursor protein, proopiomelanocortin (POMC). Interestingly, another POMC-derived peptide, endorphin, is also produced by leukocytes concomitantly with the ACTH, which further supports the similarities between the neuroendocrine and immune systems (21). Westley et al. (33) have been able to extend these findings by isolating POMC messenger RNA from virus-infected murine splenocytes. Lolait et al. (22) have similarly reported finding POMC mRNA in unstimulated spleen cells. Zurawski et al. (36) have found abundant preproenkephalin mRNA in mitogen-activated mouse T-helper cells as well as immunoreactive Met-enkephalin in the culture media from such cells. From these studies, it seems conclusive that cells of the immune system can produce ACTH and related peptides.

The immune system can also be shown to differentiate among various stimuli and respond in turn with a specific neuropeptide signal. For example, Smith et al. (29) have been able to detect thyroid-stimulating hormone (TSH) but not ACTH in mouse spleen lymphocyte cultures stimulated by a T-cell mitogen, staphylococcal enterotoxin A (SEA). The TSH was detected by immunofluorescence and isolated by affinity chromatography using rabbit anti-TSH β-chain antibody. The immuno-reactive TSH (irTSH) could be endogenously labeled with tritiated amino acids, so the source of the material was clearly the spleen cells. Electrophoresis indicated three radioactive bands of 26, 50, and 80 kilodaltons, which may correspond to monomer, dimer, and trimers of irTSH. The irTSH could also be acid treated and reduced to give bands corresponding to the 12-kilodalton α subunit and 14-kilodalton β subunit of *bona fide* TSH. Finally, the irTSH was shown to be a glycoprotein by binding to a ConA–sepharose column. Thus, in several aspects, the irTSH shows extensive identification with neuroendocrine-derived TSH. It should be noted that the irTSH has not been assayed for TSH activity, nor have sequencing studies been done. There is, however, evidence as to the possible function of lymphocyte-produced TSH, since TSH can be shown to enhance the production of specific antibody-producing B cells in an *in vitro* immunization (Mishell–Duton) assay. This enhancement appears to depend on the presence of T cells and so is probably an indirect effect on the B cells (20).

Another example of a stimulus-specific neuropeptide response is that chorionic gonadotropin (CG) has been found in mixed lymphocyte cultures but not in response to other stimuli (16). As before, the techniques used to characterize this peptide have been immunofluorescence, affinity chromatography, endogenous labeling, exclusion gel chromatography, electrophoresis, and *in vitro* testosterone induction. The biological ramifications of possible CG synthesis are interesting, particularly in terms of reproductive biology, since many aspects of a mixed lymphocyte reaction (MLR) may occur at the site of embryo implantation, where maternal immune cells are challenged by foreign antigens of paternal origin on the embryo cells. It is known that CG synthesis is necessary for maintenance of the embryo and also that closely matched HLA types between the parents can, in some instances, be shown to be involved in spontaneous abortion (12).

Finally, there is the question of the physiological significance of these varied observations. In support of the concept that immune-derived ACTH may function to signal the neuroendocrine system and as a demonstration of the *in vivo* physiological relevance of the ACTH produced, it was shown that virus-infected hypophysectomized mice (mice with surgically removed pituitaries and deprived of a neuroendocrine source of ACTH) elicit sufficient ACTH to produce increased circulating corticosterone levels. The spleens of the infected mice were shown by immunofluorescence to be synthesizing ACTH (28). This experiment clearly demonstrated that functionally the immune system can provide an alternative and sufficient source of ACTH to induce an adrenal gland response. The relative contributions of the two sources in intact animals during an immune response remains to be determined. Production of ACTH by lymphocytes can also have pathological implications, as was shown by Dupont et al. (8). They described a patient who presented characteristics of ectopic ACTH syndrome. Although no ACTH-producing tumor was found, ACTH levels returned to normal after removal of an inflammatory mass in which normal immune cells were positive for ACTH by immunofluorescence.

In conclusion, these observations of production of neuroendocrine hormones by cells of the immune system, presence of receptors for neuroendocrine hormones on cells of the immune system, and similar mechanisms of control at the cellular and molecular levels all suggest that the neuroendocrine and immune systems may function as a larger integrated system. We are beginning to establish the molecular basis of neuroimmunoendocrinology, and these advances in turn hold promise for new approaches to problems in both clinical and basic sciences. For example, Bernton et al. (2) have reported on the use of an opiate antagonist, naloxone, to block symptoms of gram-negative sepsis and endotoxic shock. Another example is that the presence of neuroendocrine hormone receptors on lymphocytes may provide a peripheral source of these receptors for the investigation of the role of defective binding sites in neuroendocrine disorders such as adrenal insufficiency.

Considering the recent demonstration that human immunodeficiency virus (HIV) can infect macrophage-like cells derived from brain tissue (11) and the previously quoted reports of macrophage-derived β-endorphin (21), as well as the viral induction of this peptide (20), it is tempting to speculate on the contribution of this hormone to AIDS-associated dementia and the possible therapeutic effects of naloxone in such patients. In the future, we anticipate that the list of neuroendocrine peptides having immunoregulatory activities will lengthen, as will the number of lymphokines found to have neuroendocrine functions. Investigation of the function and physiological significance of these "immunotransmitters" (14) promises to be an interesting area of research.

ACKNOWLEDGMENTS

The authors are supported in part by the National Institutes of Health (7 R01 DK38024-01).

REFERENCES

1. Beach, J. E., Bernton, E. W., Holaday, J. W., Smallridge, R. C., and Fein, H. G. (1986): Interleukin-1 modulates secretion by rat pituitary cells in monolayer culture. In: *Proceedings 1st International Congress of Neuroendocrinology,*
2. Bernton, E. W., Long, J. B., and Holaday, J. W. (1985): Opioids and neuropeptides: Mechanisms in circulatory shock. *Fed. Proc.*, 44:290–299.
3. Besedovsky, H., Del Ray, A., Sorkin, E., Prada, M. D., Burri, R., and Honegger, C. (1983): The immune response evokes changes in brain noradrenergic neurons. *Science*, 221:564–566.
4. Besedovsky, H. O., Del Ray, A., Sorkin, E., Lotz, W., and Schwulera, U. (1985): Lymphoid cells produce an immunoregulatory glucocorticoid increasing factor (GIF) acting through the pituitary. *Clin. Exp. Immunol.*, 59:622–628.
5. Besedovsky, H., Del Ray, A., Sorkin, E., and Dinarello, E. A. (1986): Immunoregulatory feedback between interleukin-1 and glucocorticoid hormones. *Science*, 233:652–654.
6. Blalock, J. E. (1984): The immune system as a sensory organ. *J. Immunol.*, 132:1067–1070.
7. Bost, K. K., and Blalock, J. E. (1986): Molecular characterization of a corticotropin (ACTH) receptor. *Mol. Cell. Endocrinol.*, 44:1–9.
8. Dupont, A. G., Somers, G., Van Steirteghem, A. C., Warson, F., and Vanhaelst, L. (1984): Ectopic adrenocorticotropin production: Disappearance after removal of inflammatory tissue. *J. Clin. Endocrinol. Metab.*, 58:654–658.
9. Felton, D. L., Felton, S. Y., Carlson, S. L., Olschowska, J. A., and Livnat, S. (1985): Noradrenergic and peptidergic innervation of lymphoid tissue. *J. Immunol.*, 135s:755s–765s.
10. Fontana, A., Weber, E., and Dayer, J. M. (1984): Synthesis of interleukin-1/endogenous pyrogen in the brain of endotoxin treated mice: A step in fever induction? *J. Immunol.*, 133:1696–1698.
11. Gartner, S., Markovits, P., Markovitz, D. M., Kaplan, M. H., Gallo, R. C., and Popovic, M. (1986): The role of mononuclear phagocytes in HTLV-III/LAV infections. *Science*, 233:215–219.
12. Gill, J. J. (1983): Immunogenetics of spontaneous abortions in humans. *Transplantation*, 35:1–6.
13. Gilman, S. C., Schwartz, J. M., Milner, R. J., Bloom, F. E., and Feldman, J. D. (1982): β-Endorphin enhances lymphocyte proliferative responses. *Proc. Natl. Acad. Sci. U.S.A.*, 79:4226–4230.
14. Hall, N. R., McGillis, J. P., Spangelo, B. L., and Goldstein, A. L. (1985): Evidence that thymosins and other biologic response modifiers can function as neuroactive immunotransmitters. *J. Immunol.*, 135s:806s–811s.

15. Harbour-McMenamin, D., Smith, E. M., and Blalock, J. E. (1985): Bacterial lipopolysaccharide induction of leukocyte-derived ACTH and endorphins. *Infect. Immun.*, 48:813–817.
16. Harbour-McMenamin, D., Smith, E. M., and Blalock, J. E. (1986): Production of lymphocyte-derived chorionic gonadotropin in a mixed lymphocyte reaction. *Proc. Natl. Acad. Sci. U.S.A.*, 83:6834–6838.
17. Johnson, H. M., Smith, E. M., Torres, B. A., and Blalock, J. E. (1982): Neuroendocrine hormone regulation of *in vitro* antibody production. *Proc. Natl. Acad. Sci. U.S.A.*, 79:4171–4174.
18. Johnson, H. M., Torres, B. A., Smith, E. M., Dion, L. D., and Blalock, J. E. (1984): Regulation of lymphokine (interferon-γ) production by corticotropin. *J. Immunol.*, 132:246–250.
19. Kehrer, P., Gaillard, R. C., Dayer, J. M., and Muller, A. F. (1986): Human interleukin-1 β stimulates ACTH release from rat anterior pituitary cells in a cAMP and prostaglandin E_2 independent manner. In: *Proceedings 1st International Congress of Neuroendocrinology.*
20. Kruger, T. E., and Blalock, J. E. (1986): Cellular requirements for thyrotropin enhancement of in vitro antibody production. *J. Immunol.*, 137:197–200.
21. Lolait, S. J., Lim, A. T. W., Toh, B. H., and Funder, J. W. (1984): Immunoreactive β-endorphin in a subpopulation of mouse spleen macrophages. *J. Clin. Invest.*, 73:277–280.
22. Lolait, S. J., Clements, J. A., Markwick, A., Cheng, C., McNally, M., Smith, A. I., and Funder, J. W. (1986): Pro-opiomelanocortin messenger ribonucleic acid and posttranslational processing of beta endorphin in spleen macrophages. *J. Clin. Invest.*, 77:1776–1779.
23. Mann, J. J., Brown, R. P., Halper, J. P., Sweeney, J. A., Kocsis, J. H., Stokes, P. E., and Bilezikian, J. P. (1985): Reduced sensitivity of lymphocyte beta-adrenergic receptors in patients with endogenous depression and psychomotor agitation. *N. Engl. J. Med.*, 313:715–720.
24. Plotnikoff, N. P., Murgo, A. J., Miller, G. C., Corder, C. R., and Faith, R. F. (1985): Enkephalins: Immunomodulators. *Fed. Proc.*, 44:118–122.
25. Riley, V. (1981): Psychoneuroendocrine influences on immunocompetence and neoplasia. *Science*, 212:1100–1109.
26. Siegel, H. S., Gould, N. R., and Latimer, J. W. (1985): Splenic leukocytes from chickens injected with *Salmonella pullorum* antigen stimulate production of corticosteroids by isolated adrenal cells (42037). *Proc. Soc. Exp. Biol. Med.*, 178:523–530.
27. Smith, E. M., and Blalock, J. E. (1981): Human lymphocyte production of ACTH and endorphin-like substances: Association with leukocyte interferon. *Proc. Natl. Acad. Sci. U.S.A.*, 78:7530–7534.
28. Smith, E. M., Meyer, W. J., and Blalock, J. E. (1982): Virus-induced increases in corticosterone in hypophysectomized mice: A possible lymphoid adrenal axis. *Science*, 218:1311–1312.
29. Smith, E. M., Phan, M., Kruger, T. E., Coppenhaver, D. H., and Blalock, J. E. (1983): Human lymphocyte production of immunoreactive thyrotropin. *Proc. Natl. Acad. Sci. U.S.A.*, 80:6010–6013.
30. Smith, E. M., Brosman, P., Meyer, W. J., and Blalock, J. E. (1987): A corticotropin receptor on human mononuclear lymphocytes: Correlation with adrenal ACTH receptor activity. *N. Engl. J. Med.*, 317:1266–1269.
31. Smith, E. M., Morrill, A. C., Meyer, W. J. III, and Blalock, J. E. (1986): Corticotropin releasing factor induction of leukocyte-derived immunoreactive ACTH and endorphins. *Nature*, 321:881–882.
32. Weber, R. J., and Pert, C. B. (1984): Opiatergic modulation of the immune system. In: *Central and Peripheral Endorphins: Basic and Clinical Aspects*, edited by E. E. Muller and A. R. Genazzani, pp. 35–42. Raven Press, New York.
33. Westley, H. J., Kleiss, A. J., Kelley, K. W., Wong, P. K. Y., and Yuen, P. H. (1986): Newcastle disease virus-infected splenocytes express the proopiomelanocortin gene. *J. Exp. Med.*, 163:1589–1594.
34. Woloski, B. M. R. N. J., Smith, E. M., Meyer, W. J., Fuller, G. M., and Blalock, J. E. (1985): Corticotropin-releasing factor activity of monokines. *Science*, 230:1035–1037.
35. Wybran, J., Appelboom, T., Famaey, J. P., and Govaerts, A. (1979): Suggestive evidence for receptors for morphine and methionine-enkephalin on normal blood T lymphocytes. *J. Immunol.*, 123:1068–1070.
36. Zurawski, G., Benedik, M., Kamb, B. J., Abrams, J. S., Zurawski, S. M., and Frank, F. D. (1986): Activation of mouse T-helper cells induces abundant pre-proenkephalin mRNA synthesis. *Science*, 232:772–775.

Psychological, Neuropsychiatric, and
Substance Abuse Aspects of AIDS,
edited by T. Peter Bridge et al.
Raven Press, New York © 1988.

Molecular Components Common to the Immune System and Neurons: Growth Factors and Their Receptors

*Joanna M. Hill, †Michael R. Ruff, ‡Maxine A. Lesniak,
‡Jesse Roth, and *Candace B. Pert

*Section on Brain Biochemistry, Clinical Neuroscience Branch, Intramural Research
Program, National Institute of Mental Health, Alcohol, Drug Abuse, and Mental Health
Administration; †Cellular Immunology Section, Laboratory of Microbiology and
Immunology, National Institute of Dental Research, National Institutes of Health,
Bethesda, Maryland 20892; and ‡Diabetes Branch, National Institute of Diabetes,
Digestive and Kidney Diseases, National Institutes of Health, Bethesda, Maryland 20892*

The growth factors are a heterogeneous group of substances that coordinate different aspects of the activation, replication, growth, differentiation, repair, and maintenance of cells. Growth factors are typically polypeptides and are often well studied in their roles as hormones (e.g., insulin and the insulin-like growth factors), transport molecules (e.g., transferrin), or cytokines (e.g., interleukin-1).

The emergence of autoradiographic techniques has made possible the determination of the regional distribution of receptors for hormones, neurotransmitters, neuromodulators, drugs, and viruses. This technique is especially useful for the determination of the regional distribution of receptors in the brain (9), a structure with rich anatomical complexity.

Recent studies have revealed that numerous growth factors and their receptors are present in brain. This chapter summarizes our recent progress in the distribution of selected growth factor receptors in brain.

TRANSFERRIN

Transferrin is well known as the chief iron-carrying serum protein of the body. Cells take up iron after transferrin binds to a specific cell surface receptor (17,35,42) and the receptor is internalized (3,19,21). Transferrin receptor expression is associated with cell growth (28,37,41,42) and differentiation (4,6,38–40), and they have been found on a wide variety of cell types (27) including those of the brain (1). The recent localization of transferrin receptors on brain capillary en-

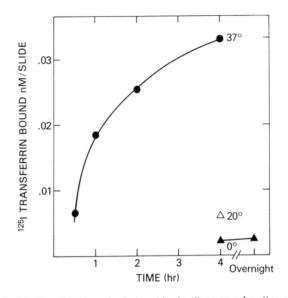

FIG. 1. Specific binding of ^{125}I-transferrin to rat brain slices as a function of time and temperature. Slide-mounted sections were incubated in 0.5 nM ^{125}I-transferrin. Nonspecific binding in the presence of 10 μM transferrin has been subtracted from all points. Values are the means of three or more determinations.

dothelial cells (18) suggests a route through which iron can be transported into the brain. Iron is widespread and unevenly distributed in the brain (14), increases with age (5,10,36), and accumulates in some regions of the human brain to levels reached in the liver (5).

With autoradiographic methods (9) on fresh frozen rat brain, we have demonstrated that specific binding of ^{125}I-transferrin occurs throughout the brain with a pattern of distribution related to the underlying cytoarchitecture (13). This study also showed that between 70 and 75% of the total binding of ^{125}I-transferrin was displaceable by 10 μM transferrin and that the binding of transferrin was both time and temperature dependent (Fig. 1). The saturation curve and Scatchard analysis (Fig. 2) reveal a single class of transferrin receptor with an apparent K_d of $\sim 1 \times 10^{-9}$ M, which is similar to that reported for rat (6), mouse (19), and human (21) cells. Binding of ^{125}I-transferrin was also found to be reversible with a $t_{1/2}$ of 7 min (Fig. 3).

Immunoprecipitation of the transferrin receptor with an antibody directed against the rat transferrin receptor (Fig. 4, lane C) but not with an antibody directed against the human transferrin receptor (Fig. 4, lane D) further characterizes these binding sites as transferrin receptors.

The pattern of distribution of ^{125}I-transferrin is illustrated in Fig. 5 (A, C,E,G,I,K,M,O). Transferrin receptors are widespread and unevenly distributed throughout the brain, with the medial habenula having the highest concentration of

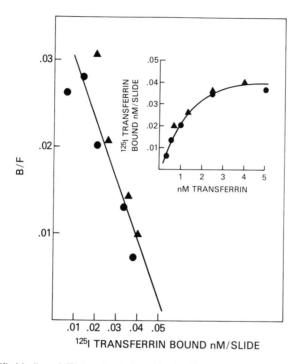

FIG. 2. Specific binding of ^{125}I-transferrin to rat brain slices as a Scatchard analysis and as a function of the concentration of transferrin (**inset**). Slide-mounted sections were incubated in various concentrations of ^{125}I-transferrin. Nonspecific binding in the presence of 10 μM transferrin has been subtracted from all points. Values are the means of four or more determinations, and the results from two separate experiments (● and ▲) are given.

receptors. Transferrin receptors are typically more dense in the molecular layers of laminated structures, as can be seen in the olfactory bulb (Fig. 5A), hippocampal formation (Fig. 5J,L), and cerebellum (Fig. 5O). Iron-stained sections at approximately the same levels as the sections labeled with ^{125}I-transferrin are shown in Fig. 5 (B,D,F,H,J,L,N,P). There is little overlap in the distribution of iron and the transferrin receptor. [For a complete description of iron in the brain, see Hill and Switzer (14).] Additional evidence that ^{125}I-transferrin binding reveals transferrin receptor distribution is afforded by the distribution pattern achieved by localizing the antibody to the rat transferrin receptor with radioimmunocytochemistry. The pattern produced is almost identical with that obtained with ^{125}I-transferrin binding (Fig. 6).

Although the role of transferrin in iron transport is well established, of current interest is its correlation with cell activation and proliferation (28,35,42). The brain regions with dense transferrin receptors could reveal brain areas with activated and/ or dividing glial cells. This explanation, however, does not account for the lack of correspondence of transferrin receptors with iron localization in the brain. With the

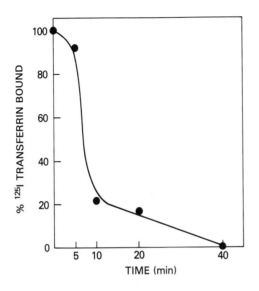

FIG. 3. Specific binding of ^{125}I-transferrin to rat brain slices after the addition of excess (10 μM) transferrin, showing the reversibility of binding with time under these conditions.

FIG. 4. Sodium dodecylsulfatepolyacrylamide gel analysis of transferrin receptor immunoprecipitates prepared from brain slices preincubated with ^{125}I-transferrin. Lanes: **A**, native labeled ^{125}I-transferrin; **B**, material recovered from brain slices after standard incubation conditions; **C**, immunoprecipitate prepared from brain slices using an antirat transferrin receptor antibody; **D**, immunoprecipitate prepared using an antihuman transferrin receptor antibody. The specific binding to section shown in Fig. 5C was 1,930 cpm. Saturating amounts of antirat transferrin receptor (2 μg per reaction) recovered 28% of the total slice bound activity prior to solubilization and immunoprecipitation. Total samples for each immunoprecipitate (lanes **C**, **D**, and **E**) as well as total slice bound radioactivity (lane **B**) were resolved on 8% NaDodSO$_4$/polyacrylamide gels in the presence of 2-mercaptoethanol. Autoradiographs of dried gels are presented.

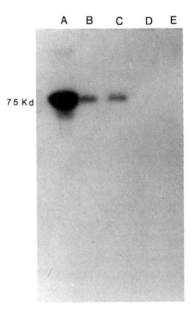

exception of the interpeduncular nucleus, which has both large numbers of trans-ferrin receptors and abundant iron (14), no high-iron areas of the brain are enriched with transferrin receptors. However, most high-iron brain regions receive axonal input from regions with abundant transferrin receptors (13). This suggests that iron is taken up in regions enriched with transferrin receptors and transported by axonal flow to those regions where iron is stored.

It is not clear how the transport of iron or of an iron–transferrin complex may function in brain chemistry; however, the iron-rich regions of the brain are sites where GABAergic systems terminate (11). In addition, recent evidence suggests that iron accumulation in the brain may be related to γ-aminobutyric acid (GABA) metabolism (11). Thus, iron or the iron–transferrin complex may be involved in some aspect of GABA transport or metabolism.

Many brain regions enriched with transferrin receptors are not known to be in-volved in iron storage or transport. The distribution pattern formed by these regions is "neuropeptide-like" insofar as it reveals abundant transferrin receptors in limbic regions such as the hippocampus, amygdala, and septum (30). The neuropeptide-like pattern of distribution of the transferrin receptor, along with the fact that trans-ferrin is synthesized in brain (24), suggests that transferrin, like other neuropep-tides, may be involved in the modulation of behavior.

INSULIN

Insulin, a well-studied polypeptide hormone, is known to regulate the synthesis, transport, and uptake of substances essential for growth as well as to regulate met-abolic pathways for carbohydrates, fats, and proteins. Although the liver, apido-cytes, and skeletal muscle are the main target tissues for insulin action, both insulin and insulin receptors have recently been demonstrated throughout brain (7, 8,31,46). Using autoradiographic methods, we have found that ^{125}I-insulin binds specifically throughout the brain in a pattern related to well-known anatomical structures (12).

Specific binding of ^{125}I-insulin decreased when brain slices were incubated with a modest amount of unlabeled insulin (Fig. 7) and was completely displaced in the presence of 1 μM insulin (Fig. 7). Quantitation of binding under these conditions revealed that specific binding accounted for 70 to 95% of the total binding.

We further characterized the insulin receptor of brain on tissue slices from olfac-tory bulb and cerebellum. The binding of ^{125}I-insulin on these tissue sections showed dose-dependent competition by unlabeled insulins according to their bioac-tivity (Fig. 8): chicken insulin $\cong$ pork insulin $>$ human proinsulin $>$ mixture of chemically modified A and B chains. The pattern of competitive binding achieved on brain sections is the same as that found in membrane studies from both target and nontarget cell tissue as well as from membranes dissected from brain regions. Insulin binding on brain sections was both time and temperature dependent. As is typical of the insulin receptor, binding was directly related to temperature at early times and inversely related to temperature at steady state (Fig. 9).

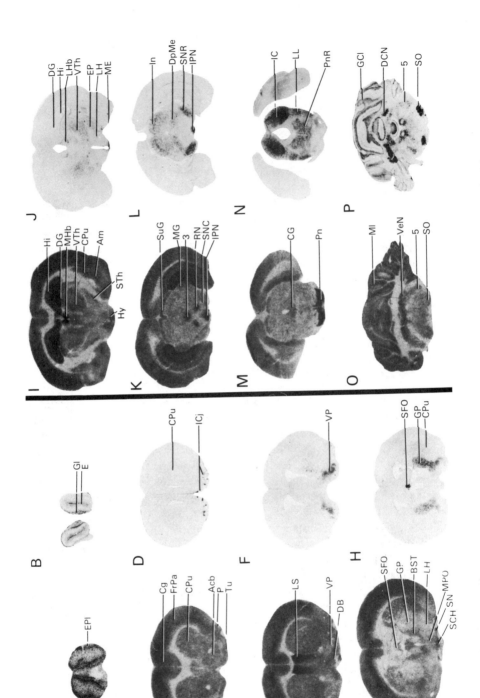

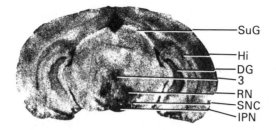

FIG. 6. Film autoradiograph of monoclonal antibody to rat transferrin receptor binding through the level of the interpeduncular nucleus. Rat brain sections were incubated in mouse monoclonal antibody to rat transferrin receptor followed by incubation in ^{125}I-labeled goat antimouse immunoglobulin. For abbreviations, see Fig. 5.

The pattern of distribution of the insulin receptor is illustrated in Fig. 10. The highest number of insulin receptors occurs in the external plexiform layer of the olfactory bulb (Fig. 10c,d), but many other olfactory and limbic structures are enriched with receptors. Insulin receptors are also notably present on several motor areas including the caudate/putamen (Fig. 10a,c,d), cerebellum, and throughout the neocortex (Fig. 10a,c,d). In laminated regions of the brain, insulin receptors were prominent in plexiform or molecular layers, where afferent input arrives and where the dendrites of principle neurons branch.

Among auxiliary brain structures, the choroid plexus demonstrates prominent binding (Fig. 10a,b,c).

Although the roles of insulin receptors and insulin in the brain are not clear, insulin has been shown to modulate neuronal firing (29) and stimulate the release of neurotransmitters (26). In addition, insulin is reported to influence food intake (43,44). Interestingly, the olfactory and limbic regions, which are enriched with insulin receptors, play an important part in feeding (25). Like insulin, the receptors

---

FIG. 5. Film autoradiographs (**A,C,E,G,I,K,M,O**) of ^{125}I-transferrin receptor distribution in rat brain and photomicrographs of sections stained for iron histochemistry (**B,D,F,H,J,L,N,P**) at approximately the same levels of the brain. Acb, nucleus accumbens; Am, amygdala; Bst, bed nucleus of the stria terminalis; Cg, cingulate cortex; CG, central gray; CPu, caudate putamen; DB, diagonal band; DG, dentate gyrus; DpMe, deep mesencephalic nucleus; E, ependymal and subependymal layer of olfactory bulb; EP, entopeduncular nucleus; EPl, external plexiform layer of the olfactory bulb; FrPa, frontoparietal cortex; GCl, granule cell layer of the cerebellar cortex; Gl, glomerular layer of olfactory bulb; GP, globus pallidus; Hi, hippocampus; Hy, hypothalamus; IC, inferior colliculus; ICj, islands of Calleja; In, intermediate layer of the superior colliculus; IPN, interpeduncular nucleus; LH, lateral hypothalamus; LHb, lateral habenula; LL, lateral lemniscus; LS, lateral septum; ME, median eminence; MHb, medial habenula; MG, medial geniculate; Ml, molecular layer of the cerebellar cortex; MPO, medial preoptic area; P, pyriform cortex; Pn, pontine nuclei; PnR, pontine reticular nucleus; RN, red nucleus; SCH, suprachiasmatic nucleus; SFO, subfornical organ; SN, supraoptic nucleus; SNC, substantia nigra, pars compacta; SNR, substantia nigra, pars reticulata; SO, superior olive; STh, subthalamus; SuG, superficial gray layer of the superior colliculus; Tu, olfactory tubercle; VeN, vestibular nucleus; VP, ventral pallidum; VTh, ventral thalamus; 3, oculomotor nucleus; 5, trigeminal nucleus.

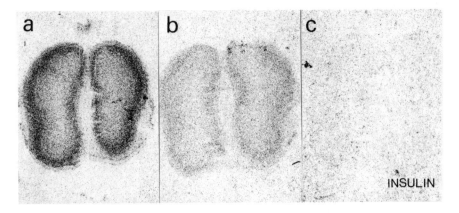

FIG. 7. Autoradiographs of olfactory bulb where ^{125}I-labeled insulin binding was inhibited by a modest amount or an excess of unlabeled insulin. Tissue slices (36 μm) were incubated 90 min at 15°C as described (12). **(a)** ^{125}I-Insulin binding with no unlabeled insulin; **(b)** with insulin at 25 ng/ml (comparable to a stimulated level *in vivo*); and **(c)** with insulin at 5 μg/ml.

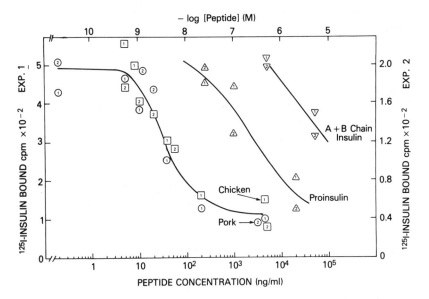

FIG. 8. Inhibition of ^{125}I-labeled insulin binding by insulin and related peptides. Olfactory bulb slices (36 μm) were incubated with ^{125}I-labeled insulin (0.3 nM) in absence or presence of varying concentrations of insulin (pork or chicken), proinsulin (human), or a mixture of A and B chain (oxidized beef insulin). Data from two separate experiments are shown; the experiment number is noted inside each symbol. The data are plotted as labeled insulin bound as a function of peptide concentration. Each data point is a mean of triplicate samples.

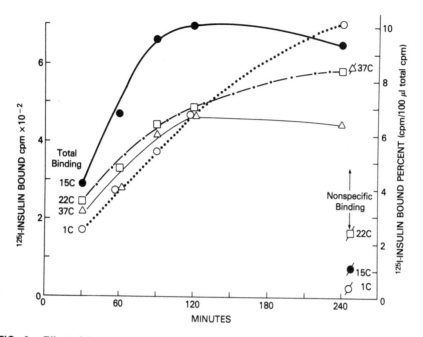

FIG. 9. Effect of time and temperature on insulin binding. Olfactory bulb tissue slices (36 μm) were incubated in 5 ml HEPES buffer, pH 7.8, with ¹²⁵I-labeled insulin (~0.3 nM) in absence (total binding) or presence of 1 μM insulin (nonspecific binding) for times indicated.

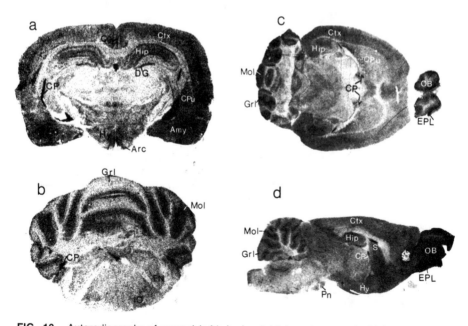

FIG. 10. Autoradiographs of coronal (**a,b**), horizontal (**c**), and parasagittal (**d**) sections of rat brain incubated with ¹²⁵I-insulin. Abbreviations used: Amy, amygdala; Arc, arcuate nucleus; Cg, cingulate gyrus; CP, choroid plexus; CPu, caudate/putamen; Ctx, cortex; DG, dentate gyrus; EPL, external plexiform layer; FN, facial nucleus; Grl, granule cell layer; Hip, hippocampus; Hy, hypothalamus; IO, inferior olive; Mol, molecular layer; OB, olfactory bulb; Pn, pontine nucleus; S, septum.

for other neuropeptides are enriched in limbic and associated structures (30), suggesting that insulin, although best known as a hormone, may function as other neuropeptides to modulate behavior.

THE INSULIN-LIKE GROWTH FACTORS

The insulin-like growth factors I and II are structurally closely related to insulin (31–33) and cross react at the receptor level (15,20). The IGFs share with insulin similar biochemical activities but with different degrees of activity, i.e., relatively weak insulin-like metabolism effects but potent growth-promoting effects (47). The IGFs differ from insulin in that they are coupled to specific carrier proteins in blood and other body fluids (48).

Our use of autoradiographic techniques has revealed the binding patterns of ^{125}I-IGF-I and ^{125}I-IGF-II in brain and allowed a comparison with the binding pattern of ^{125}I-insulin (23). Like insulin, receptors for the two IGFs were found throughout the brain localized in regions corresponding to the cytoarchitecture of the region. However, within each area the three growth factors bound to different loci. This was especially evident in laminated structures such as the olfactory bulb, hippocampus, and neocortex, where each of the three peptides had different densities of receptors localized in different laminae (Table 1). Thus, except for the choroid plexus, where all three receptors are abundant, each of the receptors are apparently on nearby but distinctly different structures.

Competition studies were performed on brain slices from the olfactory bulb and cerebellum. From these studies the IGF-I receptor in brain appears to be a typical IGF-I receptor; unlabeled IGF-I competes for labeled IGF-I better than IGF-II, better than insulin. However, in the presence of low concentrations of IGF-II or insulin, there is an increase in ^{125}I-IGF-I binding. This phenomenon is reproducible but not, as yet, completely understood.

TABLE 1. *Relative density of binding of labeled insulin,*
IGF-I, and IGF-II to select brain regions

Binding regions[a]	Receptors[b]		
	Insulin	IGF-I	IGF-II
Olfactory	+ + + +	+ + + +	+ +
Hypothalamus	+ +	+ + +	+ +
Cerebellum	+ +	+ +	+ +
Median eminence	*	+ + + +	+ + + +
Choroid plexus	+ + + +	+ + + +	+ + + +

[a]Table shows only a few of several regions studied.
[b]Preliminary computer densitometry scoring: + + + +, high; + + +, moderately high; + +, moderate; *, present but density not determined.

The binding of ^{125}I-IGF-II is competed for by unlabeled IGF-II better than IGF-I, and, in our assay system, insulin also occasionally competes for the IGF-II receptor, albeit very weakly.

As with transferrin and insulin, the IGFs and their receptors are present in brain. Although their function in brain is obscure, recently several peptides with well-known functions outside the brain have been localized in the CNS [e.g., cholecystokinin (2,16), vasoactive intestinal peptide (22,34)]. It has been postulated that, in brain, these hormones function to modulate neuronal activity and thus function as neuropeptides in addition to their role at other target organs. The growth factors may function similarly, and, in addition to regulating and promoting growth activities, they may modulate neuronal activity and behavior.

ACKNOWLEDGMENTS

The authors gratefully acknowledge Mrs. Sharon Morgan for her careful preparation of the manuscript.

REFERENCES

1. Angelova-Gateva, P. (1980): Iron transferrin receptors in rat and human cerebellum. *Agressologie*, 21:27–80.
2. Beinfeld, M. C., Meyer, D. K., Eskay, R. L., Jensen, R. T., and Brownstein, M. J. (1981): The distribution of cholecystokinin immunoreactivity in the central nervous system of the rat as determined by radioimmunoassay. *Brain Res.*, 212:51–57.
3. Dautry-Versat, A., Ciechanover, A., and Lodisk, H. F. (1983): pH and the recycling of transferrin during receptor-mediated endocytosis. *Proc. Natl. Acad. Sci. U.S.A.*, 80:2258–2262.
4. Ekblom, P., Thesleff, I., Sanen, I., Meittinen, A., and Timple, R. (1983): Transferrin as a fetal growth factor: Acquisition of responsiveness related to embryonic induction. *Proc. Natl. Acad. Sci. U.S.A.*, 80:2651–2655.
5. Hallgren, B., and Sourander, P. (1958): The effect of age on the nonhaem iron in the human brain. *J. Neurochem.*, 3:41–51.
6. Hamilton, T. A. (1982): Regulation of transferrin receptor expression in concanavalin A stimulated and gross virus transformed rat lymphoblasts. *J. Cell. Physiol.*, 113:40–46.
7. Havrankova, J., Roth, J., and Brownstein, M. J. (1978): Insulin receptors are widely distributed in the central nervous system. *Nature*, 272:827–829.
8. Havrankova, J., Schmichel, D., Roth, J., and Brownstein, M. J. (1978): Identification of insulin in rat brain. *Proc. Natl. Acad. Sci. U.S.A.*, 75:5737–5741.
9. Herkenham, M., and Pert, C. B. (1982): Light microscopic localization of brain opiate receptors: A general autoradiographic method which preserves tissue quality. *J. Neurosci.*, 2:1129–1149.
10. Hill, J. M. (1981): *Brain Iron in the Rat: Distribution Sex Differences and Effects of Sex Hormones.* Ph.D. Thesis, Michigan State University, East Lansing.
11. Hill, J. M. (1985): Iron concentration reduced in ventral-pallidum, globus pallidus, and substantia nigra by GABA-transaminase inhibitor gamma vinyl GABA. *Brain Res.*, 342:18–25.
12. Hill, J. M., Lesniak, M. A., Pert, C. B., and Roth, J. (1986): Autoradiographic localization of insulin receptors in rat brain: Prominence in olfactory and limbic areas. *Neuroscience*, 17:1127–1138.
13. Hill, J. M., Ruff, M. R., Weber, R. J., and Pert, C. B. (1985): Transferrin receptors in rat brain: neuropeptide-like pattern and relationship to iron distribution. *Proc. Natl. Acad. Sci. U.S.A.*, 82:4553–4557.

14. Hill, J. M., and Switzer, R. C. III (1984); The regional distribution and cellular localization of iron in the rat brain. *Neuroscience,* 11:595–603.
15. Hintz, R. L., Clemmons, D. R., Underwood, L. E., and Van Wyk, J. J. (1972): Competitive binding of somatomedin to the insulin receptors of adipocytes, chondrocytes and liver membranes. *Proc. Natl. Acad. Sci. U.S.A.,* 69:2351–2353.
16. Innis, R. B., Correa, F. M. A., Uhl, G. R., Schneider, B., and Snyder, S. H. (1979): Cholecystokinin octapeptide-like immunoreactivity: Histochemical localization in rat brain. *Proc. Natl. Acad. Sci. U.S.A.,* 76:521–525.
17. Jandl, J. H., and Katz, J. H. (1963): The plasma-to-cell cycle of transferrin. *J. Clin. Invest.,* 42:314–326.
18. Jefferies, W. A., Brandon, M. R., Hunt, S. V., Williams, A. F., Gatter, K. C., and Mason, D. Y. (1984): Transferrin receptor on endothelium of brain capillaries. *Nature,* 312:162–163.
19. Kavin, M., and Mintz, B. (1981): Receptor-mediated endocytosis of transferrin in developmentally totipotent mouse teratocarcinoma stem cells. *J. Biol. Chem.,* 256:3245–3252.
20. King, G. L., Kahn, C. R., Rechler, M. M., and Nissley, S. P. (1980): Direct demonstration of separate receptors for growth and metabolic activities of insulin and multiplication-stimulating activity (an insulin-like growth factor) using antibodies for the insulin receptor. *J. Clin. Invest.,* 66:130–140.
21. Klausner, R. D., Ashwell, G., van Renswonde, J., Harford, J. B., and Bridge, K. R. (1983): Binding of apotransferrin to K562 cells: Explanation of the transferrin cycle. *Proc. Natl. Acad. Sci. U.S.A.,* 80:2263–2266.
22. Larsson, L. I., Fahrenkrag, L., Schaffalitsky de Muckadell, O. B., Sundler, F., Hakanson, R., and Rehfeld, J. F. (1976): Localization of vasoactive intestinal polypeptide (VIP) to central and peripheral neurons. *Proc. Natl. Acad. Sci. U.S.A.,* 73:3197–3200.
23. Lesniak, M. A., Hill, J. M., Roth, J., and Pert, C. B. (1986): Autoradiographic localization of ^{125}I-IGF-I and ^{125}I-IGF-II receptors in rat brain: Comparison with insulin receptors. *Diabetes,* 35:58A.
24. Levin, M. J., Tuil, D., Uzan, G., Dreyfus, J. C., and Kahn, A. (1984): Expression of the transferrin gene during development of non-hepatic tissues: high level of transferrin in mRNA in fetal muscle and adult brain. *Biochem. Biophys. Res. Commun.,* 122:212–217.
25. MacLean, P. D., and Delgado, J. M. R. (1953): Electrical and chemical stimulation of frontotemporal portion of limbic system in the waking animal. *Electroencephalogr. Clin. Neurophysiol.,* 5:91–100.
26. McCaleb, M. L., Myers, R. D., Singer, G., and Willis, G. (1979): Hypothalamic norepinephrine in the rat during feeding and push–pull perfusion with glucose, 2DG or insulin. *Am. J. Physiol.,* 236:R312–R321.
27. Newman, R., Schneider, C., Sutherland, R., Vodineleck, L., and Greaves, M. (1982): The transferrin receptor. *Trends Biochem. Sci.,* 7:397–400.
28. Omary, M. B., Trowbridge, I. S., and Minowada, J. (1980): Human cell-surface glycoprotein with unusual properties. *Nature,* 286:888–891.
29. Oomura, Y., and Kita, H. (1981): Insulin acting as a modulator of feeding through the hypothalamus. *Diabetologia,* 20:290–298.
30. Pert, C. B., Ruff, M. R., Weber, R. J., and Herkenham, M. (1985): Neuropeptides and their receptors: a psychosomatic network. *J. Immunol.,* 135:820s–826s.
31. Rinderknecht, E., and Humbel, R. E. (1976): Amino-terminal sequences of two polypeptides from human serum with nonsuppressible insulin-like and cell-growth-promoting activities: Evidence for structural homology with insulin B chain. *Proc. Natl. Acad. Sci. U.S.A.,* 73:4379–4381.
32. Rinderknecht, E., and Humbel, R. E. (1978): The amino acid sequence of human insulin-like growth factor I and its structural homology with proinsulin. *J. Biol. Chem.,* 253:2769–2775.
33. Rinderknecht, E., and Humbel, R. E. (1978): Primary structure of human insulin-like growth factor II. *FEBS Lett.,* 89:283–286.
34. Said, S. I., and Rosenberg, R. N. (1976): Vasoactive intestinal polypeptide: abundant immunoreactivity in neural cell lines and normal nervous tissue. *Science,* 192:907–908.
35. Seligman, P. A., Schleicher, R. B., and Selen, R. H. (1979): Isolation and characterization of the transferrin receptor from human placenta. *J. Biol. Chem.,* 254:9943–9946.
36. Spatz, H. (1922): Eisennachweis im Gehirn, besonders in Zentren des extrapyramidalen Systems. *Z. Ges. Neurol. Psychiatr.,* 77:261–390.

37. Sutherland, R., Della, D., Schneider, C., Newman, R., Kemshead, J., and Greaves, M. (1981): Ubiquitous cell-surface glycoprotein on tumor cells is proliferation-associated receptor for transferrin. *Proc. Natl. Acad. Sci. U.S.A.*, 78:4515–4519.

38. Tei, I., Makino, Y., Sakagam, H., Kanamaru, I., and Konno, K. (1982): Decrease of transferrin receptor during mouse myeloid leukemia (M1) cell differentiation. *Biochem. Biophys. Res. Commun.*, 107:1419–1424.

39. Testa, V., Thomopoulos, P., Vinci, G., Titura, M., Bettaieb, A., Vainchenker, M., and Rochant, H. (1982): Transferrin binding to K562 cell line, effect of heme and sodium butyrate induction. *Exp. Cell. Res.*, 140:251–260.

40. Trowbridge, I. S., Lesley, J., and Schutte, R. (1982): Murine cell surface transferrin receptor: Studies with an anti-receptor monoclonal antibody. *J. Cell. Physiol.*, 112:403–410.

41. Trowbridge, I. S., and Lopez, F. (1982): Monoclonal antibody to transferrin receptor blocks transferrin binding and inhibits human tumor cell growth *in vitro*. *Proc. Natl. Acad. Sci. U.S.A.*, 79:1175–1179.

42. Trowbridge, I. S., and Omary, M. B. (1981): Human cell surface glycoprotein related to cell proliferation is the receptor for transferrin. *Proc. Natl. Acad. Sci. U.S.A.*, 78:3039–3043.

43. Woods, S. C., Lotter, E. C., McKay, L. D., and Porte, D., Jr. (1979): Chronic intracerebroventricular infusion of insulin reduces food intake and body weight of baboons. *Nature*, 282:503–505.

44. Woods, S. C., and Porte, D., Jr. (1978): The central nervous system pancreatic hormones, feeding and obesity. *Adv. Metab. Disord.*, 9:283–311.

45. Young, W. S. III, Kuhar, M. J., Roth, J., and Brownstein, M. J. (1980): Radiohistochemical localization of insulin receptors in the adult and developing rat brain. *Neuropeptides*, 1:15–22.

46. Zahniser, N. R., Goens, M. B., Hanaway, P. J., and Vinych, J. V. (1984): Characterization and regulation of insulin receptors in rat brain. *J. Neurochem.*, 42:1354–1362.

47. Zapf, J., Schoenle, E., and Froesch, E. R. (1978): Insulin-like growth factors I and II: Some biological actions and receptor binding characteristics of two purified constituents of nonsuppressible insulin-like activity of human sera. *Eur. J. Biochem.*, 87:285–296.

48. Zapf, J., Waldvogel, M., and Froesch, E. R. (1975): Binding of nonsuppressible insulin-like activity to human serum: Evidence for a carrier protein. *Arch. Biochem. Biophys.*, 168:638–645.

Psychological, Neuropsychiatric, and
Substance Abuse Aspects of AIDS,
edited by T. Peter Bridge et al.
Raven Press, New York © 1988.

Characterization of Interleukin 1 Receptors in Brain

*William L. Farrar, †Patricia L. Kilian, ‡Michael R. Ruff,
§Joanna M. Hill, and §Candace B. Pert

*Laboratory of Molecular Immunoregulation, Biological Response Modifiers Program,
Division of Cancer Treatment, National Cancer Institute, Frederick Cancer Research
Facility, Frederick Maryland 21701; †Department of Immunopharmacology, Hoffman-
LaRoche, Nutley, New Jersey 07110; ‡Cellular Immunology Section, Laboratory of
Microbiology and Immunology, National Institute of Dental Research, National Institutes
of Health, Bethesda, Maryland 20892; and §Section of Brain Biochemistry, Clinical
Neuroscience Branch, Intramural Research Program, National Institute of Mental Health,
Alcohol, Drug Abuse, and Mental Health Administration, National Institutes of Health,
Bethesda, Maryland 20892

Interleukin 1 (IL-1) is a 17,500 M_r polypeptide synthesized by a variety of cell types including those of hematological, dermasomal, and neuronal histological origins (2,6,7,9,10,21,23). The ubiquitous distribution of IL-1 in diverse tissues has accordingly suggested an equally pleiotypic range of biological activities attributed to the molecule. The most rigorously studied biological effects of IL-1 have been its proposed role as an immunomodulatory molecule (20,21), in promotion of fibroblast growth (24), as a regulatory of hepatic acute-phase glycoprotein synthesis (2), and as a principal mediator of fever in mammalian species (endogenous pyrogen) (2). Because of its highly conserved phylogenetic activity, potentially broad tissue distribution, and biological action, rapid progress has been made in the elucidation of primary structure, deduced from cDNA clones, of human and murine IL-1 (1,8,16,17). Moreover, recent evidence has characterized high-affinity receptors for IL-1 on fibroblasts and lymphocytes (13–15).

Among the potent biological activities ascribed to IL-1 are its effects on the central nervous system. In addition to the regulation of febrile responses, intracerebroventricular (ICV) administration of IL-1 induces acute-phase glycoprotein synthesis (13), slow-wave sleep, and loss of appetite (15,19). Moreover, IL-1 has been shown to stimulate astrocyte growth and is detected following cerebral trauma (10). The biological evidence suggests that IL-1 participates in the modulation of CNS physiology and behavior in a fashion characteristic of neuroendocrine hormones. Here, we present data that describe the neuroanatomical distribution of IL-1 receptors in rat brain. Furthermore, antipyretic neuroendocrine hormones that modulate febrile responses do not competitively displace IL-1 from its high-affinity receptor. Initial characterization of the IL-1 receptor in brain reveals two major binding sites with molecular weights that correspond to that observed on fibroblasts and lymphocytes.

MATERIALS AND METHODS

Interleukin 1α Radioiodination

Recombinant murine IL-1α was obtained by expression of murine IL-1 cDNA in *E. coli* as described (16) with the exception that 17 amino acids were deleted from the *N* terminus of the IL-1α protein (14). The truncated analog, which corresponds to amino acids 131 through 270 of the precursor protein, retains the complete spectrum of biological activity of the 156-amino-acid protein and binds to the same receptor recognized by IL-1β (14). Since both IL-1α and -β apparently bind to the same recognition site in murine T cells (14,18), for the purposes of this study, IL-1α analog will be referred to as IL-1. The recombinant IL-1 analog was purified to homogeneity and was labeled with ^{125}I by utilizing enzymobead iodination reagent according to instructions from the manufacturer (Bio-Rad, Richmond, CA). The ^{125}I-IL-1 was readily separated from unreacted ^{125}I by use of Biogel PG-DG (Bio-Rad) and assayed for biological activity as described previously (14).

Preparation of Rat Brain Membrane and Autoradiography

As described by Herkenham and Pert (12), 24-μm-thick sections of adult male Sprague–Dawley rat brain, cut in either the coronal or the horizontal plane, were mounted onto gelatin-coated slides. Sections were stored under vacuum at 4°C at least 16 hr before use.

The brain sections were preincubated 15 min in each of two changes of RPMI with 1 mg/ml BSA and 20 mM Hepes at room temperature followed by 4 hr of incubation in the same buffer at 37°C with ^{125}I-IL-1 (98,000–100,000 cpm/ml) with or without 1 μM nonradioactive IL-1, 1 μM control fragment with biological activity, 1 μM melanocyte-stimulating hormone, 1 μM substance P, 1 μM arginine vasopressin, 1 μM thyrotropin-releasing hormone, or 1 μM vasoactive intestinal peptide (Penninsula Labs). Following incubation, the slides were transferred through five rinses, 1 min each, of phosphate-buffered saline, pH 7.4, on ice and rapidly dried under a stream of cold air. Some sections were scraped off the slides, and the radioactivity was counted in an auto γ counter. Specific binding was calculated as the difference in counts bound in the absence and presence of 1 μM nonradioactive IL-1. The above conditions provided optimum specific binding as determined by experiments varying preincubation and incubation conditions.

The remaining sections were used for receptor visualization and localization. Sections were fixed in hot paraformaldehyde vapors (12) and placed in a cassette with LKB Ultrofilm for 4 days. After exposure, the film was developed in Kodak D-19 at 20°C for 4 min, and the densities of the film were quantified (11). Some sections were then defatted in xylene, dipped into liquid emulsion (Kodak NTB-2), and exposed for 2 weeks at 4°C, developed in Kodak D-19 at 20°C for 2 min, and stained with thionin. Microscopic examination of these sections facilitated the identification of receptor distribution in relation to underlying cytoarchitecture.

Affinity Cross Linking of ^{125}I-IL-1 to Rat Membranes

Fresh rat brain membranes were prepared as described (12), washed, and resuspended in binding buffer. The ^{125}I-IL-1, 200,000 cpm, was bound to 3.0 mg brain membranes (net weight) in 0.5 ml at 4°C for 60 min. At the end of this incubation period, membranes were pelleted in a microfuge, washed with 1.0 ml cold binding buffer by pelleting, then resuspended in 0.5 ml cold buffer containing the homobifunctional cross linker disuccinimidyl suberate (DSS) at 0.2 mM. Cross linking was done for 15 min on ice. Membranes were collected by centrifugation and then resuspended in Laemlli sample buffer, boiled, and recentrifuged prior to electrophoresis on 8% SDS-polyacrylamide gels. Reaction products were visualized by autoradiography.

RESULTS

Autoradiography emerged in the mid 1970s as a powerful tool with which to determine the precise localization of neurotransmitter and drug receptors in brain. As described by Herkenham and Pert (12), 24-μm-thick sections of adult male Sprague–Dawley rat brain, cut in either coronal or horizontal plane, were mounted onto gelatin-coated slides. Pure, *E. coli*-derived recombinant murine IL-1 was labeled with ^{125}I and used for receptor binding studies. The coordinate addition of 1 μM "cold" unlabeled IL-1 revealed that almost 80% of total saturable binding could be inhibited at 37°C and was, therefore, specific. In contrast, a number of antipyretic neuroendocrine hormones, including α-melanocyte-stimulating hormone (MSH), substance P, Arg-vasopressin, thyrotropin-releasing hormone (TRH), and vasoactive intestinal peptide (VIP) added at concentrations of 1 μM failed to displace competitively ^{125}I-IL-1 binding from various areas of brain incubated under optimal conditions (data not shown).

^{125}I-Interleukin-1 binding is widespread throughout the rat brain and was detectable in numerous discrete brain areas. The pattern of distribution of ^{125}I-IL-1 binding sites is illustrated in Fig. 1, and Table 1 lists the brain areas groups according to receptor density of specific binding.

In the olfactory bulb (Fig. 1A), grain densities were highest in the mitral cell layer (MCL) and the glomerular layer (GL). In forebrain regions (Fig. 1B), binding was moderate in the caudate putamen (CPu), diagonal band (not shown), anterior preoptic region (AP), and septum (S), somewhat more dense in the deeper layers

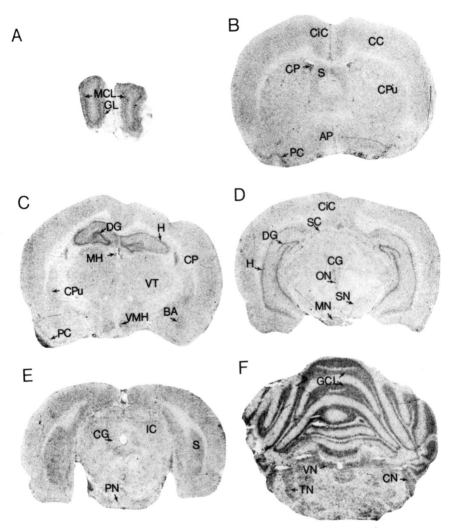

FIG. 1. Autoradiographs of ¹²⁵I-IL-1 binding in rat brain. **A**, Olfactory bulb; **B**, forebrain; **C**, thalamus; **D**, midbrain; **E**, posterior midbrain; **F**, cerebellum. AP, anterior preoptic region; BA, basolateral amygdala; CC, cerebral cortex; CG, central gray; CiC, cingulate cortex; CN, cochlear nucleus; CP, choroid plexus; CPu, caudate putamen; DG, dentate gyrus; GCL, granule cell layer; GL, glomerular layer; H, hippocampus; IC, inferior colliculus; MCL, mitral cell layer; MH, medial habenula; MN, mammillary nuclei; ON, oculomotor nuclei; PC, pyriform cortex; PN, pontine nuclei; S, subiculum; SC, superior colliculus; Se, septum; SN, substantia nigra; TN, trigeminal nucleus; VMH, ventromedial hypothalamic nucleus; VN, vestibular nucleus; VT, ventral thalamus.

TABLE 1. *Distribution of ^{125}I-IL-1 binding in rat brain*[a]

Very high	Olfactory bulb, mitral cell layer, and glomerular layer
	Dentate gyrus, granule cell layer
	Hippocampus, pyramidal cell layer
	Cerebellar cortex, granule cell layer
	Choroid plexus
High	Cingulate cortex, layer II/III
	Dentate gyrus, molecular layer
	Hippocampus, molecular layers
	Pyriform cortex, pyramidal cell layer
	Medial habenula
	Anterior dorsal thalamus
	Cerebral cortex, intermediate layers
	Ventromedial hypothalamus, oculomotor complex
	Dorsal tegmental nucleus
	Vestibular nuclei
	Cochlear nuclei
Moderate	Olfactory tubercle, superficial layers
	Caudate/putamen
	Diagonal band
	Septum
	Anterior preoptic area
	Ventral thalamus
	Basolateral amygdaloid nucleus
	Substantia nigra, pars compacta
	Medial geniculate nucleus
	Superior colliculus, superficial gray
	Central gray
	Posterior cingulate cortex
	Inferior colliculus
	Subiculum
	Entorhinal cortex, pyramidal layer
	Cerebellar cortex, molecular layer
	Trigeminal nucleus
	Facial nucleus
Low	Nucleus accumbens
	Median eminence
	Anterior hypothalamus
	Mammillary nuclei
	Olfactory tubercle, deep layers
	Pontine nuclei

[a]The density of ^{125}I-IL-1 binding to rat brain was determined by computer-assisted densitometry (11) of LKB films exposed to sections from several levels of rat brain. Within each group listed (e.g., high, moderate), differences in density were slight. Therefore, within groups, brain areas are listed in rostral–caudal position rather than rank order.

of the anterior cingulate cortex (CiC), frontal parietal cortex (FrPa), and the pyramidal cell layer of the pyriform cortex (Pc), but most dense in the choroid plexus (CP). At the level of the thalamus (Fig. 1C), the densest binding occurred in the granule cell layer of the dentate gyrus (DG), the pyramidal cell layer of the hippocampus (H), and the medial habenula (MH). Moderately high binding occurred in the anterior dorsal thalamus (not shown) and ventromedial hypothalamus

(VMH). Moderate density of ^{125}I-IL-1 bound to the basolateral amygdaloid nuclei (BA), ventral thalamic nuclei (VT), and subthalamus (not shown). At midbrain regions (Fig. 1D), the hippocampal binding is very evident, and the subiculum (not shown) and oculomotor complex (ON) also express moderately high binding. In this region, moderate binding occurs in the superficial gray of the superior collicus (SC), central gray (CG), substantia nigra (SN), medial geniculate (not shown), raphe nuclei (not shown), and mammillary nuclei (MN). The inferior collicus (Fig. 1E) has moderate binding, the pontine nuclei (PN) low, and the subiculum (S) and the dorsal tegmental nucleus moderately high at more posterior midbrain levels. At the level of the cerebellum (Fig. 1F), very high binding can be found in the granule cell layer of the cerebellar cortex (GCL), moderately high levels in the vestibular nuclei (VN) and cochlear nuclei (CN), but only moderate levels in the molecular layer of the cerebellar cortex, trigeminal nucleus, and facial nucleus (FN).

Affinity Cross Linking of ^{125}I-IL-1 to Rat Brain

Rat forebrain membranes were prepared and incubated for 60 min with ^{125}I-IL-1. The ^{125}I-IL-1 was cross linked to binding proteins via the addition of disuccimidyl suberate, and products were visualized on 8% SDS-PAGE. Membranes revealed two major products migrating with apparent molecular weights of 97,000 and 75,000 (Fig. 2A). These products are candidates for an IL-1 receptor since their formation was blocked in the presence of unlabeled IL-1 (Fig. 2B). The relationship of these products to one another is currently unknown, although they could indicate heterogeneity of brain IL-1 receptors. Alternatively, they may share a product/precursor relationship, as degradation is a complication of analyses of this type. Minor reaction products can be observed at higher M_rs as well. The two major identified cross-linked products suggest subunit sizes for brain IL-1 receptor(s) of approximately 80 kd and 58 kd, observations that are in accord with Dower et al. (5), who found ^{125}I-IL-1 binding proteins at approximately 80 kd in murine lymphocytes (5) and fibroblasts (4). Additionally, Matsushima et al. (18) has recently observed a 60-kd binding protein in human B lymphocytes.

DISCUSSION

The best-known effect of IL-1 on the central nervous system is its ability to cause fever (2). Recently, IL-1 has been shown to stimulate slow-wave sleep (15), food intake (19), and growth of astrocytes (10), suggesting further multiple levels by which IL-1 may modify neural cell function or behavior. Furthermore, IL-1 has recently been found to be synthesized in murine brain as well as by glioblastoma cell lines (6,10). The available data suggest that IL-1 may possess neuroendocrine functions as well as immunomodulatory activities.

Brain sections incubated in ^{125}I-IL-1 demonstrated a distinctive pattern of IL-1 receptor distribution, which was widespread throughout the brain. Figure 1 is a

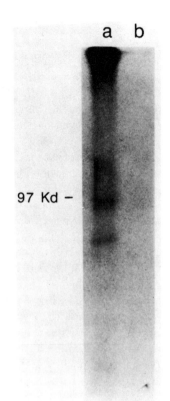

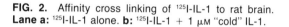

FIG. 2. Affinity cross linking of ^{125}I-IL-1 to rat brain. **Lane a:** ^{125}I-IL-1 alone. **b:** ^{125}I-IL-1 + 1 μM "cold" IL-1.

coronal view of IL-1 binding through the hippocampal region of the rat brain. The greatest amount of binding (darkest in the autoradiograph) occurs in areas where neurons are grouped in tight clusters such as the granule cells of the dentate gyrus (Fig. 1C), the pyramidal cells of the hippocampus (Fig. 1D), and the neurons of the oculomotor nucleus (Fig. 1D). The cerebral cortex, with more dispersed neurons, has less dense IL-1 binding.

The fact that both IL-1 binding and neuron-stained sections are densest in regions where cell bodies are clustered, such as in the granule cell layers of the dentate gyrus and the cerebellar cortex, suggests that IL-1 binding might occur in neurons throughout the brain. Binding is dense where neurons are dense and pale where neurons are sparse. However, there are several features of the IL-1 binding pattern that differ from that of a cell stain pattern, supporting the idea that the receptors are localized on only a subset of neurons. For example, binding is low in the granule cell layer of the olfactory bulb, a region composed of densely clustered neurons. Although the IL-1 binding pattern is similar to that of a cell stain typically used to identify the boundaries of nuclei, we cannot exclude the possibility that IL-1 is bound to neuron-associated glial cells in these regions.

Affinity cross linking of ^{125}I-IL-1α to rat brain revealed two potential binding proteins that may represent binding proteins of heterogeneity or possibly degradation products typical of this form of analysis. Nevertheless, the two species discerned are in accordance with described binding proteins for T lymphocytes (5,14), fibroblasts (80 kd) (4), and β lymphocytes (60 kd) (18). Both IL-1 species, α and β, are believed to bind to the same receptor (14,18) as well as to generate febrile responses. Further analysis of the function of brain IL-1 receptors await *in vitro* evaluation of IL-1 receptors on cell lines of neurological origins.

The preoptic region of the brain, an area important for the febrile response to IL-1, has only low to moderate IL-1 binding. The current view of the regulation of fever by endogenous pyrogen is that IL-1 enters the brain from the blood. It is not known, however, whether the entire molecule enters or only an active fragment, or how IL-1 reaches or otherwise signals receptors. For that matter, IL-1 may not cross the blood–brain barrier at all; labeled IL-1 injected intravenously into rabbits does not localize in brain even though fever is produced (3). The most anterior end of the hypothalamus with the posterior preoptic area below the anterior commissure in proximity to the ventricle is the region in all species studied from which the most rapid and intense febrile response to locally injected IL-1 is elicited (25). Injection of IL-1 into this site also augments the hepatic synthesis of acute-phase glycoproteins. Interestingly, antipyretic hormones such as α-MSH, TRH, β-endorphin, etc. had no competitive activity for IL-1 binding to rat brain (Fig. 1), supporting the notion that the IL-1 receptor is unique among hormone receptors that modulate fever.

It has also been recently demonstrated that intracerebroventricular administration of IL-1 promotes slow-wave sleep, although the area of the brain mediating this effect has not been identified. It is not clear how peripheral IL-1 may mediate many of the effects observed on intracerebral administration; nevertheless, perhaps the most provocative role of IL-1 in CNS is derived from the generation of the molecule within the brain itself (6,7,10). The widespread distribution of IL-1 receptors throughout the brain and their association with clusters of neurons suggest a potentially broader role of IL-1 in brain than previously suggested. The observations of Fontana et al. (6,7) and Giulian and Lachman (10) that IL-1 may be synthesized following cerebral trauma and promote astrocyte growth have suggested a potential role for IL-1 in brain cell repair or viability. Other neuroendocrine properties of IL-1 remain to be elucidated.

Shared antigenic structures between the immune and central nervous systems have recently been described by Pert et al. (23). Furthermore, a number of studies have shown that immune cells are functionally modulated by neurohormones previously believed to be restricted to other physiological systems. Such studies have led to the proposal that a biochemical network, a sharing and reciprocity of chemical messengers, exists between the two physiological systems. The data presented here provide a unique example of a common receptor for a cytokine produced by both immune and central nervous systems. Although a similar receptor is identified in both physiological systems, the biological role of IL-1 may be quite distinctive in the respective systems. The autoradiographic technique allows a quantitative and qualitative evaluation of receptor distribution, which may provide clues to physiological behavior and neuroendocrine activities of IL-1 previously not appreciated.

REFERENCES

1. Auron, P. E., Webb, A. C., Rosenwasser, L. J., Mucci, S. F., Rich, A., Wolff, S. M., and Dinarello, C. A. (1984): Nucleotide sequence of human monocyte interleukin 1 precursor cDNA. *Proc. Natl. Acad. Sci. U.S.A.*, 81:7907–7910.
2. Dinarello, C. A. (1984): Interleukin 1. *Rev. Infect. Dis.*, 6:51–78.
3. Dinarello, C. A., Weiner, P., and Wolff, S. M. (1978): Radiolabeling and disposition in rabbits of purified human leukocyte pyrogen. *Clin. Res.*, 26:522A–524A.
4. Dower, S. A., Call, S. M., Gillis, S., and Urdal, D. L. (1986): Similarity between IL 1 receptors on murine T lymphome and a murine fibroblast cell line. *Proc. Natl. Acad. Sci. U.S.A.*, 83:1060–1065.
5. Dower, S. K., Kronheim, S. R., March, C. J., Conlon, P. J., Hopp, T. P., Gillis, S., and Urdal, D. L. (1985): Detection and characterization of high affinity plasma membrane receptors for human interleukin 1. *J. Exp. Med.*, 162:501–505.
6. Fontana, A., Kristensen, F., Dubs, R., Gemsa, D., and Weber, E. (1982): Production of prostaglandin E and an interleukin 1-like factor by cultured astrocytes and C6 glioma cells. *J. Immunol.*, 129:2413–2416.
7. Fontana, A., Weber, E., and Dayer, J. M. (1984): Synthesis of interleukin 1/endogenous pyrogen in the brain of endotoxin-treated mice: A step in fever induction? *J. Immunol.*, 133:1696–1698.
8. Furutani, Y., Notake, M., Yamayoshi, M., Yamagishi, J., Nomura, H., Onue, M., Furutz, R., Fukui, T., Yamada, M., and Nakamura, S. (1985): Cloning and characterization of the cDNAs for human and rabbit interleukin 1 precursor. *Nucleic Acid Res.*, 13:5869–5872.
9. Gery, I., and Waksman, B. H. (1972): Potentiation of the T-lymphocyte response to mitogen. *J. Exp. Med.*, 137:143–147.
10. Giuliam, D., and Lachman, L. B. (1985): Interleukin 1 stimulation of astroglial proliferation after brain injury. *Science*, 228:497–499.
11. Goochee, C., Rasband, W., and Sokoloff, L. (1980): Computerized demitometry and color coding of [^{14}C]deoxyglucose autoradiographs. *Ann. Neurol.*, 7:359–361.
12. Herkenham, M., and Pert, C. B. (1982): Light microscopic localization of brain opiate receptors: A general autoradiographic method which preserves tissue quality. *J. Neurosci.*, 2:1129–1132.
13. Kampschmidt, R. F. (1984): The numerous postulated biological manifestations of interleukin 1. *J. Leukocyte Biol.*, 36:341–344.
14. Kilian, P. L., Kuffka, K. L., Stern, A. S., Woehle, D., Benjamin, W. R., Dechiara, T. M., Gubler, U., Farrar, J. J., Mizel, S. B., and Lomedico, P. T. (1986): Interleukin 1 α and interleukin β bind to the same receptor on T cells. *J. Immunol.*, 136:4509–4512.
15. Krueger, J. M., Walter, J., Dinarello, C. A., Wolff, S. M., and Chedid, L. (1984): Sleep-promoting effects of endogenous pyrogen (interleukin 1). *Am. J. Physiol.*, 246:R994–997.
16. Lomedico, P. T., Gubler, U., Hellman, C. F., Dukovich, M., Giri, J. G., Pan, Y. -C. E., Collier, K., Semionow, R., Chua, A. O., and Mizel, S. B. (1984): Cloning and expression of murine interleukin 1 cDNA in *Escherichia coli*. *Nature*, 312:458–461.
17. March, C. J., Mosley, B., Larsen, A., Cerretti, D. P., Braedt, G., Price, V., Gillis, S., Henney, C. S., Kronheim, S. R., Gradbstein, K., Conlon, P. J., Hopp, T. P., and Cosman, D. (1985): Cloning, sequence, and expression of two distinct human interleukin 1 complementary DNAs. *Nature*, 315:641–644.
18. Matsushima, K., Akahoshi, T., Yamada, M., Furutani, Y., and Oppenheim, J. J. (1986): Properties of a specific interleukin 1 (IL 1) receptor on human Epstein Barr virus transformed B lymphocytes. Identity of the receptor for ILl α and IL 1 β. *J. Immunol.*, 136:4496–4499.
19. McCarthy, D. O., Kluger, M. J., and Vander, A. J. (1985): The effect of peripheral and intracerebroventricular administration of interleukin 1 on food intake of rats. In: *The Physiologic*,

Metabolic, and Immunologic Actions of Interleukin 1, edited by M. J. Kluger, J. J. Oppenheim, and M. C. Powanda, p. 171–173. Alan R. Liss, New York.

20. Mizel, S. B. (1982): Interleukin 1 and T cell activation. *Immunol. Rev.,* 63:51.
21. Oppenheim, J. J., and Gery, I. (1983): Interleukin 1 is more than an interleukin. *Immunol. Today,* 3:113–114.
22. Paxinos, G., and Watson, C. (1982): *The Rat Brain in Sterotaxic Coordinates,* pp. 131–134. Academic Press, New York.
23. Pert, C. B., Ruff, M. R., Weber, R. J., and Herkenham, M. (1985): Neuropeptides and their receptors: A psychosomatic network. *J. Immunol.,* 135:8208–8211.
24. Schmidt, J., Mizel, S. B., Cohen, D., and Green, I. (1982): Interleukin 1, a potential regulator of fibroblast proliferation. *J. Immunol.,* 128:2177–2180.
25. Stitt, J. T. (1981): Neurophysiology of fever. *Fed. Proc.,* 40:2835–2836.

Psychological, Neuropsychiatric, and Substance Abuse Aspects of AIDS,
edited by T. Peter Bridge et al.
Raven Press, New York © 1988.

raf Protooncogene Expression in Neural and Immune Tissues

*George E. Mark, *Andrea Pfeifer, *Dean L. Mann,
*Curtis C. Harris, †Rob Berman, and †Candace B. Pert

Laboratory of Human Carcinogenesis, National Cancer Institute, National Institutes of Health, Bethesda, Maryland 20892; and †Section on Brain Biochemistry, Clinical Neuroscience Branch, Intramural Research Program, National Institute of Mental Health, Alcohol, Drug Abuse, and Mental Health Administration, National Institutes of Health, Bethesda, Maryland 20892

Protooncogenes represent normal genes that encode proteins whose actions control cellular growth and differentiation (2,3,10,11); simply stated, they are the normal counterparts of the oncogene.

It follows that these normal cellular genes must be "activated" to oncogenes before their cellular fomenting potential may be realized. This process of activation may be accomplished via multiple mechanisms, all of which involve somatic cell mutations as a consequence of DNA-damaging events. The present concepts of cellular transformation and carcinogenesis recognize the need for several discrete steps in the progression from normality to a fully malignant phenotype (8,26). Experimentally, cellular transformation may be achieved by introducing into a cell one gene whose product imparts to the cell an infinite proliferative capacity in addition to one gene whose expression may short circuit the cell's ability to differentiate terminally and die (1,14,18,25). Thus, more than one oncogene is needed. To date more than four dozen oncogenic sequences have been recognized. Most oncogenes thus far identified encode receptors (see Table 1, Class I).

Protooncogene receptors, like other cellular receptors, collect information from other cells and the environment and set in motion biochemical events. These events are essential or pivotal to the initiation of cell proliferation or the maintenance of cellular viability.

Three and a half years ago my laboratory cloned and sequenced a new oncogene, termed *raf*, which was snatched from a mouse cell by a passing retrovirus (22). The amino acid sequence of this oncogene revealed both the unique character of this protein and its familiar relationship to the *src* family of tyrosine kinases (16)—enzymes capable of transferring a phosphate from ATP to a tyrosine amino acid residue of some associated protein (7,13).

TABLE 1. *Potential oncogenes*

Class I	Class II	Others
fps	Ha-*ras*	*rel*
fes	ki-*ras*	erb A
yes	N-*ras*	*ets*
fgr		*dbl*
lyt	Class III	*bcl*-1
slk/sny (fyn)	*sis*/PDGF-B	*bcl*-2
lck	PDGF-A	*tcl*-1
trk	IL-3	*tcl*-2
met	NGF	*hst*
kit		*mcf*.2
sea	Class IV	*mas*
abl	*fos*	*jun*
src	*myb*	
ros/mcf3	*ski*	
Insulin-R	c-*myc*	
IGF1-R	N-*myc*	
PDGF-R	L-*myc*	
erb-B/EGF-R	B*lym*	
neu/EGF2-R	p53	
fms/CSF1-R		
raf/mil		
pkC1		
pkC2		
pkC3		
mos		

We have applied two basic approaches in our investigations into the functioning and malfunctioning of the *raf* sequence. First, we are using molecular biologic techniques to disassemble the *raf* oncogenic sequence to discover those domains of the protein that are essential for malignant transformation. Second, we are attempting to determine under what circumstances this protooncogene is physiologically expressed—in which cells, under what conditions. Naturally, we are also interested in identifying tumors in which *raf* is pathologically expressed. We hope that the normal will lead us to the abnormal. The data presented show the expression of the *raf* protooncogene in proliferating B and T lymphocytes as well as in small cell lung carcinomas (cells with a definite lymphoid characteristic), in cells of the limbic system and cerebellum in normal rat brain, and in two malignancies of neural origin. Finally, the commonality between the immune and nervous systems suggested that the specific recombination mechanisms (30) employed by both T and B cells to create unique receptor–ligand interactions may be active in neuronal cells. We have, I believe, observed this phenomenon in at least one neural tumor.

PROTOONCOGENES, ONCOGENES, AND *raf*

A list of genes whose oncogenic potential has been experimentally determined or can be inferred based on their known enzymatic activities may be compiled

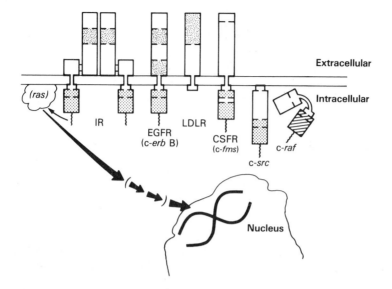

FIG. 1. Schematic representation of various types of cellular receptors. Depicted are the α (external) and β (cytoplasmic tyrosine kinase) subunit structures of the insulin receptor (IR); the epithelial growth factor receptor (EGFR, a truncated version of this receptor has been found to be identical to the *src* family oncogene v-*erb* B) which shares structural elements with the low-density lipid receptor (LDLR) and the IR; the colony-stimulating factor 1 receptor (CSFR), homologous to the v-*fms* oncogene of the *src* family; and the c-*src* and c-*raf* receptors, whose functions are unknown. All but the c-*raf* receptor and the LDLR appear to transmit their proliferative signal to the nucleus by way of the *ras* gene product (28). The structural homologies we have found between the c-*raf* receptor and protein kinase C suggest that these receptors employ related mechanisms of signal transduction, and the "activated" form of the c-*raf* receptor may represent membrane associations other than the transmembrane one depicted here.

(Table 1). Four classes of oncogenes have been identified; the largest is composed of the *src* family of protein kinases (Class I). The other classes represent the *ras* family of G-like proteins (Class II), the small peptide growth factors such as those derived from platelets (Class III), and a group of proteins that share the characteristic of being found predominantly intranuclearly (Class IV).

How is *raf* related to the other *src* family oncogenes? A cartoon depicting several of the *src* family receptors is shown in Fig. 1. Each is composed of an amino-terminally located ligand-binding domain, many of which contain cysteine-rich regions (lightly shaded in Fig. 1), and a kinase domain (darkly shaded in Fig. 1). In addition, the extreme carboxy end of each polypeptide seems to carry unique sequences that may account for the functioning of these proteins in a tissue-specific manner. Alterations that transform the benign protein into an oncogene usually result from the loss of domains that are necessary for the controlled, metered function of the receptor. To date, very little is known about the mechanism by which extracellular signals are converted by these receptors to changes in the program of the cell.

New light has recently been shed on the potential pathway of signal transduction

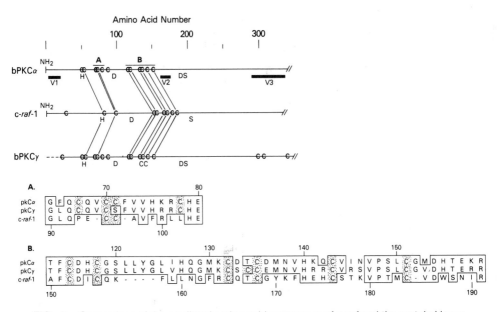

FIG. 2. Comparison of the predicted amino acid sequences of c-*raf* and the protein kinase C family of receptors. Cysteine residues (C) are connected by lines or shaded. V1, V2, and V3 represent variable regions within the pkC family of kinases.

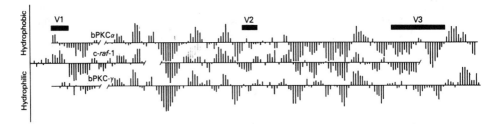

FIG. 3. Comparison of the hydrophobic and hydrophilic regions within the amino-terminal protein domains of the human c-*raf*-1 and bovine protein kinase C α and γ polypeptides.

resulting from activation of the c-*raf* "receptor." The DNA sequences for the family of phorbol ester receptors (protein kinase C, pkC) have been determined (6,14,19–21), and the predicted amino acid composition of these serine/threonine kinases reveals regions homologous to *raf* within their respective receptor domains. This is most notable in the sequences including and surrounding their cysteine residues (Fig. 2), which comprise a possible nucleic acid binding domain. The similarity between pkC and c-*raf* is also apparent when the secondary structures of their ligand-binding domains are compared by hydropathy measurements (Fig. 3). Finally, pkC has been found to transit from the cytosolic fraction to the plasma membrane

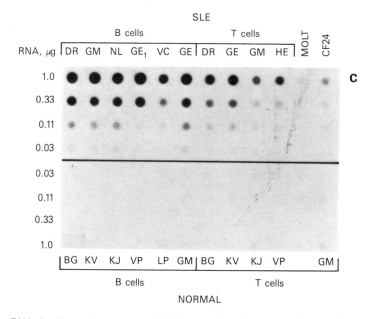

FIG. 4. RNA dot blot analysis of c-*raf* RNA expression in peripheral blood lymphocytes obtained from normal and diseased individuals. Molt 4 and CF 24 are T and B cell lines used as controls. The most undiluted dot represents 1 μg of total cell RNA. Blotting and hybridization conditions were as previously described (5).

fraction in response to its activation by ligand and calcium binding. We have found c-*raf* capable of such associations when it is "activated," as has occurred in peripheral neuroepitheliomas.

We have examined a wide variety of cell types and found the expression of the *raf* "receptor" to be limited to proliferating hematopoietic cells (4,5) and regenerating cells of the liver and pancreas. Recently we have extended this list to include cells of both the CNS and peripheral nervous system (see below). Although other tissues may express *raf* during specific stages in their differentiation, we have not seen this gene expressed in either epithelial cells or connective tissue.

The expression of the *raf* gene in the proliferating lymphoid cells of patients suffering from systemic lupus erythematosus is illustated in Fig. 4. Nonproliferating lymphoid cells obtained from normal donors showed little evidence of *raf* expression, whereas "activated" T and B cells from the peripheral blood of diseased individuals expressed significant levels of *raf* RNA. We have observed following mitogen treatment of normal lymphoid the transcription of the *raf* protooncogene in a controlled and regulated fashion prior to, or simultaneous with, the initiation of S phase.

We have also documented (10) the expression of *raf* in cells obtained from a very aggressive type of human lung cancer, small cell lung carcinoma (SCLC). Whereas most non-SCLCs are not expressors, all SCLCs are (Fig. 5). This is particularly

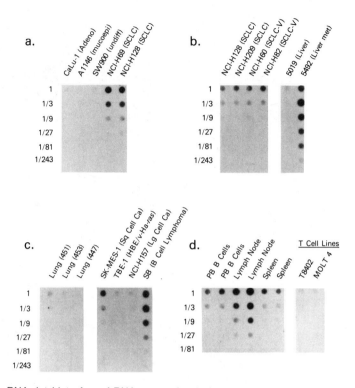

FIG. 5. RNA dot blot of c-*raf* RNA expression in human cell lines and primary tissues. Panels **a** and **b** contain RNAs isolated from small cell lung carcinoma cell lines (SCLC) of a SCLC liver metastasis and its corresponding normal liver tissue. Panel **c** shows expression in normal lung parenchymal tissues, *ras* oncogene-transformed human bronchial epithelium (31), and a cell line derived from a B-cell lymphoma (SB). Panel **d** reveals c-*raf* expression in normal human lymphoid tissues. Methods are as described in Fig. 2; top dot represents 1 μg of total cell RNA.

evident in the metastases of the primary tumor (Fig. 5, panel b). In 1984, Ruff and Pert (23) reported that cells of this malignancy carried surface characteristics of hematopoietic cells, specifically monocytes. Our observations of *raf* expression in SCLCs and lymphoid cells are not inconsistent with their finding. Consequently, we examined the surface components of a series of malignant and nonmalignant cells for specific lymphoid proteins. We have found two markers (Table 2) representing early monomyelocytic surface antigens (MY4 and MY9) that were expressed by all SCLCs. These cells also expressed presumed B-cell-specific and macrophage-specific antigens detected by monoclonal antibodies B1 and OKM1, respectively. These latter markers were not, however, found exclusively on SCLC cells. We tentatively conclude, as have Ruff and Pert (23,24), that the cells of this malignancy appear to be of monocytic origin.

With increasing frequency, elements responsible for signal transduction between neuronal cells—that is, neuropeptides and their receptors—are being found associated with lymphoid cells. Conversely, several lymphoid cell surface receptors

TABLE 2. *Expression of surface antigens on normal and neoplastic human lung cells: Percentage of cells showing positive fluorescence*[a]

Cell		Monoclonal antibody							
		W6/32 (I)	3.1 (II)[b]	OKB2	B1	OKM1	MY4	MY7	MY9
				B-cell			Monocytic markers		
Small cell lung carcinomas									
H128	C[c]	44	6	46	15	19	8	0	15
H69	C	22	7	71	29	39	32	0	24
N417	V	28	5	56	8	16	29	0	10
H82	V	20	10	7	10	6	8	ND	8
N592	C	9	9	75	22	22	24	0	10
UMC-1	C	10	0	76	10	14	10	0	12
UMC-5	C	13	6	60	14	22	19	0	14
UMC-6	V	13	12	62	12	15	11	0	15
UMC-7	C	18	9	27	10	13	13	0	15
TUMOR1[d]		12	11	45	8	7	9	0	14
TUMOR2		4	30	71	8	18	12	0	17
Normal epithelial cells									
NHBE[e]		83	13	37	2	10	0	0	0
NHBE		75	5	55	5	14	0	0	0
NHBE		71	8	43	7	8	0	0	0
"Transformed" NHBE									
TBE-1SA		63	5	4	0	0	0	0	14
Non-SCLC lung carcinomas									
H292	mucoepiderm[f]	50	7	38	19	15	13	0	18
A1146	mucoepiderm	12	0	30	5	7	0	1	5
SW900	undiffer.	72	23	25	7	4	1	0	2
A2182	adeno.	75	1	40	4	5	2	0	0
Calu-1	squamous	64	56	6	2	2	0	0	0
H157	large cell	82	40	9	ND	ND	0	0	2

[a]Percentage of cells showing greater fluorescence than negative control MoAb-stained cells; ND, not done.
[b]HLA class detected by this monoclonal antibody.
[c]"Classic" or "Variant" SCLC morphology.
[d]Fresh small cell tumor biopsies from which single cell suspensions were prepared.
[e]Normal human bronchial epithelial primary cell cultures initiated from three different donors without noted lung pathologies.
[f]Histologic type of tumor.

have been identified on neuronal cells (i.e., the T4 antigen). It was, therefore, logical to investigate brain tissue for *raf* expression.

In collaboration with Rob Berman of Dr. Pert's laboratory, we used affinity-purified *raf*-specific antibodies to examine rat brain for the existence and distribution of the *raf* protein. Brain slices were incubated with an antipeptide polyclonal rabbit antibody, SP63, specific for the carboxy-terminal 12 amino acids of the *raf* protooncogene (27). The binding of iodinated protein A to these rabbit antibodies was visualized by autoradiography (9). The density of the exposure was ultimately translated into color by computer enhancement (the highest density of silver grains is represented by white, and the lowest density is colored blue). Figure 6 shows the localization of the *raf* protooncogene in normal rat brain. The largest concentration of immunoreactive protein was observed in the cerebellum, both cortex and nuclei, with lesser amounts in hippocampus, septum, thalamus, and cerebral cortex. We conclude from these studies that the antibody binding was specific, since it was not directly related to neural cell density. In some areas fiber tracts were stained, whereas in other areas it was the neuron bodies that contained the *raf* protein. The distribution seen corresponds to specific cytoarchitectural sites; areas of the limbic system are especially enriched for the *raf* "receptor." We further conclude that the *raf* protein must be membrane associated within those cells where it is visualized, since cytosolic components would be removed during the extensive washing procedures that are part of this *in situ* technique. We interpret the distribution pattern as possibly being that of a widely disseminated potential neuropeptide receptor. Recently, the IP_3 receptor has been similarly localized (29). We are presently investigating the possibility that *raf* may bind IP_3.

Understanding the physiological role of many protooncogenes has been hampered by the lack of knowledge of the tissue or specific cell type in which the gene normally presents itself. We have identified *raf* as a significant product in both lymphoid and neural tissues. We have also found this gene associated with embryonic development in the fruitfly (17), implying that *raf* may be essential during the early stages of cellular differentiation.

As a direct consequence of the localization of the *raf* "receptor" in normal brain, we sought to determine if *raf* could be found associated with any neuronal-derived malignancy. We have been able to demonstrate, by immunofluorescent staining and northern blot analysis of transcribed RNA, the *raf* protein and mRNA in peripheral neuroepitheliomas (an extremely aggressive tumor of adolescents) and neuroblastomas. We believe the *raf* utilization leads to pathological consequences only in the neuroepitheliomas. In collaboration with Dr. Maria Tsokos in the Division of Cancer Biology and Diagnosis at the NCI, a comparison of three malignancies arising from cells of the neural crest was undertaken (Table 3). Until recently individuals with neuroepitheliomas were believed to have neuroblastomas and were treated accordingly—most died. Ewing's sarcoma, on the other hand, has a very good recovery rate. As a result of the molecular similarities between neuroepithelioma cells and Ewing's sarcoma cells, patients presenting with a cholinergic malignancy that exhibits nonneuroblastic characteristics were treated as though they had Ewing's

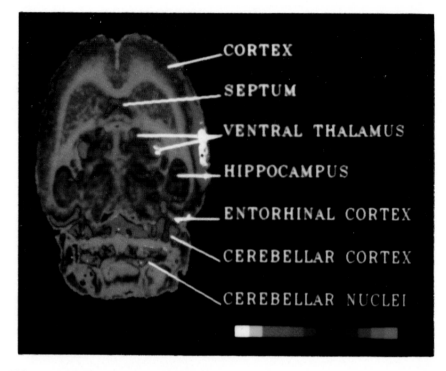

FIG. 6. Regions of normal rat brain that contain membrane-bound c-*raf* receptor. Frozen sections of brain were incubated with an affinity-purified rabbit antipeptide specific for the carboxy terminus of the c-*raf* polypeptide. ^{125}I-labeled second antibody was employed to amplify the detection. The density of the resulting silver grains in the emulsion was translated into colors by a computer enhancement program.

TABLE 3. *Comparison of three malignancies arising from cells of the neural crest*

	Ewing's sarcoma	Neuroepithelioma	Neuroblastoma
Innervation	Cholinergic	Cholinergic	Adrenergic and mixed
Chromosomal aberrations	t(11;22)	t(11;22)	—
Protooncogene expression elevated	c-*myc* and c-*raf*	c-*myc* and c-*raf*	N-*myc* and c-*raf*
c-*raf* location	?	Plasma membrane	Cytosolic
Chemotherapy	Responsive to Ewing protocol	Responsive to Ewing protocol	Responsive to neuroblastoma protocol

sarcoma. To date, 13 of 14 children are alive and recovering. The role of the *raf* "receptor" in this disease has been under investigation.

NEURONAL RECEPTORS

The diversity and specificity of the antigen-binding receptors of the T and B lymphoid cells are made possible because of the mechanism used by these cells to assemble these receptors. A specific DNA recombination system (30) rearranges the immunoreceptor genetic information within a cell in such a way that widely separated sequences are brought together. Recognition of this mechanism required that this process of juxtaposition of subunits had occurred identically in all cells under scrutiny. Tumors initiated from the unbridled proliferation of a single cell should therefore be genetically homogeneous. The similarities between the immune and neural systems prompted us to look in homogeneous neural tumors for evidence of this very specific recombination system. Southern blot analysis of Hind-III-digested genomic DNA was examined for rearrangements of the κ light chain immunoglobulin locus. The germ line unaltered locus was observed in most of the nonlymphoid cells examined (Fig. 7). The exception was the rearrangement identified in the DNA obtained from a biopsy of a human ganglioneuroma. Further studies of this DNA have shown that the immunoglobulin heavy chain locus, whose rearrangement usually precedes that of the light chain locus, was in the germ line configuration. We believe this is evidence—a footprint, if you will—of this specific recombinatory mechanism malfunctioning in these neuronal cells. We speculate that there may exist neuronal receptors that necessarily employ the inherent plasticity this system allows. Those events that occur during the development of long-term memory, requiring *de novo* protein synthesis, may employ this mechanism of gene rearrangement to alter specific receptors so as to commit the neuron to a permanent cell–cell association.

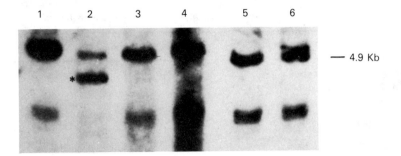

FIG. 7. Southern blot analysis of human DNAs for rearrangements in the immunoglobulin κ light chain J region gene. The human DNAs were restricted by Hind III endonuclease, electrophoresed, transferred to nitrocellulose, and probed with a 1.95-kilobase Sac I fragment representing the five germ line J regions of the κ light chain gene. The expected unaltered allele (4.9-kilobase Hind III fragment) can be seen in all lanes, and the lane representing the ganglioneuroma **(lane 2)** shows a novel 4.5-kilobase fragment. The presence of a rearrangement of this allele was also observed in this tissue when the Eco R1 restriction endonuclease was employed. The DNAs were isolated from ganglioneuromas **(lanes 1 and 2)**, ganglioneuroblastomas **(lanes 3, 5, and 6)**, and a sphenoid meningioma **(lane 4)**.

REFERENCES

1. Bechade, C., Calothy, G., Pessac, B., Martin, P., Coll, J., Saule, S., Ghysdael, J., and Stehelin, D. (1985): Induction of proliferation or transformation of neuroretina cells by *mil* and *myc* viral oncogenes. *Nature*, 316:559–562.
2. Bishop, J. M. (1983): Cellular oncogenes and retroviruses. *Annu. Rev. Biochem.*, 52:301–354.
3. Bishop, J. M. (1985): Viral oncogenes. *Cell*, 42:23–38.
4. Boumpas, D. T., Mark, G. E., and Tsokos, G. C. (1986): Oncogenes and autoimmunity. *Anticancer Res.*, 6:491–498.
5. Boumpas, D. T., Tsokos, G. C., Mann, D. L., Eleftheriades, E. G., Harris, C. C., and Mark, G. E. (1986): Increased proto-oncogene expression in peripheral blood lymphocytes from patients with systemic lupus erythematosus and other autoimmune diseases. *Arthritis Rheum.*, 29:755–760.
6. Coussens, L., Parker, P. J., Rhee, L., Yang-Feng, T. L., Chen, E., Waterfield, M. D., Francke, U., and Ullrich, A. (1986): Multiple, distinct forms of bovine and human protein kinase C suggest diversity in cellular signaling pathways. *Science*, 233:859–866.
7. Cross, F. R., and Hanafusa, H. (1983): Local mutagenesis of Rous sarcoma virus: The major sites of tyrosine and serine phosphorylation of p60[src] are dispensable for transformation. *Cell*, 34:597–607.
8. Farber, E. (1984): The multistep nature of cancer development. *Cancer Res.*, 44:4217–4223.
9. Gaudreau, P., Quirion, R., St.-Pierre, S., and Pert, C. B. (1983): Characterization and visualization of cholecystokinin receptors in rat brain using [³H]pentagastrin. *Peptides*, 4:755–762.
10. Graziano, S. L., Cowan, B. Y., Carney, D. N., Bryke, C. R., Mitter, N. S., Johnson, B., Mark, G. E., Planas, A. T., Davis, B., Poiesz, B. J., and Comis, R. L. (1987): Small cell lung cancer cell line derived from a primary tumor with a characteristic deletion of 3p. *Cancer Res.*, 47:2148–2155.
11. Hunter, T. (1984): The proteins of oncogenes. *Sci. Am.*, 251:70–79.
12. Hunter, T., and Cooper, J. A. (1985): Protein-tyrosine kinases. *Annu. Rev. Biochem.*, 54:897–930.
13. Kamps, M. P., Taylor, S. S., and Sefton, B. M. (1984): Direct evidence that oncogenic tyrosine kinases and cyclic AMP-dependent protein kinase have homologous ATP-binding sites. *Nature*, 310:589–592.

14. Knopf, J. L., Lee, M.-H., Sultzman, L. A., Kritz, R. W., Loomis, C. R., Hewick, R. M., and Bell, R. M. (1986): Cloning and expression of multiple protein kinase C cDNAs. *Cell,* 46:491–502.
15. Land, H., Parada, L. F., and Weinberg, R. A. (1983): Tumorigenic conversion of primary embryo fibroblasts requires at least two cooperating oncogenes. *Nature,* 304:596–602.
16. Mark, G. E., and Rapp, U. R. (1984): Primary structure of v-*raf* predicts relatedness to the "*src*-family" of oncogenes. *Science,* 224:285–289.
17. Mark, G. E., MacIntyre, R., Digan, M. E., Ambrosio, L., and Perrimon, N. (1987): Characterization of two loci in *Drosophila melanogaster* related to the *raf* oncogene. *Mol. Cell. Biol. (in press).*
18. Muller, R. (1986): Proto-oncogenes and differentiation. *Trends Biochem. Sci.,* 11:128–131.
19. Ohno, S., Kawasaki, H., Imajoh, S., Suzuki, K., Inagaki, M., Yokokura, H., Sakoh, T., and Hidaka, H. (1987): Tissue-specific expression of three distinct types of rabbit protein kinase C. *Nature,* 325:161–166.
20. Ono, Y., Kurokawa, T., Fujii, T., Kawahara, K., Igarashi, K., Kikkawa, U., Ogita, K., and Mishizuka, Y. (1986): Two types of complementary DNAs of rat brain protein kinase C. *FEBS Lett.,* 206:347–352.
21. Parker, P. J., Coussens, L., Totty, N., Rhee, L., Young, S., Chen, E., Stabel, S., Waterfield, M. D., and Ullrich, A. (1986): The complete primary structure of protein kinase C—the major phorbol ester receptor. *Science,* 233:853–859.
22. Rapp, U. R., Goldborough, M. D., Mark, G. E., Bonner, T. I., Groffen, J., Reynolds, F. H., Jr., and Stephenson, J. R. (1983): Structure and biological activity of v-*raf*, a novel oncogene transduced by a retrovirus. *Proc. Natl. Acad. Sci. U.S.A.,* 80:4218–4222.
23. Ruff, M. R., and Pert, C. B. (1984): Small cell carcinoma of the lung: Macrophage-specific antigens suggest hemopoietic stem cell origin. *Science,* 225:1034–1036.
24. Ruff, M. R., Farrar, F. W., and Pert, C. B. (1986): Interferon gamma and granulocyte/macrophage colony stimulating factor inhibit growth and induce antigens characteristic of myeloid differentiation in small cell lung cancer lines. *Proc. Natl. Acad. Sci. U.S.A.,* 83:6613–6617.
25. Ruley, E. (1983): Adenovirus early region IA enables viral and cellular transforming genes to transform primary cells in culture. *Nature,* 304:602–606.
26. Salomon, D. S., and Perroteau, I. (1986): Growth factors in cancer and their relationship to oncogenes. *Cancer Invest.,* 4:43–60.
27. Schultz, A. M., Copeland, T. D., Mark, G. E., Rapp, U. R., and Oroszlan, S. (1985): Detection of the myristylated gag-*raf* transforming protein with *raf*-specific antipeptide sera. *Virology,* 146:78–89.
28. Smith, M. R., DeGudicibus, S. J., and Stacey, D. W. (1986): Requirement for c-*ras* proteins during viral oncogene transformation. *Nature,* 320:540–543.
29. Worley, P. F., Baraban, J. M., Colvin, J. S., and Snyder, S. H. (1987): Inositol trisphosphate receptor localization in brain: Variable stoichiometry with protein kinase C. *Nature,* 325:159–161.
30. Yancopoulos, G. D., Blackwell, T. K., Suh, H., Hood, L., and Alt, F. W. (1986): Introduced T cell receptor variable region gene segments recombine in pre-B cells: Evidence that B and T cells use a common recombinase. *Cell,* 44:251–259.
31. Yoakum, G. H., Lechner, J. F., Gabrielson, E. W., Korba, B. E., Malan-Shibley, L., Willey, J. C., Valerio, M. G., Shamsuddin, A. M., Trump, B. F., and Harris, C. C. (1985): Transformation of human bronchial epithelial cells transfected by Harvey *ras* oncogene. *Science,* 227:1174–1179.

Psychological, Neuropsychiatric, and Substance Abuse Aspects of AIDS, edited by T. Peter Bridge et al. Raven Press, New York © 1988.

Synthetic Peptides in the Study of the Interaction of Rabies Virus and the Acetylcholine Receptor

Thomas L. Lentz, Edward Hawrot, Diana Donnelly-Roberts, and Paul T. Wilson

Departments of Cell Biology and Pharmacology, Yale University School of Medicine, New Haven, Connecticut 06510

Infectivity by many viruses is restricted to certain hosts and tissue types. Factors responsible for the tropisms of viruses include the specificity, number, and distribution of cell surface viral receptors. Enveloped viruses attach to cells by means of the glycoprotein comprising the surface spikes of the viral envelope (11,40). The glycoprotein binds to components of the cell surface, which are thereby utilized as receptors by the virus. These receptors may include any normal cell membrane constituent, including carbohydrates, lipids, or proteins such as enzymes, ion channels, or hormone receptors. Neurotropic viruses infect the nervous system and include viruses such as poliovirus, herpesvirus, rabies virus, reovirus, encephalitis viruses, and lentiviruses including acquired immune deficiency syndrome (AIDS) or human immunodeficiency viruses (HIV) (LAV, HTLV-III, ARV) (17,18). It seems likely that some of these viruses attach to receptors that are present on or, in some cases, largely restricted to neurons.

Two such neuronal molecules that may act as host cell receptors for viruses are the acetycholine receptor (AChR), which has been suggested to serve as a rabies virus receptor (24,26), and the β-adrenergic receptor, which may represent a reovirus type 3 receptor (6). Other viral receptors that have been identified are the epidermal growth factor receptor, which is utilized by vaccinia virus (12), the complement receptor type 2 (CR2) of B lymphocytes, which is an Epstein–Barr virus receptor (14), and the T4 (CD4) antigen of T lymphocytes, which is a component of the HIV receptor (7,23,30). Evidence has been presented that brain membranes contain a T4 antigen indistinguishable from that found on T lymphocytes (35). This chapter reviews the nature of the receptors for the highly neurotropic virus, rabies virus, and focuses particularly on the possibility that the AChR serves as a receptor for rabies virus. The interaction of synthetic peptides of the rabies virus glycoprotein with the AChR has been investigated.

RABIES VIRUS PATHOGENESIS AND RECEPTORS

Rabies virus is an enveloped, negative-strand RNA rhabdovirus. Infection in nature results from inoculation into tissues of saliva containing virus from the bites of infected animals. During the variable and relatively long incubation period, viral replication in striated muscle has been observed (31). Virus subsequently enters peripheral nerves, including those at neuromuscular junctions, neuromuscular spindles, and neurotendinal spindles (31), and is carried to the spinal cord by retrograde axonal transport (42). Infection rapidly ascends in the spinal cord to the brain, where early infection is highly selective for certain neuronal populations (16). Virus is transferred from neuron to neuron at synapses, where presynaptic axon terminals endocytose virus particles, both those free in the intercellular space and those budding from the postsynaptic surface (3). Later in the disease, virus spreads centrifugally over peripheral nerves but does not appear to infect cells of most parenchymal organs. One exception is in the salivary glands, where virus replicates and buds from the apical cell surface into the duct system carrying saliva (10).

The pathogenesis of rabies, in which infection is restricted to a few specific cell types (muscle fibers, neurons, salivary gland acinar cells), indicates the existence of highly specific host cell receptors. However, the situation is complicated by the fact that although infection occurs in only a few cell types *in vivo*, a large number of cell types can be infected *in vitro*. Available evidence, in fact, suggests that a number of different cell surface constituents may act as attachment determinants for rabies. Phosphatidylserine could be a rabies virus receptor because rabies virus and vesicular stomatitis virus share a receptor site on cultured baby hamster kidney (BHK) cells (45) and there is evidence that phosphatidylserine serves as a binding site for vesicular stomatitis virus (38). In addition, it has been proposed that carbohydrate moieties, phospholipids, and highly sialylated gangliosides contribute to a receptor complex for rabies virus (39). Finally, as noted above, the AChR has been proposed as a host cell receptor for rabies virus.

RABIES VIRUS AND THE ACETYLCHOLINE RECEPTOR

The suggestion that the AChR might serve as a rabies virus receptor was based on observations that rabies virus antigen could be localized by immunofluorescence at neuromuscular junctions, which contain a high density of AChR, shortly after immersion of mouse diaphragm in a suspension of rabies virus (26). Similarly, in cultured embryonic chick myotubes infected with rabies virus, viral antigen was distributed in patches on the cell surface in a pattern similar to that of high-density AChR as demonstrated by rhodamine-labeled α-bungarotoxin (α-BTX) staining. Pretreatment of myotubes with the nicotinic cholinergic antagonists α-BTX and *d*-tubocurarine resulted in a reduction in the number of myotubes that became infected after exposure to rabies virus. Finally, it was shown that the binding of rabies virus to membrane preparations from embryonic chick myotubes of increasing developmental age closely paralleled the AChR content of these membranes (27). Together, these findings provided indirect evidence that rabies virus might bind to the AChR. More recently, Tsiang et al. (43) have shown that α-BTX inhibits rabies virus infection of cultured primary rat myotubes.

The nicotinic AChR is one of the best characterized receptor molecules (29,33,36). It is a macromolecular complex composed of four homologous subunits with a stoichiometry of α_2, β, γ, and δ. The α subunits bear the binding site for acetylcholine and snake venom curaremimetic neurotoxins. These neurotoxins, such as α-BTX, block binding of cholinergic agonists and antagonists and, therefore, are believed to bind at or near the acetylcholine binding site on the α subunit (21,22). The subunits span the lipid bilayer, and some of the transmembrane segments form the wall of the ion channel (Fig. 1) (13). The subunits have a large

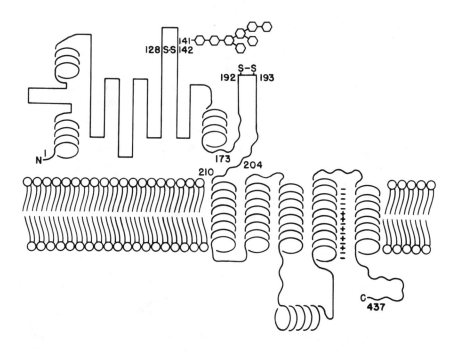

FIG. 1. Schematic diagram illustrating the secondary structure and transmembrane structure of the α subunit of the AChR [based on Finer-Moore and Stroud (13)]. A potential site of glycosylation occurs at asparagine 141. Cysteines 192 and 193 form a disulfide (19) and bind the affinity alkylating agent 4-(N-maleimido)benzyltrimethylammonium iodide (20). A 32-residue peptide comprising residues 173 to 204 binds α-bungarotoxin with the same affinity as the isolated α subunit (44). This model proposes four hydrophobic transmembrane segments and a fifth amphipathic transmembrane helix, which may contribute to the wall of the ionic channel (13).

ectodomain, which in the case of the α subunit bears the acetylcholine binding site. It has been shown that a 32-residue peptide comprising residues 173 to 204 of the α subunit binds α-BTX with the same affinity as the intact isolated subunit (44). In addition, a peptide corresponding to residues 185 to 196 binds α-BTX (32). These findings indicate that a major determinant of the BTX-binding site lies within this region of the α subunit. However, it is possible that other, nonadjacent sequences contribute to the overall high-affinity binding of α-BTX observed with intact AChR.

Direct binding of labeled rabies virus to purified AChR has been demonstrated (25). The AChR from the electric organ of *Torpedo californica* was affinity-purified on a cobratoxin–Sepharose column. Rabies virus (CVS strain) was labeled with ^{125}I- or ^{35}S-methionine. Binding of labeled virus was demonstrated by a dot blot assay in which receptor was adsorbed onto nitrocellulose and by solid-phase radioassays in which receptor was immobilized on the plastic of 96-well microtest plates. For the dot blot assay, nitrocellulose filters containing increasing amounts of AChR were incubated with a constant amount of ^{125}I-labeled rabies virus. Autoradiography of the filter showed that virus binding increased as a function of AChR amount (Fig. 2).

In order to determine whether the binding of virus to the AChR was saturable, wells of polystyrene microtest plates were coated with a constant amount of AChR and incubated with increasing amounts of ^{125}I-labeled virus. Nonspecific binding was considered the amount of labeled virus bound at each point in the presence of a 100-fold excess of native unlabeled virus. This value was subtracted from the total labeled virus bound in the absence of native unlabeled virus to determine the amount specifically bound. Specific binding increased linearly at the lower concentrations of virus, but at higher concentrations, progressively smaller increments in binding were observed (Fig. 3). Scatchard analysis of the data from the saturation experiment yielded a nonlinear curve, so no definite conclusions could be drawn concerning the nature of the binding event. Nonlinear plots could result from multiple binding sites, cooperativity, or nonequilibrium binding conditions. In addition to saturability of binding with respect to receptor, evidence for specificity included

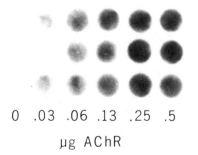

0   .03 .06 .13 .25 .5

μg AChR

FIG. 2. Dot blot assay of rabies virus binding to AChR. Circles of nitrocellulose were incubated with increasing amounts of AChR purified from *Torpedo* electric organ (0 to 0.5 μg) in 0.05 M carbonate/bicarbonate buffer, pH 9.6, overnight. The filters were washed three times in phosphate-buffered saline and quenched in 10% dry nonfat milk overnight. The filters were washed and were then incubated with ^{125}I-labeled rabies virus (147,000 cpm) in phosphate buffer, pH 5.5, containing 0.1% Triton X-100 overnight. The filters were washed six times and autoradiographed.

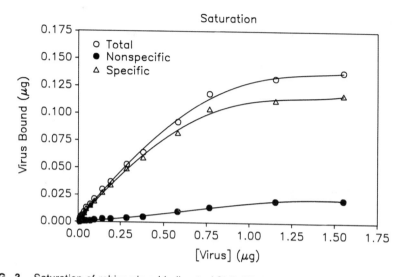

FIG. 3. Saturation of rabies virus binding to AChR. Wells of polystyrene microtiter plates were coated with 0.1 μg AChR and incubated with increasing amounts of ¹²⁵I-labeled rabies virus (0 to 1.55 μg) for 20 hr at room temperature. Bound virus was solubilized with sodium dodecylsulfate, and radioactivity was measured in a γ counter. Total represents the total amount of radioactivity bound at each concentration. Nonspecific is the amount of radioactivity bound in the presence of a 100-fold excess of cold virus. Specific binding was determined by subtracting the nonspecific bound from total bound. Values represent means of three replicates.

inhibition of labeled virus binding by increasing amounts of native unlabeled virus particles. Finally, autoradiography after SDS-PAGE analysis of the labeled material bound to the AChR revealed the same viral proteins as in the starting preparation. Thus, the radioactivity attached to the AChR represented labeled viral proteins.

Attachment of rabies virus to the AChR may explain some aspects of the pathogenesis of the disease. After inoculation of virus and during the incubation period, viral replication in striated muscle has been observed and suggested to be important in amplifying the inoculum prior to uptake by peripheral nerves (31). The high density of AChR at the neuromuscular junction could concentrate virus particles at this site. Because the virus particle with its numerous glycoprotein spikes represents a multivalent ligand, it could cross link receptors and induce endocytosis and internalization by muscle. Virus particles localized at the neuromuscular junction could also be endocytosed by the adjacent nerve terminal, although it is not known if this is a process mediated by attachment to specific receptors. In the central nervous system, α-BTX-binding proteins of unknown function (5,34) and a protein homologous to the α subunit of muscle nicotinic AChR (2) have been identified. Binding of rabies virus to these neuronal receptors could play a role in the transsynaptic transfer of virus.

SEQUENCE SIMILARITY BETWEEN RABIES VIRUS GLYCOPROTEIN AND NEUROTOXINS

The experiments described above demonstrate direct binding of rabies virus to the nicotinic AChR. The molecular basis for the virus–AChR interaction may lie in a structural similarity between the snake venom neurotoxins and a portion of the rabies virus glycoprotein. A large number of snake venom neurotoxins have been

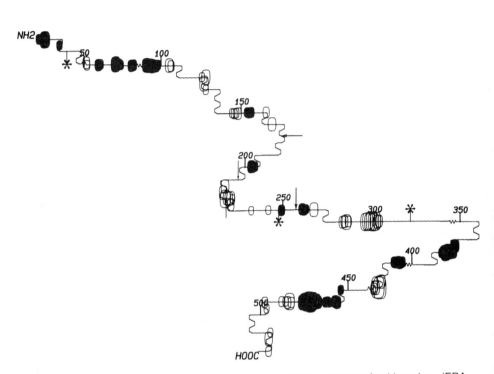

FIG. 4. Predicted secondary structure and hydrophilicity pattern of rabies virus (ERA strain) glycoprotein. Predictions were performed using the programs CHOUFAS and PLOTCHOU of the Sequence Analysis Software Package of the University of Wisconsin Genetics Computer Group (9). The programs were prepared by B. Foertch of the Max-Planck Institut. These programs produce a graphic representation of Chou and Fasman (4) protein secondary structure predictions with hydrophilicity values (15) superimposed. Positions of α helices are indicated by *coils*, β sheets by *narrow zigzags*, random coils as *wide zigzags*, and β turns by *turns of the chain*. *Open ovals* denote hydrophilic regions, and *filled ovals* indicate hydrophobic regions. The size of the oval is proportional to the average hydrophilicity as calculated over seven residues. Numbering is that of the glycoprotein precursor, although the signal peptide is not included in the analysis. The hydrophobic region between residues 459 and 480 is most likely the transmembrane segment. Sites of *N*-linked glycosylation on the ectodomain are indicated by *asterisks*. The segment of the glycoprotein showing an amino acid similarity to the neurotoxins (residues 176–257 of precursor glycoprotein) is bracketed by *large arrows*. *Small arrows* delineate the 13-residue region that was synthesized and tested for ability to inhibit neurotoxin binding to the AChR.

RV Gp (157–238) GKC–SGVAVSSTYCSTNHD––YT–IWMPENPRLGMS
Ntx (1–73)   TKCYVTPDATSQTCPDGQDICYTKTW–––––––––––
Common   KC   S C   D YT W

CDIFTNSRGKRASKG–SETCGFVDERGLYKSLKGACKLKLCGVLGLRLMDG
CDGFCSSRGKRIDLGCAATCPKVK–PGV––DIK–CCSTDNCNPFPTWKRKH
CD F SRGKR   G   TC V   G   K C   C

FIG. 5. Alignment of a long neurotoxin (*Ophiophagus hannah* toxin b) (Ntx) with a segment (residues 157–238) of rabies glycoprotein (ERA strain). Alignment was performed using the program ALIGN of the Protein Identification Resource (PIR) of the National Biomedical Research Foundation. ALIGN was prepared by B. C. Orcutt, M. O. Dayhoff, D. G. George, and W. C. Barker. The mutational data matrix for 250 point-accepted mutations (PAMs), a matrix bias of +3, and a gap penalty of 6 were used. Alignment score was derived from the standard deviation obtained with alignments made with 100 scrambled sequences having the same lengths and compositions as the neurotoxin and glycoprotein. The above alignment has 24 identities (35%), eight gaps, and an alignment score of 5.28 SD.

sequenced, and there is considerable information on their structure–function relationships (22). For two strains of rabies virus, the amino acid sequence of the glycoprotein has been deduced from the nucleotide sequence of cloned cDNA (1,46). The glycoprotein is composed of 505 amino acids and has three carbohydrate attachment sites on the ectodomain. The predicted secondary structure of the rabies virus glycoprotein (ERA strain) is shown in Fig. 4.

The sequences of the toxins and the virus were compared (28) with the computer program ALIGN as described by Dayhoff and co-workers (8). These analyses revealed a significant sequence similarity between the entire long neurotoxin sequence of 71 to 74 residues and a segment of the rabies virus glycoprotein, namely, residues 157 to 238 (Fig. 5). This segment of the rabies glycoprotein lies on the ectodomain of the molecule and includes a highly hydrophilic region (Fig. 4).

Most importantly, the greatest similarity between the glycoprotein and neurotoxins occurs with those amino acids that are highly conserved or invariant among all of the neurotoxins. These residues are considered to be the most important for toxicity and include those residues believed to bind to the acetylcholine binding site on the AChR. The latter are located at the end of loop 2, the "toxic" loop, a long central loop protruding from the toxin molecule. It has been proposed that the guanidinium group of arginine-37 may be the counterpart of the quaternary ammonium group of acetylcholine and that a hydrogen-bonded ion pair between the side chain carboxylate of aspartate-31 and the guanidinium group of arginine-37 may form a stereochemical analog of acetylcholine (41). Rabies virus shows identity with all of the residues in loop 2 that are highly conserved or invariant among all the neurotoxins (Tyr[25], Trp[29], Asp[31], Arg[37], Gly[38], Gly[44]) (Fig. 5). In contrast, the glycoprotein sequence of vesicular stomatitis virus, a rhabdovirus whose overall sequence is homologous to the overall rabies virus glycoprotein sequence (37), shows little similarity to the rabies glycoprotein and the neurotoxins in this particular region.

COMPETITION BETWEEN GLYCOPROTEIN PEPTIDES AND
NEUROTOXINS

Because of the similarity of the rabies virus glycoprotein with the toxic loop of the neurotoxins, this region of the glycoprotein may interact with the same site on the AChR as do the neurotoxins. To test this, experiments have been performed to determine whether neurotoxin can compete with rabies for binding to the receptor and whether viral peptides can inhibit toxin binding. Competition would be predicted if viral glycoprotein and neurotoxins indeed share a common binding site. A constant amount of ^{35}S-labeled virus was incubated with AChR in the presence of increasing concentrations of α-BTX. α-Bungarotoxin was found to have an inhibitory effect on virus binding, inhibiting binding up to 50% (Fig. 6). The concentration of α-BTX that produced a half-maximal effect was 3×10^{-9}M.

Peptides within the region of the rabies virus glycoprotein that is homologous to the tip of loop 2 of the neurotoxins have been synthesized (Fig. 7). This region of the glycoprotein is hydrophilic, and its structure is primarily β sheet with β turns (Fig. 4). Thirteen-residue peptides for the ERA and CVS strains of rabies virus (ERA 13-mer, CVS 13-mer) matching in sequence residues 187 to 199 of the glycoprotein and a CVS 10-mer comprising residues 190 to 199 were synthesized. In addition, a BTX 13-mer and a BTX 10-mer comprising toxin positions 28 to 40

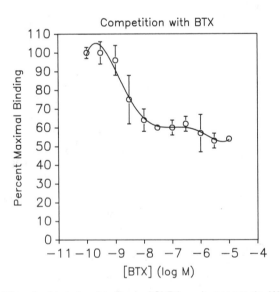

FIG. 6. Competition of rabies virus binding to AChR by α-bungarotoxin. Wells of microtiter plates were coated with 0.5 μg AChR and incubated with constant ^{35}S-labeled rabies virus (3 μg, 23,000 cpm) in 0.05 M phosphate buffer, pH 5.5, and protease inhibitors in the presence of increasing amounts of α-bungarotoxin at 37°C. After 8 hr of incubation, wells were washed, bound virus solubilized, and radioactivity measured in a scintillation counter. Values represent the means of three replicates.

α−Bungarotoxin, 28−40 (BTX 13−mer)
α−Bungarotoxin, 31−40 (BTX 10−mer)
Rabies Virus ERA Strain, 187−199 (ERA 13−mer)
Rabies Virus CVS Strain, 187−199 (CVS 13−mer)
Rabies Virus CVS Strain, 190−199 (CVS 10−mer)

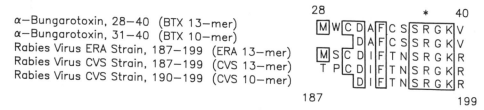

FIG. 7. Sequences and alignments of synthetic peptides of α-bungarotoxin and rabies virus glycoprotein. Sequence homologies are boxed. The toxin peptides are located at the end of loop 2 of the neurotoxins. The position of the virus peptides on the glycoprotein is shown in Fig. 4. The *asterisk* is arginine-37, which may represent the counterpart of the quaternary ammonium of acetylcholine.

and 31 to 40, respectively, were synthesized. The CVS 10-mer and CVS 13-mer were synthesized by the Children's Hospital Corporation Peptide Facility, Boston, Massachusetts, and the BTX 10-mer, BTX 13-mer, and ERA 13-mer were synthesized by the Protein Chemistry Facility, Department of Molecular Biophysics and Biochemistry, Yale University. Composition of peptides was verified by amino acid analysis. Crude peptides were purified by column chromatography on a Sephadex G-25 column equilibrated with 10 mM phosphate buffer, pH 7.2.

The viral peptides were compared with other cholinergic ligands and with the toxin peptides for their ability to compete with α-BTX binding to the AChR in a solid-phase assay (Figs. 8 and 9). Increasing amounts of ligand were incubated with 1 nM ^{125}I-labeled α-BTX for 30 min, and bound α-BTX was measured. The concentration of ligand that produced 50% inhibition of α-BTX binding was determined. The IC_{50} values allow the relative affinities of the various ligands to be compared (Table 1). The BTX 13-mer and ERA 13-mer inhibited toxin binding with affinities comparable to *d*-tubocurarine. The CVS 13-mer inhibited toxin binding with an efficiency intermediate between *d*-tubocurarine and nicotine. The BTX 10-mer and the CVS 10-mer had approximately the same affinity as nicotine. These findings show that the rabies virus glycoprotein peptides compete with α-BTX for binding to the AChR, indicating that they bind at or near the acetylcholine binding site on the receptor. Although the affinity of the virus peptides is considerably less than that of intact toxin, it is comparable to that of other cholinergic antagonists or agonists and to corresponding toxin peptides. These studies also indicate that short synthetic peptides are capable of interacting specifically with proteins. Since small peptides in solution may exist in dynamic equilibrium with a multiplicity of conformational states, it would be expected that the peptides would at least transiently adopt a conformation capable of interacting with a binding site on a receptor. It is also possible that in some cases a relatively short stretch of amino acids can adopt the conformation found in the native protein. The ability of peptides to interact with a receptor indicates that they could be potentially useful as antiviral agents.

Antibody was raised in rabbits against the CVS 10-mer coupled to keyhole limpet hemocyanin. The reactivity of the antibody against the CVS 10-mer was tested by

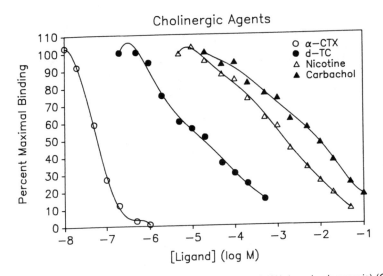

FIG. 8. Binding-inhibition assay. The abilities of α-cobratoxin (*Naja naja siamensis*) (CTX), *d*-tubocurarine (*d*-TC), nicotine, and carbachol to compete with binding of [125]-labeled α-bungarotoxin to the AChR were compared. Wells of microtiter plates were coated with 0.15 μg AChR and incubated for 10 min with 1 nM labeled toxin and increasing concentrations of ligand. After washing, bound radioactivity was removed and measured. Values represent means of three replicates.

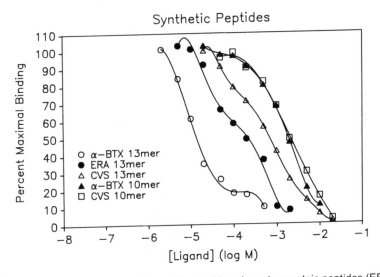

FIG. 9. Binding-inhibition assay. The ability of rabies virus glycoprotein peptides (ERA 13-mer, CVS 13-mer, and CVS 10-mer) and α-bungarotoxin peptides (BTX 13-mer, BTX 10-mer) to compete binding of [125]-labeled α-bungarotoxin were compared. Assays were performed as described in Fig. 8.

TABLE 1. *Binding-inhibition assay*[a]

	IC_{50} (M)
Cholinergic ligands	
α-Cobratoxin	6.0×10^{-8}
d-Tubocurarine	2.1×10^{-5}
Nicotine	1.5×10^{-3}
Carbamylcholine	8.4×10^{-3}
Synthetic peptides	
BTX 13-mer	1.7×10^{-5}
ERA 13-mer	9.2×10^{-5}
CVS 13-mer	3.0×10^{-4}
BTX 10-mer	1.8×10^{-3}
CVS 10-mer	1.9×10^{-3}

[a]The concentrations of agents that produced 50% inhibition (IC_{50}) of 1 nm ^{125}I-α-bungarotoxin to AChR are listed. Values are determined from experiments and data shown in Figs. 8 and 9.

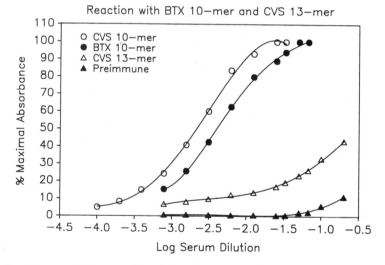

FIG. 10. Cross reactivity of antibody raised against a rabies virus glycoprotein peptide (CVS 10-mer) with the CVS 10-mer, a CVS 13-mer, and an α-bungarotoxin peptide (BTX 10-mer). See Fig. 7 for sequences of peptides. Wells of microtiter plates were coated with 5 μg of peptide and incubated with serial dilutions of polyclonal antibody (log serial dilution) raised in rabbits against the CVS 10-mer coupled to keyhole limpet hemocyanin. The reaction of preimmune serum against the CVS 10-mer was measured (preimmune). Bound antibody was determined by ELISA using alkaline phosphatase-conjugated goat antirabbit IgG (1 : 750), reacting for alkaline phosphatase, and reading absorbance at 405 nm.

enzyme-labeled immunosorbent assay (ELISA) (Fig. 10). The anti-CVS 10-mer cross reacted with the BTX 10-mer and the CVS 13-mer. The affinity of binding to the CVS 13-mer was reduced, even though this peptide includes the sequence of the 10-mer, indicating that conformation plays an important role in antibody binding to these peptides. Cross reaction between the CVS 10-mer and BTX 10-mer provides additional evidence for the structural similarity between the glycoprotein and neurotoxin peptides.

SIGNIFICANCE FOR VIRAL DISEASES

These studies provide evidence that binding of rabies virus to the AChR is mediated by a portion of the rabies glycoprotein bearing a structural similarity to the region of snake venom neurotoxins that binds near the acetylcholine binding site on the AChR. The regions of other viruses that bind to host cell molecules may in many cases also be similar to the binding domains of proteins or other ligands that normally bind to these molecules. If viral infection is followed by production of antibodies to the idiotypes, these antiidiotypic antibodies would have the ability to react with the cellular receptors. In the case of viruses binding to neuronal molecules or receptors, such a mechanism could lead to chronic diseases of the nervous system, autoimmune responses to neural elements, or impaired neural function, including mental illness.

Identification of either the viral domains involved in binding to cellular receptors or the domains comprising the binding sites of the receptors could be important in forming a basis for certain types of treatment. These sites could be the target of chemical agents that might prove effective in inhibiting viral binding. Synthetic peptides comprising the binding domains might themselves act as competitive inhibitors and prevent attachment of virus to cell surface receptors. In fact, it has been shown that synthetic decapeptides of vaccinia virus protein and transforming growth factor α inhibit vaccinia virus infection of murine L fibroblasts (12), and an octapeptide of HIV gp120 inhibits HIV infection of human T cells (35). The binding domains of the virus could be used as immunogenic agents in the development of safe and specific subunit vaccines. Such novel strategies for therapy may be necessary for viruses that infect the central nervous system or that evade immune clearance by frequent mutation. In the case of such viruses, which appear to include the AIDS virus (18), antiviral agents must be able to cross the blood–brain barrier, and the immunogenic regions of the virus used to develop vaccines should be highly conserved and not undergo genetic drift. It might be expected that the receptor-binding domain of the viral glycoprotein is less variable. It has been noted that if all pathogenic strains of AIDS virus display T4$^+$ T-cell tropism, then the region of the gp110 protein interacting with the T4 molecules is likely to be conserved, and antibodies directed against this epitope should be broadly reactive against different AIDS virus isolates (30).

SUMMARY

The neurotropism of some viruses may be explained in part by the attachment of these viruses to host cell receptors that are present on or even largely restricted to neurons. Rabies virus is an RNA virus that, after a period of replication in muscle, gains access to the central nervous system, where it selectively infects certain neuronal populations. The nicotinic acetylcholine receptor occurs in high density at the neuromuscular junction and is present in the central nervous system. Although several different cell surface constituents may act as attachment determinants for rabies, direct binding of radioactively labeled virus to affinity-purified acetylcholine receptor has been demonstrated. Binding of virus to the receptor was saturable and inhibited by up to 50% by α-bungarotoxin, a snake venom neurotoxin that binds at or near the acetylcholine binding site on the receptor.

The molecular basis for the virus–receptor interaction may lie in an amino acid sequence similarity between the snake venom neurotoxins and a segment of the rabies virus glycoprotein. Two peptides (10 and 13 residues) of the rabies virus glycoprotein and homologous bungarotoxin peptides were synthesized and tested for ability to compete with labeled α-bungarotoxin for binding to the acetylcholine receptor. The peptides were found to compete with toxin binding with affinities comparable to those of the cholinergic ligands *d*-tubocurarine and nicotine. These findings indicate that a segment of the rabies virus glycoprotein interacts with the acetylcholine receptor at or near the acetylcholine binding site of the receptor. The similarity between the virus glycoprotein and the neurotoxin was further evidenced by the cross reaction of antibody raised against the virus 10-mer with the bungarotoxin 10-mer. Binding of rabies virus to the acetylcholine receptor or to other neuronal bungarotoxin-binding proteins may be related to the neurotropism of this virus. In addition, knowledge of both the region of the virus involved in binding and the binding domain on the receptor may be helpful in developing new strategies for treatment, especially for viruses that infect the central nervous system or evade the immune response through genetic drift. These strategies include development of antiviral agents that cross the blood–brain barrier and inhibit viral binding and the utilization as immunogens the regions of viruses, such as their binding domains, that are highly conserved among different strains.

ACKNOWLEDGMENTS

This research was supported by NSF grant BNS 85-06404, NIH grants NS 21896 and GM 32629, the Muscular Dystrophy Association, and USAMRAA Contract DAMD17-86-C-6043.

REFERENCES

1. Anilionis, A., Wunner, W. H., and Curtis, P. J. (1981): Structure of the glycoprotein gene in rabies virus. *Nature*, 294:275–278.

2. Boulter, J., Evans, K., Goldman, D., Martin, G., Treco, D., Heinemann, S., and Patrick, J. (1986): Isolation of a cDNA clone coding for a possible neural nicotinic acetylcholine receptor α-subunit. *Nature,* 319:368–374.
3. Charlton, K. M., and Casey, G. A. (1979): Experimental rabies in skunks. Immunofluorescence light and electronic microscopic studies. *Lab. Invest.,* 41:36–44.
4. Chou, P. Y., and Fasman, G. D. (1974): Prediction of protein conformation. *Biochemistry,* 13:222–245.
5. Clarke, P. B. S., Schwartz, R. D., Paul, S. M., Pert, C. B., and Pert, A. (1985): Nicotinic binding in rat brain: Autoradiographic comparison of [³H]acetylcholine, [³H]nicotine, and [¹²⁵I]-α-bungarotoxin. *J. Neurosci.,* 5:1307–1315.
6. Co, M. S., Gaulton, G. M., Tominaga, A., Homcy, C. J., Fields, B. N., and Greene, M. I. (1985): Structural similarities between the mammalian β-adrenergic and reovirus type 3 receptors. *Proc. Natl. Acad. Sci. U.S.A.,* 82:5315–5318.
7. Dalgleish, A. G., Beverley, P. C. L., Clapham, P. R., Crawford, D. H., Greaves, M. F., and Weiss, R. A. (1984): The CD4(T4) antigen is an essential component of the receptor for the AIDS retrovirus. *Nature,* 312:763–768.
8. Dayhoff, M. O., Barker, W. C., and Hunt, L. T. (1983): Establishing homologies in protein sequences. *Methods Enzymol.,* 91:524–545.
9. Devereux, J., Haeberli, P., and Smithies, O. (1984): A comprehensive set of sequence analysis programs for the VAX. *Nucleic Acids Res.,* 12:387–395.
10. Dierks, R. E., Murphy, F. A., and Harrison, A. K. (1969): Extraneural rabies virus infection. Virus development in fox salivary gland. *Am. J. Pathol.,* 54:251–274.
11. Dimmock, N. J. (1982): Initial stages in infection with animal viruses. *J. Gen. Virol.,* 59:1–22.
12. Eppstein, D. A., Marsh, Y. V., Schreiber, A. B., Newman, S. R., Todaro, G. J., and Nestor, J. J., Jr. (1985): Epidermal growth factor receptor occupancy inhibits vaccinia virus infection. *Nature,* 318:663–665.
13. Finer-Moore, J., and Stroud, R. M. (1984): Amphipathic analysis and possible formation of the ion channel in an acetylcholine receptor. *Proc. Natl. Acad. Sci. U.S.A.,* 81:155–159.
14. Fingeroth, J. D., Weis, J. J., Tedder, T. F., Strominger, J. L., Biro, P. A., and Fearon, D. T. (1984): Epstein–Barr virus receptor of human B lymphocytes is the C3d Receptor CR2. *Proc. Natl. Acad. Sci. U.S.A.,* 81:4510–4514.
15. Hopp, T. P., and Woods, K. R. (1981): Prediction of protein antigenic determinants from amino acid sequences. *Proc. Natl. Acad. Sci. U.S.A.,* 78:3824–3828.
16. Johnson, R. T. (1965): Experimental rabies. Studies of cellular vulnerability and pathogenesis using fluorescent antibody staining. *J. Neuropath. Exp. Neurol.,* 24:662–674.
17. Johnson, R. T. (1982): *Viral Infections of the Nervous System.* Raven Press, New York.
18. Johnson, R. T., and McArthur, J. C. (1986): AIDS and the brain. *Trends Neurosci.,* 9:91–94.
19. Kao, P. N., and Karlin, A. (1986): Acetylcholine receptor binding site contains a disulfide cross-link between adjacent half-cystinyl residues. *J. Biol. Chem.,* 261:8085–8088.
20. Kao, P. N., Dwork, A. J., Kaldany, R.-R. J., Silver, M. L., Wideman, J., Stein, S., and Karlin, A. (1984): Identification of the α subunit half-cystine specifically labeled by an affinity reagent for the acetylcholine receptor binding site. *J. Biol. Chem.,* 259:11662–11665.
21. Karlin, A. (1980): Molecular properties of nicotinic acetylcholine receptor. In: *The Cell Surface and Neuronal Function,* edited by C. W. Cotman, G. Poste, and G. L. Nicolson, pp. 191–260. Elsevier/North-Holland Biomedical Press, New York.
22. Karlsson, E. (1979): Chemistry of protein toxins in snake venoms. *Handb. Exp. Pharmacol.,* 52:159–212.
23. Klatzmann, D., Champagne, E., Chamaret, S., Gruest, J., Guetard, D., Hercend, T., Gluckman, J.-C., and Montagnier, L. (1984): T-lymphocyte T4 molecule behaves as the receptor for human retrovirus LAV. *Nature,* 312:767–768.
24. Lentz, T. L. (1985): Rabies virus receptors. *Trends Neurosci.,* 8:360–364.
25. Lentz, T. L., Benson, R. J. J., Klimowicz, D., Wilson, P. T., and Hawrot, E. (1987): Binding of rabies virus to purified *Torpedo* acetylcholine receptor. *Mol. Brain Res,* 1:211–219.
26. Lentz, T. L., Burrage, T. H., Smith, A. L., Crick, J., and Tignor, G. H. (1982): Is the acetylcholine receptor a rabies virus receptor? *Science,* 215:182–184.
27. Lentz, T. L., Chester, J., Benson, R. J. J., Hawrot, E., Tignor, G. H., and Smith, A. L. (1985):

Rabies virus binding to cellular membranes measured by enzyme immunoassay. *Muscle Nerve,* 8:336–345.

28. Lentz, T. L., Wilson, P. T., Hawrot, E., and Speicher, D. W. (1984): Amino acid sequence similarity between rabies virus glycoprotein and snake venom curaremimetic neurotoxins. *Science,* 226:847–848.

29. McCarthy, M. P., Earnest, J. P., Young, E. F., Choe, S., and Stroud, R. M. (1986): The molecular biology of the acetylcholine receptor. *Annu. Rev. Neurosci.,* 9:383–413.

30. McDougal, J. S., Kennedy, M. S., Sligh, J. M., Cort, S. P., Mawle, A., and Nicholson, J. K. A. (1986): Binding of HTLV-III/LAV to T4$^+$ T cells by a complex of the 110K viral protein and the T4 molecule. *Science,* 231:382–385.

31. Murphy, F. A. (1977): Rabies pathogenesis. Brief review. *Arch. Virol.,* 54:279–297.

32. Neumann, D., Barchan, D., Safran, A., Gershoni, J. M., and Fuchs, S. (1986): Mapping of the α-bungarotoxin binding site within the α subunit of the acetylcholine receptor. *Proc. Natl. Acad. Sci. U.S.A.,* 83:3008–3011.

33. Numa, S., Noda, M., Takahashi, H., Tanabe, T., Toyosato, M., Furutani, Y., and Kikyotani, S. (1983): Molecular structure of the nicotinic acetylcholine receptor. *Symp. Quant. Biol.,* 48:57–69.

34. Oswald, R. E., and Freeman, J. A. (1981): α-Bungarotoxin binding and central nervous system nicotinic acetylcholine receptors. *Neuroscience,* 6:1–14.

35. Pert, C. B., Hill, J. M., Ruff, M. R., Berman, R. M., Robey, W. G., Arthur, L. O., Ruscetti, F. W., and Farrar, W. L. (1986): Octapeptides deduced from the neuropeptide receptor-like pattern of antigen T4 in brain potently inhibit human immunodeficiency versus receptor binding and T-cell infectivity. *Proc. Natl. Acad. Sci. U.S.A.,* 83:9254–9258.

36. Popot, J.-L., and Changeux, J.-P. (1984): Nicotinic receptor of acetylcholine: Structure of an oligomeric integral membrane protein. *Physiol. Rev.,* 64:1162–1239.

37. Rose, J. K., Doolittle, R. F., Anilionis, A., Curtis, P. J., and Wunner, W. H. (1982): Homology between the glycoproteins of vesicular stomatitis virus and rabies virus. *J. Virol.,* 43:361–364.

38. Schlegel, R., Tralka, T. S., Willingham, M. C., and Pastan, I. H. (1983): Inhibition of VSV binding and infectivity by phosphatidylserine: Is phosphatidylserine a VSV-binding site? *Cell,* 32:639–646.

39. Superti, F., Hauttecoeur, B., Morelec, M.-J., Goldoni, P., Bizzini, B., and Tsiang, H. (1986): Involvement of gangliosides in rabies virus infection. *J. Gen. Virol.,* 67:47–56.

40. Tardieu, M., Epstein, R. L., and Weiner, H. L. (1982): Interaction of viruses with cell surface receptors. *Int. Rev. Cytol.,* 80:27–61.

41. Tsernoglou, D., Petsko, G. A., and Hudson, R. A. (1978): Structure and function of snake venom curarimimetic neurotoxins. *Mol. Pharmacol.,* 14:710–716.

42. Tsiang, H. (1979): Evidence for an intraaxonal transport of fixed and street rabies virus. *J. Neuropathol. Exp. Neurol.,* 38:286–296.

43. Tsiang, H., de la Porte, S., Ambroise, D. J., Derer, M., and Koenig, J. (1986): Infection of cultured rat myotubes and neurons from the spinal cord by rabies virus. *J. Neuropathol. Exp. Neurol.,* 45:28–42.

44. Wilson, P. T., Lentz, T. L., and Hawrot, E. (1985): Determination of the primary amino acid sequence specifying the α-bungarotoxin binding site on the α subunit of the acetylcholine receptor from *Torpedo californica. Proc. Natl. Acad. Sci. U.S.A.,* 82:8790–8794.

45. Wunner, W. H., Reagan, K. J., and Koprowski, H. (1984): Characterization of saturable binding sites for rabies virus. *J. Virol.,* 50:691–697.

46. Yelverton, E., Norton, S., Obijeski, J. F., and Goeddel, D. V. (1983): Rabies virus glycoprotein analogs: Biosynthesis in *Escherichia coli. Science,* 219:614–620.

Psychological, Neuropsychiatric, and
Substance Abuse Aspects of AIDS,
edited by T. Peter Bridge et al.
Raven Press, New York © 1988.

HIV Receptor in Brain and Deduced Peptides That Block Viral Infectivity

*Candace B. Pert, *Michael R. Ruff, †Frank Ruscetti,
†William L. Farrar, and *Joanna M. Hill

*Section on Brain Biochemistry, Clinical Neuroscience Branch, Intramural Research
Program, National Institute of Mental Health, Alcohol, Drug Abuse, and Mental Health
Administration, National Institutes of Health, Bethesda, Maryland 20892; and
†Laboratory of Molecular Immunoregulation, Biological Response Modifiers Program,
National Cancer Institute, Frederick, Maryland 21701

The acquired immune deficiency syndrome (AIDS) is a cellular immunodeficiency disorder that is characterized by malignancies and opportunistic infections with a variety of pathogens (9,23,35).

Central nervous system involvement is a common feature in AIDS patients, as evidenced by intellectual and cognitive impairment (14), language disorders, movement dysfunction, stroke symptoms (39), delirium, and dementia (21,36). Neuropathological complications such as encephalitis, neoplasms, and vascular lesions also frequently occur (36).

The retrovirus HIV (human immunodeficiency virus) has been identified as the causative agent in AIDS (3,20,29). AIDS infection is found to deplete the helper/ inducer T-lymphocyte subset, which is characterized by the presence of the T4 (CD4) surface antigen (17). Since HIV binding, absorption, and replication in human (5,17,24) T cells is inhibited by anti-T4 Mab, it appears that the T4 antigen complex acts as the viral entry protein or receptor.

Spurred by the realization that immune cells and brain cells frequently share common antigens (28), as well as the report that HIV-associated retrovirus has been isolated from brain tissue (34), we recently demonstrated that similar T4 antigen structures are present on lymphoid and brain structures (32).

The HIV envelope protein, gp120, was iodinated and specifically bound to membranes from human T cells and human, monkey, and rat brain membranes. A single radiolabeled cross-linking product of $\approx$180 kDa was obtained from all three preparations (25). These results show that ^{125}I-gp120 can be coupled to a $\approx$60-kDa protein, the approximate molecular weight of CD4 (32), on human, monkey, and rat brain that is indistinguishable from the molecule on human T cells. In addition, we found a $\approx$60-kDa protein precipitated by a monoclonal antibody to T4 (OKT4)

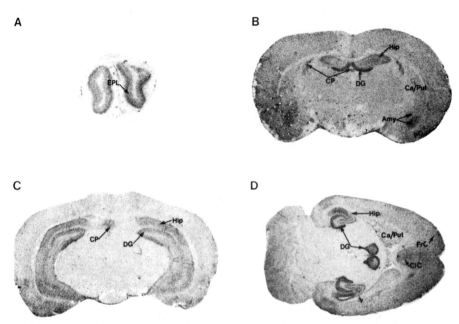

FIG. 1. Autoradiograph of T4 antigen in rat brain: (**A**) olfactory bulb level, (**B**) thalamus level, (**C**) hippocampus/midbrain level, (**D**) horizontal view. Amy, amygdala; Ca/Put, caudate/putamen; CiC, cingulate cortex; CP, choroid plexus; DG, dentate gyrus; EPL, external plexiform layer; FrC, frontal cortex; Hip, hippocampus; PC, pyriform cortex. (From Hill et al., ref. 12.)

on monkey brain and human T4 T cells (25,32), but a similar monoclonal antibody to another human T-cell surface antigen (OKT8) did not recognize any brain antigens (25).

Using a novel autoradiographic method and OKT4, the Mab to T4, we have mapped the distribution pattern of the AIDS virus receptor in rat, monkey (12), and human brain (13). Figures 1, 2, and 3 of T4 binding in the rat, monkey, and human brain, respectively, demonstrate that the binding pattern is similar in all three of these diverse mammals.

The highest density of binding occurred in the molecular layer of the dentate gyrus in the rat (Fig. 1B,C,D), monkey (Fig. 2D,E), and human brain (Fig. 3D). High density also occurred in the hippocampus (Fig. 1B,C,D, rat; Fig. 2D,E, monkey; Fig. 3D, human). Receptors were prominent in the nuclei of the amygdala of all three brains (rat, Fig. 1B; monkey, Fig. 2C,D; and human, not shown) and in the superficial layers of the primate cortex, especially in the cingulate (Fig. 2A,C,D,E; Fig. 3A), insular (Fig. 2A,C,D; Fig. 3D), opercular (Fig. 2A,C,D), temporal (Fig. 2C,D,E; Fig. 3C,D), medial temporal (Fig. 2A,C,D,E; Fig. 3C), and striate cortex (Fig. 2F). In the rat the frontal cortex (Fig. 1D), pyriform cortex (Fig. 1B) (especially near the rhinal fissure), cingulate cortex (Fig. 1D), and striate

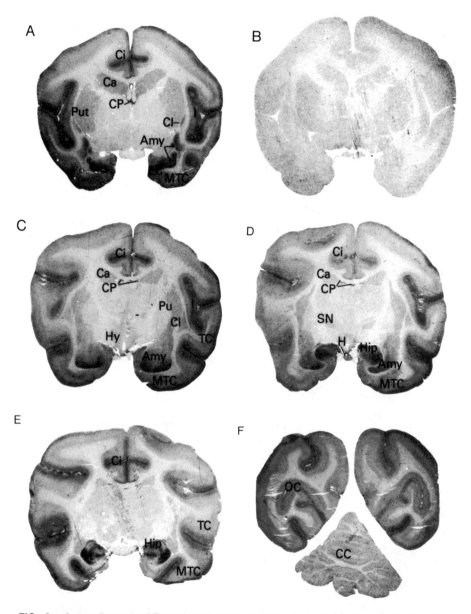

FIG. 2. Autoradiograph of T4 antigen in monkey brain. **A, C, D, E,** and **F** were incubated in OKT4 followed by ^{125}I-immunoglobulin; **B**, a no-primary-antibody control, was incubated in ^{125}I-immunoglobulin alone. Amy, amygdala; Ca, caudate; CC, cerebellar cortex; Ci, cingulate cortex; Cl, claustrum; CP, choroid plexus; EC, entorhinal cortex; H, hypophysis; Hip, hippocampal formation; Hy, hypothalamus; I, insula; MTC, medial temporal cortex; OC, occipital cortex; Put, putamen; SN, substantia nigra; TC, temporal cortex. (From Hill et al., ref. 12.)

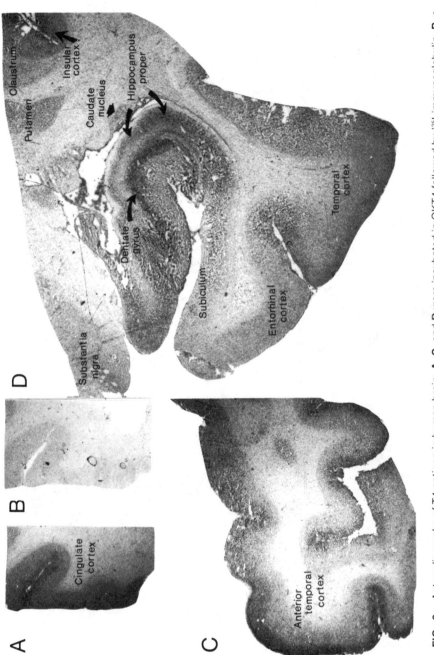

FIG. 3. Autoradiographs of T4 antigen in human brain. **A**, **C**, and **D** were incubated in OKT4 followed by ^{125}I-immunoglobulin. **B**, a no-primary-antibody control, was incubated in ^{125}I-immunoglobulin alone. (From Hill et al., ref. 13.)

cortex had a higher density of binding than other cortical areas. A moderate density of binding occurred in the deep layers of the cortex, claustrum (Fig. 2A,C,D; Fig. 3D), caudate (Fig. 2A,C,D; Fig. 3D), putamen (Fig. 2A,C,D), hypothalamus (Fig. 2C,D), and substantia nigra (Fig. 2D; Fig. 3D) of the monkey and human and the accumbens, caudate/putamen (Fig. 1B), claustrum, and lateral septum of the rat. Among ancillary brain structures, the choroid plexus (Fig. 1B,C, rat; Fig. 2A,C,D, monkey) and hypophysis (Fig. 2C,D), had a high density of binding.

Sections incubated in radiolabeled secondary antibody without prior incubation in the anti-T4 monoclonal antibody show no pattern and merely a low level of "background" optical density (Fig. 2B; Fig. 3B). Specificity is further demonstrated by our previous work in which a monoclonal antibody to the transferrin receptor revealed a different distribution pattern in rat brain with similar methods (11).

Most of the brain regions with a high density of T4 antigen are laminated cortical structures in which the prominent binding occurs in the superficial layers. This is evident in the hippocampal formation, where binding is greatest in the molecular layer of the dentate gyrus and hippocampus, and in the olfactory bulb external plexiform layer. In addition, in the neocortex of the monkey and human, greatest binding is localized to superficial layers. These superficial layers are composed primarily of the dendritic and axonal branches of neurons, the cell bodies of which are in different laminae or structures. Consistent with this observation, microscopic examination of emulsion-coated slides revealed that receptor binding sites occur primarily throughout the neuropil; however, they were also observed over neurons and glial cells.

^{125}I-gp120 was also bound to brain sections, and it produced a pattern of distribution similar to that achieved with OKT4 (25). Other Mabs that recognize other T-cell surface antigens, e.g., OKT8 and OKT11, apparently did not recognize any brain antigens (25).

Since the T4 antigen acts as the receptor for the AIDS retrovirus, those brain areas with high densities of T4 antigen are at greatest risk as the targets of AIDS virus binding. T4 antigen is especially prominent in the cortical areas of the brain, being abundant in the hippocampus, amygdala, and many subdivisions of the neocortex. The area of highest binding, the hippocampal formation, plays an important role in learning and memory and, in addition, is a major component of the limbic system, which functions in the mediation of emotion. The amygdala, a second limbic structure, is also especially enriched with T4 antigen and is concerned with a variety of behaviors including agonistic behavior, feeding activities, and sexual behavior (15). Other limbic sites that have a moderate to high density of T4 antigen include the cingulate cortex, which is involved in maternal behaviors and vocalization (22), the hypothalamus, a center for the coordination of visceral functions, and the insular cortex, which functions in gustatory integration as well as being the highest waystation of somatosensory integration (8).

A high concentration of T4 antigen is also found in the temporal and occipital cortices, which are involved in auditory and visual integration, and in the caudate, putamen, and substantia nigra, brain areas that govern motor functions.

It should be emphasized that dense concentrations of T4 antigen are localized in all of the several cortical areas specialized for processing information from each sensory modality, i.e., olfactory, gustatory, visual, somatosensory, and auditory. Generally, it is the regions subserving "higher" cortical functions, i.e., progressively more highly processed sensory information (37), that we would predict to be most susceptible to viral damage.

The predominantly cortical brain areas characterized by the presence of T4 antigen are thus involved in extensive and varied brain functions. The fact that these areas are the potential sites for AIDS virus infection could explain the variety of psychiatric and neuropathological abnormalities seen in AIDS patients.

To date, however, it has not been demonstrated that neurons in brain areas with the greatest HIV virus receptor density are the most susceptible to viral infections or that viral perturbation of neuronal cell surface molecules can modulate brain activity, cognition, and mood. Much recent evidence indicates that the latter may indeed be the case. The HIV receptor distribution is similar to that of neuropeptide receptors, and, additionally, the receptor is shared by both the nervous and immune systems. It is thus potentially a cell surface recognition molecule for an informational substance subserving emotion (28; M. R. Ruff, *personal communication*).

The neuropathology of AIDS has revealed a shrunken cortex, and PET studies suggest reduced metabolism in this area (R. W. Price, Second International Conference on AIDS, June 1986). The missing components have yet to be identified, but a careful analysis of the T4 distribution pattern of brains of AIDS victims should reveal if loss of neurons with HIV receptors underlies the clinical picture of dementia and apathy. Visualization of core viral protein in "large multinucleated cells" (macrophages) lodged in both white and gray matter of the brains of AIDS victims (2) suggests that concentrations of degraded viral debris occur during the mounting of an inflammatory biological response.

The demonstrated preference of the HIV virus for humans, with nonhuman primate infection thus far proving difficult (G. Mark, *personal communication*), suggests that the possession of cellular HIV receptors is not sufficient for infection to occur. Whether they are indeed necessary will be revealed by future studies.

Within the last several years it has become possible to identify the recognition molecules that various viruses employ as their initial cellular attachment sites. Most exciting is the realization that several of these cell surface molecules serve as receptors for well-known physiological signaling ligands. For example, the vaccinia virus employs the epidermal growth factor receptor (6), rabies the acetylcholine receptor (19), rheo virus the β-adrenergic receptor (4), and Epstein–Barr (E–B) virus the complement receptor (CR2) (7). This principle, whereby virus may exert cell and tissue tropism via initial attachment to intrinsic and discrete cell membrane receptors, encouraged us to hypothesize that viral mimicry of endogenous peptide ligands could thereby form a basis for viral infectivity.

Since the same highly conserved neuropeptide informational substances integrate immune and brain function through receptors remarkably similar to those for HIV (28), we assumed that a shared amino acid sequence between the HIV gp120 and a short peptide previously identified in another context might indicate the core peptide essential for viral receptor binding. A computer-assisted comparison of all known protein sequences with HIV gp120 revealed that the octapeptide sequence Ala-Ser-Thr-Thr-Thr-Asn-Tyr-Thr of the California HIV isolate (33) is almost identical to an envelope region of the E–B virus, which has a glutamic acid residue instead of the third threonine (1). Spurred on by this improbable coincidence ($p = 1/20^7$), we synthesized this deduced octapeptide for further study and termed it "peptide T" because half of its amino acids are threonine, whose single-letter abbreviation is T.

Before undertaking viral infectivity experiments, we examined the properties of peptide T and three rationally designed peptide analogs in a viral envelope receptor binding assay. Figure 4 shows the high (0.1 nM range) affinity and saturability (Fig. 4A) of ^{125}I-gp120 binding to freshly prepared rat brain membranes. Specificity (Fig. 4B) was demonstrated by blockade with OKT4 and OKT4A but not with OKT3 (0.1 µg/ml). Peptide T and two of its synthetic analogs (but not the irrelevant octapeptide substance P_{1-8}) significantly inhibited ^{125}I-gp120 binding in the 0.1 nM range (Fig. 4C). Substitution of a D-threonine amide in position 8 resulted in at least a 100-fold loss of receptor binding activity. The classical D-alanine substitution for

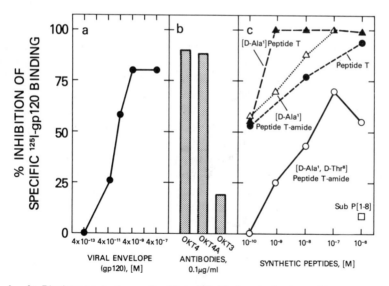

FIG. 4. A: Displacement of specific ^{125}I-gp120 binding to fresh rat hippocampal membranes. **B:** Specificity of OKT4 (*bar*), labeled T4, and OKT4a (T4a) but not OKT3 (T3). **C:** Inhibition of binding by peptide T (●) and analogs [D-Ala¹]peptide T (▲), [D-Ala¹]peptide T amide (△), and [D-Ala¹, D-Thr⁸]peptide T amide (○) compared with that of substance P_{1-8} octapeptide (□). Each determination was performed in triplicate; the results of one experiment, which was performed three times with similar results, are shown. Specific binding displaceable by 10 µg/ml of OKT4 and OKT4a ranged between 27% and 38% of total binding, which was 2,201 ± 74 cpm in the experiment shown. (From Pert et al., ref. 25.)

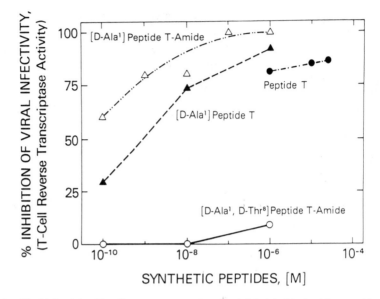

FIG. 5. Viral infectivity (T-cell reverse transcriptase activity) is blocked by peptide T (●) and its synthetic analogs [D-Ala¹]peptide T (▲), [D-Ala¹]peptide T amide (△), and [D-Ala¹, D-Thr⁸]peptide T amide (○).

L-alanine in position 1 of the octapeptide (26) resulted in a consistently more potent, presumably more peptidase-resistant (26), analog than peptide T; amidation of the C-terminal threonine also consistently produced somewhat greater potency.

The synthetic peptides then were tested independently for their ability to block viral infection of human T cells. At 100 nM the three peptides active in the binding assay were able to reduce detectable levels of reverse transcriptase activity by about ninefold (25). The less-active binding displacer [D-Ala¹,D-Thr⁸]peptide T amide was unable to block viral infection. Thus, as shown in Fig. 5, not only the rank order of potencies of the four peptides ([D-Ala¹]peptide T amide > [D-Ala¹]peptide T > peptide T > [D-Ala¹, D-Thr⁸]peptide T amide) but also their absolute concentrations in inhibiting receptor binding and viral infectivity were closely correlated. No effect of peptides on lymphocyte viability in the concentration range reported could be detected.

We do not know the relevance, if any, of the shared presence of peptide T in the E–B virus envelope. Although HIV and E–B virus are clearly both lymphotropic viruses, the E–B virus receptor (7) is considered unrelated to T4. New experiments on the effect of peptide T on E–B virus infection might prove interesting, but the shared sequence may be of historical interest only. An analysis of additional isolates suggests that the core sequence required for HIV attachment may be an even shorter pentapeptide. Both classical HIV isolates, HTLV-IIIb (30) and LAV (38), contain the sequence Thr-Thr-Ser-Tyr-Thr, which differs from peptide T by only one amino acid (serine instead of asparagine) and is quite potent (27).

The most potent of the synthetic peptides, [D-Ala^1]peptide T amide, inhibits receptor binding and T-cell infectivity in the 0.1 nM range and thus deserves further study for therapeutic potential. Certainly, the sensitivity of other strains of HIV to these peptides should be thoroughly explored. The several-orders-of-magnitude loss in apparent receptor affinity accomplished by a single amino acid enantiomeric substitution (D-Thr in position 8 of [D-Ala^1]peptide T amide) is typical of neuropeptides for which extensive structure–activity analyses have been performed, particularly for opiate peptides (18). The "threshold effect," whereby activity is lost in the bioassay but is still detectable in the receptor binding assay, is also not unusual.

The synthesis of this peptide must be reviewed as the beginning of binding-assay-assisted rational peptide drug design, with bioavailability in the central nervous system as well as further increases in potency and stability as important goals. Although it would not be unprecedented if the HIV virus had additional receptors for cellular entry, the similar brain distribution of viral envelope receptor and T4 antigen are compatible with a single entry protein. Our identification of the highly sought-after attachment portion of the viral envelope (e.g., glycoprotein 120 residues 196–200 in ref. 30) should help the production of neutralizing antibodies and vaccine development. Perhaps even more important, peptide T or a derivative might be useful clinically to halt or attenuate the spread of the virus in infected individuals.

In summary, the CNS dysfunction characteristic of AIDS patients, unrelated to secondary infections, could be caused by the binding of the virus, or shed viral envelope protein gp120, to T4 receptors in the brain, by which the normal functioning of T4-bearing cells could be disrupted. Since a mismatch between the localization of neuroactive substances and their receptors in the brain is the rule rather than the exception (10), the mismatch between the localization of the virus in macrophages in the core of the brain and the presence of the receptor in more superficial regions of the hippocampus and cortex support the view that CNS dysfunction is caused by shed viral proteins interacting at T4 sites on noncontiguous cells.

ACKNOWLEDGMENTS

We gratefully acknowledge Mrs. Sharon Morgan for her careful preparation of the manuscript and Ms. Nicole Jelesoff for excellent technical assistance.

REFERENCES

1. Baer, R., Bankier, A. T., Biggin, M. D., Deininger, P. L., Farrell, P. J., Gibson, T. J., Hatfull, G., Hudson, G. S., Satchwell, S. C., Seguin, C., Tuffnell, P. S., and Barrell, B. G. (1984): DNA sequence and expression of the B95-8 Epstein–Barr virus genome. *Nature,* 310:207–211.
2. Barnes, D. M. (1986): AIDS-related brain damage unexplained. *Science,* 232:1091–1093.
3. Barre-Sinoussi, F., Chermainn, J. C., Rey, F., Nageyre, M. T., Chamaret, S., Gruest, J., Daugeut, S., Anler-Blin, C., Vezinet-Brun, F., Rouzivux, C., Roxenbaum, W., and Montagnier, L. (1983): Isolation of a T-lymphotropic retrovirus from a patient at risk for acquired immune deficiency syndrome (AIDS). *Science,* 220:868–871.

4. Co, M. S., Gaulton, G. N., Fields, B. N., and Greene, M. I. (1985): Isolation and biochemical characterization of the mammalian reovirus type 3 cell-surface receptor. *Proc. Natl. Acad. Sci. U.S.A.*, 82:1494–1498.

5. Dalgleish, A. C., Beverley, D. C. L., Clapham, P. R., Crawford, D. H., Greaves, M. F., and Weiss, R. A. (1985): The CD4 (T4) antigen is an essential component of the receptor for the AIDS retrovirus. *Nature*, 312:763–767.

6. Eppstein, D. A., Marsh, Y. V., Schreiber, A. B., Newman, S. R., Todaro, G. J., and Nestor, J. J., Jr. (1985): Epidermal growth factor receptor occupancy inhibits vaccinia virus infection. *Nature*, 318:663–667.

7. Fingeroth, J. D., Weis, J. J., Tedder, T. F., Stroninger, J. L., Biro, D. A., and Fearon, D. T. (1984): Epstein–Barr virus receptor of human B lymphocytes in the C3D receptor CR2. *Proc. Natl. Acad. Sci. U.S.A.*, 81:4510–4514.

8. Friedman, D. P., Murray, E. A., O'Neill, J. B., and Mishkin, M. (1986): Cortical connections of the somatosensory fields in the lateral sulcus of macaques: Evidence for a corticolimbic pathway for touch. *J. Comp. Neurol.*, 252:323–347.

9. Gottlieb, M. S., Schroff, R., Schanker, H. M., Weisman, J. D., Fan, P. T., Wolf, R. A., and Saxon, A. (1981): *Pneumocystis carinii* pneumonia and mucosal candidiasis in previously healthy homosexual men. *N. Engl. J. Med.*, 305:1425–1431.

10. Herkenham, M. (1987): Mismatches between receptor and transmitter localization in the brain: Observations and implications. *Neuroscience*, 23:1–38.

11. Hill, J. M., Ruff, M. R., Weber, R. J., and Pert, C. B. (1985): Transferrin receptors in rat brain: Neuropeptide-like pattern and relationship to iron distribution. *Proc. Natl. Acad. Sci. U.S.A.*, 82:4553–4557.

12. Hill, J. M., Farrar, W. L., and Pert, C. B. (1986): Localization of the T4 antigen/AIDS virus receptor in monkey and rat brain: prominence in cortical regions. *Psychopharmacol. Bull.*, 22:686–694.

13. Hill, J. M., Farrar, W. L., and Pert, C. B. (1986): Autoradiographic localization of the T4 antigen, the HTLV-III/LAV receptor in human brain. *Int. J. Neurosci.*, 29:687–693.

14. Joffe, R. T., Rubinow, D. R., Squillace, K., Lane, C. H., Duncan, C. C., and Fauci, A. S. (1986): Neuropsychiatric manifestations of acquired immune deficiency syndrome (AIDS). *Psychopharmacol. Bull.*, 22:684–688.

15. Kaada, B. R. (1972): Stimulation and regional ablation of the amygdaloid complex with reference to functional representations. In: *The Neurobiology of the Amygdala. The Proceedings of a Symposium on the Neurobiology of the Amygdala,* edited by B. E. Eleftheriou, pp. 205–281. Plenum Press, New York.

16. Klatzman, D., Barre-Sinoussi, F., Nageyre, M. T., Dauguet, C., Vilmer, E., Griscelli, C., Brun-Vezinet, F., Rouzioun, C., Gluckman, J. C., Chermann, J., and Montagnier, L. (1984): Selective tropism of lymphadenopathy associated virus (LAV) for helper–inducer T lymphocytes. *Science*, 225:59–63.

17. Klatzman, D., Champagne, E., Chamaret, S., Gruest, J., Guetard, D., Hercend, T., Gluckman, J. C., and Montagnier, L. (1985): T-lymphocyte T4 molecule behaves as the receptor for human retrovirus LAV. *Nature*, 312:767–768.

18. Kosterlitz, H. (1976): *Opiates and Endogenous Opioid Peptides.* North Holland, Amsterdam.

19. Lentz, T. L., Burrage, T. G., Smith, A. L., Crick, J., and Tigner, G. H. (1982): Is the acetylcholine receptor a rabies virus receptor? *Science*, 215:182–184.

20. Levy, J. A., Hoffman, A. D., Kramer, S. M., Landis, J. A., Shimabukuro, J. M., and Oshiro, L. S. (1984): Isolation of lymphocytopathic retroviruses from San Francisco patients with AIDS. *Science*, 225:840–842.

21. Lowenstein, R. J., and Sharfstein, S. S. (1983–84): Neuropsychiatric aspects of acquired immune deficiency syndrome. *Int. J. Psychiatry Med.*, 13:255–260.

22. MacLean, P. D. (1985): Brain evolution relating to family, play and the separation call. *Arch. Gen. Psychiatry,* 42:405–417.

23. Masur, H., Michelis, M. A., Greene, J. B., Orarato, I., Vande Stouwe, R. A., Holzman, R. A., Wormser, G., Brettman, L., Lange, M., Murray, H. W., and Cunningham-Rundles, S. (1981): An outbreak of community acquired *Pneumocystis carinii* pneumonia. *N. Engl. J. Med.*, 305:1431–1438.

24. McDougal, J. S., Mawle, A., Cort, S. P., Nicholson, J. K. A., Cross, G. D., Scheppler-Campbell, J. A., Hicks, D., and Sligh, J. (1985): Cellular tropism of the human retrovirus

HTLV-III/LAV. Role of a T cell activation and expression of the T4 antigen. *J. Immunol.*, 135:3151–3162.

25. Pert, C. B., Hill, J. M., Ruff, M. R., Berman, R. M., Robey, W. G., Arthur, L. O., Ruscetti, F. W., and Farrar, W. L. (1986): Octapeptides deduced from the neuropeptide receptor-like pattern of antigen T4 in brain potently inhibit human immunodeficiency virus receptor binding and T-cell infectivity. *Proc. Natl. Acad. Sci. U.S.A.*, 83:9254–9258.

26. Pert, C. B., Pert, A., Chang, J.-K., and Fong, B. T. W. (1976): Opiate receptor autoradiographic localization in rat brain. *Proc. Natl. Acad. Sci. U.S.A.*, 73:3729–3733.

27. Pert, C. B., and Ruff, M. R. (1986): Peptide T[4–8]: A pentapeptide sequence in the AIDS virus envelope which blocks infectivity is essentially conserved across nine isolates. *Clin. Neuropharmacol.*, 9(S4):482.

28. Pert, C. B., Ruff, M. R., Weber, R. J., and Herkenham, M. (1985): Neuropeptides and their receptors: A psychosomatic network. *J. Immunol.*, 135:820s–826s.

29. Popovic, M., Sarngadharan, M. G., Read, E., and Gallo, R. C. (1984): Detection, isolation and continuous production of cytopathic retroviruses (HTLV-III) from patients with AIDS and pre-AIDS. *Science*, 224:497–500.

30. Ratner, L., Haseltine, W., Patarca, R., Livah, K. J., Starcich, B., Joseph, S. F., Doran, E. R., Rafalski, J. A., Whitehorn, E. A., Baumesiter, K., Ivanoff, L., Petteway, S. R., Jr., Pearson, M. L., Lautenberger, J. A., Papas, T. S., Ghrayeb, J., Chang, N. T., Gallo, R. C., and Wong-Staal, F. (1985): Complete nucleotide sequence of the AIDS virus, HTLV-III. *Nature*, 313:277–284.

31. Ruff, M. R., and Pert, C. B. (1984): Small cell carcinoma of the lung: Macrophage-specific antigens suggest hemopoietic stem cell origin. *Science*, 225:1034–1036.

32. Ruscetti, F. W., Farrar, W. L., Hill, J. M., and Pert, C. B. (1987): Visualization of the human helper T lymphocyte related antigen (T4) in primate brain: Implications for HTLV-III/LAV infection. *Peptides (in press)*.

33. Sanchez-Pescador, R., Power, M. D., Barr, P. J., Steimer, K. S., Stempien, M. M., Brown-Shimer, S. L., Gee, W. W., Renard, A., Randolph, A., Levy, J. A., Dina, D., and Luciw, P. W. (1985): Nucleotide sequence and expression of an AIDS-associated retrovirus (ARV-2). *Science*, 227:484–492.

34. Shaw, G. M., Harper, M. E., Hahn, B. H., Epstein, L. G., Gadjusek, D. C., Rue, R. W., Navia, B. A., Petito, C. K., O'Hara, C. J., Groopman, J. E., Cho, E., Oleske, J. M., Wong-Staal, F., and Gallo, R. C. (1985): HTLV-III infection in brains of children and adults with AIDS encephalopathy. *Science*, 227:177–181.

35. Siegal, F. P., Lopez, C., Hammer, G. S., Brown, A. E., Kornfeld, S. J., Gold, J., Hasset, J., Hirschman, S. Z., Cunningham-Rundles, S., and Armstrong, D. (1981): Severe acquired immunodeficiency in male homosexuals manifested by chronic perianal ulcerative *Herpes simplex* lesions. *N. Engl. J. Med.*, 305:1439–1444.

36. Snider, W. D., Simpson, D. M., Nielsen, S., Gold, S. W. M., Metroka, C. E., and Posner, J. B. (1983): Neurological complications of acquired immune deficiency syndrome: Analysis of 50 patients. *Ann. Neurol.*, 14:403–418.

37. Turner, B. H., Mishkin, M., and Krapp, M. (1985): Organization of the amygdalopetal projections from modality-specific cortical association areas in the monkey. *J. Comp. Neurol.*, 191:9–17.

38. Wain-Hobson, S., Sonigo, P., Danos, O., Cole, S., and Alizon, M. (1985): Nucleotide sequence of the AIDS virus, LAV. *Cell*, 40:9–17.

39. Wolcott, D. L., Fawzy, F. I., and Pasnau, R. D. (1987): Acquired immune deficiency syndrome (AIDS) and consultation–liaison psychiatry. *Gen. Hosp. Psychiatry (in press)*.

Psychological, Neuropsychiatric, and
Substance Abuse Aspects of AIDS,
edited by T. Peter Bridge et al.
Raven Press, New York © 1988.

Models for Understanding the Psychiatric Consequences of AIDS

David G. Ostrow

*Department of Psychiatry, University of Michigan School of Medicine, and Ann Arbor
Veterans Administration Medical Center, Ann Arbor, Michigan 48105*

The pace of the new AIDS discoveries and clinical complications is such that those actively involved in AIDS clinical research might feel caught in a vortex of events, many of which appear to be out of control. During the past 6 years, since the syndrome called AIDS was first described, I have attempted to observe and understand the response of the general public and various groups to the AIDS epidemic. The experimental work on which many of these observations is based is an ongoing study of approximately 1,000 gay and bisexual men at high risk of AIDS. These men comprise the Chicago cohort of a Multicenter AIDS Cohort Study (MACS), which is funded by NIAID and NCI. The aim of the MACS is to describe the natural history and epidemiology of AIDS and human immunodeficiency virus (HIV, formerly known as HTLV-III or LAV)-related disease. In Chicago, 95% of the MACS cohort is also participating in an NIMH-funded study of the psychosocial consequences of being at high risk for AIDS. In this chapter I present some models incorporating organizing principles to help us understand the context in which AIDS impacts on behavior. They are presented here in the hope that such organizing concepts may help us to impact in a constructive fashion on the psychological and social consequences of AIDS.

The epidemic curve of new AIDS cases (Fig. 1) combined with the well-known fate of any single person with AIDS is enough to explain the magnitude, if not the form, of these responses. No other medical event in recent history has produced the degree of public fear and private response that the AIDS epidemic has produced. With the recognition that perhaps 30 to 100 times as many persons with AIDS are already infected with a virus that represents a ticking time bomb (Curran, 1985), there has been a dramatic increase in the second epidemic, the epidemic of fear. This fear, whether it be of death, contamination, or just passivity in the face of a mortal threat, may well be the driving force behind all behavioral responses to AIDS. Certainly the fear of AIDs is the encouragement for various other campaigns that seek to exploit the public's fears for political ends and that in turn are the source of a growing sense in the affected communities that America is rapidly moving

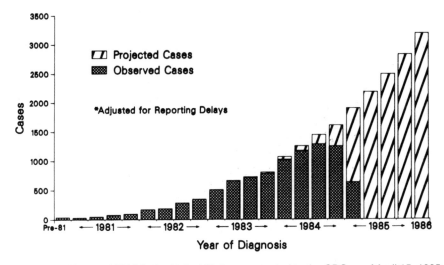

FIG. 1. Incidence of AIDS in the United States as reported to the CDC as of April 15, 1985 (*cross-hatched bars*) and projected through mid-1986 (*striped bars*). (From Curran, ref. 1.)

towards adoption of extreme measures such as mandatory HIV testing and quarantining of positive persons.

In our Chicago cohort we have seen a recent increase in fearful and angry responses to the question "Is there anything else about AIDS and how it has affected you that you would like to tell us?" These expressions of fear and anger at the reaction of general society to AIDS have shown a dramatic increase in parallel with increased media coverage of AIDS quarantine and mass HIV screening proposals (5). This observation leads to the conclusion that "fear of quarantine" is indeed a very real part of the psychiatric picture of AIDS in the United States. Whether or not such measures as quarantine are ultimately undertaken, the increasing discussion of quarantine proposals indicates the potential for negative social change and totalitarian responses to AIDS in our society.

There are, of course, many positive behavioral responses to AIDS taking place both in so-called high-risk individuals and members of that elusive group, "the general population." As early as 1983, we were seeing a dramatic reversal in direction of sexual behavioral change in prospectively examined gay men (4). These observed reductions in numbers of partners or specific sexual activities illustrate what amounts to a "sexual counterrevolution" but do not tell us anything about individual behavioral responses, which are actually quite heterogeneous. When we examined a particular sexual activity, such as receptive anal intercourse, and the change in individual frequency of this behavior at two points of observation, we saw several different behavioral responses. These ranged from adoption of abstinence to reduction in frequency and/or partner numbers to some men who did not change their behavior at all between 1982 and 1983.

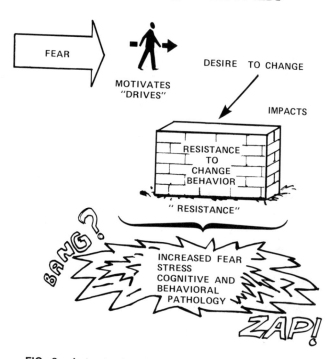

FIG. 2. A structural model of the psychiatric effects of AIDS.

In 1984 we began to ask men who were having sexual activities that were generally considered high risk why they continued such activity. The reasons given included gratification overcoming judgment, peer or partner pressure, and various rationalizations of minimal risk (6). These observations, which parallel explanations given for other types of unhealthy behavior, lead to a relatively simple model for understanding some of the psychiatric consequences of AIDS (Fig. 2). This structural model of barriers to behavioral change is simply the one first proposed by Freud and elaborated by many other proponents of psychoanalytical theory. Not only does it attempt to explain why behaviors that are known to be unhealthy do continue, it predicts a significant amount of psychological distress in persons who consciously recognize the risk involved in those behaviors but find themselves unable to reduce or stop their behavior. This helps us to understand the magnitude of the anxiety and stress being generated by the AIDS epidemic and the significant psychopathology that may result.

A PSYCHOSOCIAL MODEL OF THE BEHAVIORAL CONSEQUENCES OF AIDS

A more complex but realistic model goes beyond the intrapsychic realm to incorporate the role of social forces in shaping our responses to AIDS (Fig. 3). In

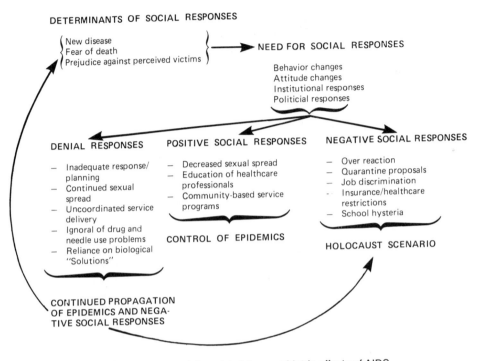

FIG. 3. A psychosocial model of the psychiatric effects of AIDS.

this model, social responses are characterized as being "positive" if they lead to containment of the physical and emotional causes of the epidemics, as "negative" if they contribute towards the negative social outcomes, and as "denial" if they continue to propagate the underlying causes of the dual epidemics of AIDS and AIDS fear through denial of their long-term consequences.

When looked at from the broader psychosocial perspective, some very basic aspects of behavioral change motivation are seen as important potential determinants of the behavioral responses to AIDS. These include an individual's belief in the efficacy of behavioral change to alter his risk of developing AIDS, his knowledge about and skills in maintaining behavioral change, perceived peer and societal support for those changes, and the availability of services that provide support for behavioral change. Recently presented cross-sectional findings in the psychosocial study indicate that knowledge about AIDS and belief in the efficacy of one's behavioral changes are strong retrospective predictors of reported sexual behavior change from "unsafe" to "safe" practices (7). We need to keep this finding and its implications in mind when considering the setting up of programs to test at-risk individuals for HIV antibodies and use those results to motivate risk reduction. According to recent findings from the Baltimore MACS, persons receiving a negative antibody test result may, in fact, experience a negative impact on their ability to maintain behavioral changes that reduce risk of exposure of their sexual partners or themselves (2). The importance of the vigorous pursuit of information regarding both cofactors for disease progression and possible therapeutic interventions is also underlined by these findings.

THE SPECTRUM OF AIDS-RELATED PSYCHIATRIC ILLNESS

In addition to the fear of developing AIDS and a feeling of inefficacy in those behavioral changes already taken, persons in AIDS risk groups may have a number of other sources of chronic stress. These include the social isolation and stigmatization that being in an AIDS risk group or having prodromal symptoms produces; the sense of helplessness one has in dealing with the disease for which there is no cure and for which there are at present no available interventions to prevent its development once infected; the significant loss of friends, lovers, and others to the disease; the giving up of sexual or drug-use behaviors and the loss of pleasure and anxiety reduction that these behavioral changes may entail; the related loss of intimacy when major forms of close social interaction are deemed "unsafe"; and the significant fear of quarantine and expectations of a "holocaust scenario" reported by many of our subjects. Given the number and magnitude of sources of chronic stress that are present in persons at high risk of AIDS, it is not surprising that we see an enormous range of psychiatric morbidity in our study population. We and others have observed a continuum of AIDS-related psychiatric problems ranging from anxiety and dysphoria to full-blown immobilization, psychosis, and even suicide (Fig. 4).

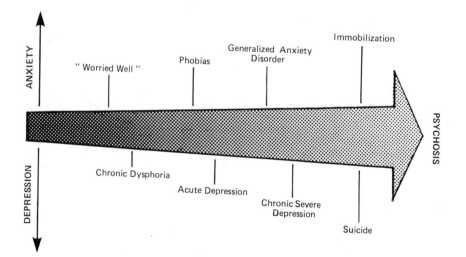

FIG. 4. The continuum of AIDS-related psychiatric problems. Problems manifesting themselves primarily in anxiety symptoms are shown above, whereas those predominantly affective are shown below the *arrow*. (From Ostrow, D. G. A psychiatric overview of AIDS. *Int. J. Neurosci.*, 1986.)

A BIOLOGICAL MODEL OF THE PSYCHIATRIC CONSEQUENCES OF AIDS

The psychological and social stresses produced by AIDS and AIDS fear are not the entire story of this epidemic and its psychiatric consequences. As other contributions to this volume describe, there is a growing recognition that HIV can directly infect the central nervous system, producing a variety of serious neurological and psychiatric complications. A biological model for the psychiatric implications of AIDS must therefore include both direct and indirect effects on behavior (Fig. 5). This model recognizes not only that the virus is a biological contributor to various psychological problems but that serologic tests for antibodies to HIV embody many psychosocial implications themselves.

Among the psychiatric problems embodied in the HIV antibody test are its ambiguities. Although developed as a test for exposure to AIDS and not AIDS itself, the test is viewed by many and used in ever increasing frequency as a "test for AIDS." There is enormous anxiety about being tested, with some persons seriously decompensating when given a positive test result. There is also denial present in the belief that a negative test result definitively indicates that one has not been exposed or will not develop AIDS. Conversely, a positive test result embodies many of the aspects of isolation and stigmatization that were discussed for the disease itself. Our subjects fear discrimination based on testing and are angry at the misuse of the test to deny them insurance, employment, and other rights. No wonder, therefore, that individuals can develop major depression as a result of the helpless-

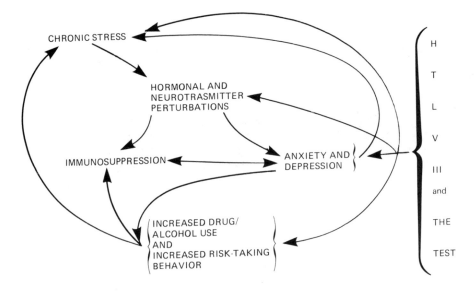

FIG. 5. A biological model for the psychiatric effects of AIDS.

ness and stress involved with the disease of AIDS and programs to test them for exposure to the virus believed necessary to produce AIDS.

THE VIRUS OF FEAR MODEL

Another model for the psychiatric effects of AIDS considers the fear of AIDS as the major vector and individual susceptibility to that fear as determining its psychiatric consequences, in a fashion analogous to the postulated effects of HIV infection on T cells (Fig. 6). By substituting the fear of AIDS for the virus itself and the media as the carrier of that agent, we see that a person can either respond positively to exposure to the various elements of AIDS and AIDS fear by developing maturing responses or develop a dedifferentiation response leading to individual decompen-

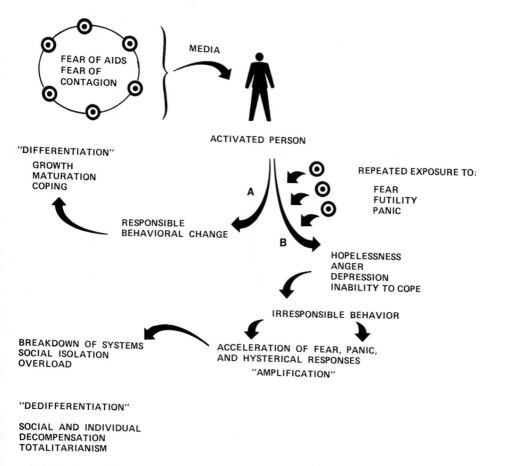

FIG. 6. A model for the potential outcomes of exposure of susceptible persons to the fear of AIDS.

sation and, ultimately, social totalitarianism. The determinants of those responses must be a variety of individual characteristics as well as the psychosocial milieu and the way in which the information is conveyed to the individual. This model is analogous to how we currently view the vulnerability to depression in persons with a positive family history of affective disorders and who have been exposed to environmental or other stressors. We do not yet know the biological, characterological, psychosocial, or other factors that determine an individual's vulnerability to decompensate given repeated exposures to AIDS fear. However, given the enormous negative implications of individual and social dedifferentiation, it is extremely important that we study, understand, and intervene to prevent such outcomes (3).

An example of the ways in which fear of AIDS can produce significant psychological distress and impair functioning in a vulnerable individual is illustrated with data obtained from the larger MACS cohort from all four cities participating in the study. We have recently reported (8,9) significantly increased scores on several subscales and total symptom scores of the Center for Epidemiological Studies-Depression (CES-D) questionnaire in men who see themselves as being at high risk for developing AIDS. This perceived high risk is manifested by individuals who report themselves as having enlarged lymph nodes or other symptoms of ARC, whether or not they actually have those symptoms on physical examination. The significant effect of perception of lymphadenopathy on psychological functioning was present in both the HIV antibody-negative and -positive men. Since we can limit the analysis to men who have remained antibody-negative for 6 to 12 months and are thus extremely unlikely to be infected with the virus, we cannot ascribe this psychological distress to the neurological or psychological effects of "hidden" viral infection. We see it instead as residing in one's perceived risk of developing AIDS and the resulting stress that produces in vulnerable individuals.

This finding was confirmed when we performed a multiple repression analysis on the CES-D factors, showing that the number of perceived AIDS-related complex (ARC) symptoms, including self-reported "glands," were highly correlated with elevated scores on all subscales and the total CES-D score (Table 1). In confirmation of our psychosocial model was the finding that a negative response to the question "Is there anyone you can talk to about important problems?" was a significant independent predictor of increased psychological distress.

CONCLUSIONS

The various models for psychiatric effects of AIDS presented here each have implications that need to be integrated into a unified psychiatric model in order to be most useful (Fig. 7). Behavior change, whether it be on an individual, group, societal, or institutional basis, is motivated by both fear and force, but also by gratification and altruism. This motivation is not sufficient in and of itself to produce positive change, which must also be facilitated by a variety of psychosocial, educational, and institutional supports and resources. The role of psychiatry in this

TABLE 1. *Relative ranking of MRA determinants of CES-D scores*

Significant MRA correlates	CES-D factor				
	Total	Depression	Enervation	Positive affect	Interpersonal sensitivities
Total number of self-reported ARC symptoms	1	1	1	1	1
No one to talk to	2	2	2	2	3
Perceived glands	3	3	4	4	—
Education level[a]	4	—	3	3	5
Perceived glands–serostatus interaction[a]	5	4	8	5	—
Number anonymous partners	6	8	6	6	4
Age[a]	7	5	5	—	2
AIDS sex partner	—	6	—	—	—

[a]These are negative correlates; i.e., increased education level, age, and positive serostatus all decreased CES-D scores.

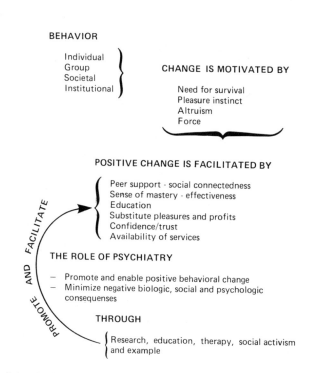

BEHAVIOR

Individual
Group
Societal
Institutional } CHANGE IS MOTIVATED BY

Need for survival
Pleasure instinct
Altruism
Force

POSITIVE CHANGE IS FACILITATED BY

{ Peer support - social connectedness
Sense of mastery - effectiveness
Education
Substitute pleasures and profits
Confidence/trust
Availability of services

THE ROLE OF PSYCHIATRY

— Promote and enable positive behavioral change
— Minimize negative biologic, social and psychologic consequenses

THROUGH

{ Research, education, therapy, social activism
and example

PROMOTE AND FACILITATE

FIG. 7. An integrated model for psychiatry's positive potential roles in meeting the mental health challenges of AIDS.

model is to promote and enable positive behavioral change while minimizing the negative biological, social, and psychological consequences of that change. As psychiatrists we can accomplish this through research, education, therapy, social activism, and even by example. The responsibilities of such a role are enormous. But the potential risks were we not to mobilize the mental health professions to pursue actively positive behavioral change in response to AID are unthinkable.

REFERENCES

1. Curran, J. W. (1985): The epidemiology and prevention of AIDS. *Ann. Intern. Med.,* 103:657–662.
2. Fox, R., Odaka, N., and Polk, B. F. (1986): Effect of learning HTLV-III/LAV antibody status on subsequent sexual activity. In: *Proceedings Second International AIDS Conference,* p. 167. Institute Pasteur, Paris.
3. Ostrow, D. G. (1985): Issues and analysis: Psychiatric implications of AIDS. *Masters Psychiatry,* 1:21–23.
4. Ostrow, D. G., Altman, N. L., Wallemark, C.-B., Goldsmith, J., Phair, J. P., and Chmiel, J. (1984): Patterns of homosexual behavior, 1979–1983. In: *Proceedings Conjoint STD Meeting,* p. 12. International STD Research Society, Montreal.
5. Ostrow, D. G., Eller, M., and Joseph, J. G. (1986): Fear of quarantine: An emerging psychosocial issue. In: *Proceedings Second International Conference on AIDS,* p. 183. Institute Pasteur, Paris.
6. Ostrow, D. G., Emmons, C. A., Altman, N. L., Joseph, J. G., Phair, J. P., and Chmiel, J. (1985): Sexual behavior change and persistence in homosexual men. In: *Proceedings First International AIDS Conference,* p. 71. UHPHS, Atlanta.
7. Ostrow, D. G., Emmons, C. A., O'Brien, K., Joseph, J. G., and Kessler, R. C. (1986): Magnitude and predictors of behavioral risk reduction as a cohort of homosexual men. In: *Proceedings Second International AIDS Conference,* p. 167. Institute Pasteur, Paris.
8. Ostrow, D. G., Joseph, J., Monjan, A., Kessler, R., Emmons, C., Phair, J. P., Fox, R., Kingsley, L., Dudley, J., and Van Raden, M. (1986): Psychosocial aspects of AIDS risk. *Psychopharmacol. Bull.,* 22:678–683.
9. Ostrow, D. G., Joseph, J., Monjan, A., and Phair, J. (1985): Psychological correlates of AIDS risk and HTLV-III exposure. In: *Proceedings Annual Meeting American College Neuropsychopharmacology,* p. 9.

Psychological, Neuropsychiatric, and Substance Abuse Aspects of AIDS, edited by T. Peter Bridge et al. Raven Press, New York © 1988.

Voodoo Death, the Stress Response, and AIDS

Sanford I. Cohen

Department of Psychiatry, Boston University School of Medicine, Boston, Massachusetts 02118; and Health and Behavior Branch, Division of Basic Science, National Institute of Mental Health, National Institutes of Health, Rockville, Maryland 20857

In 1953, an Aborigine Kinjika from Australia's northern territory was brought to a hospital in Darwin. He had not been injured or poisoned and had no known disease, but he was dying. He died after 4 days. The only information was that several days before entering the hospital he had been summoned before the tribal council (Mailli tribe) and sentenced to death for having broken the tribe's taboo against incestuous sexual relations. The bone had been pointed—the accepted method of execution (25).

A case was reported of a man raised by a very domineering mother. At age 24, he opened a night club with the help of his mother. At age 38, he decided to marry and sell the club he owned jointly with his mother. His mother warned him that if he sold the club something dire would happen to him. Two days later he had his first attack of asthma. Several months later he decided to reopen another club, this time without his mother. She told him he would be cursed for the way he ignored his obligation to his mother. One hour after this call, the patient died (41).

A mother learned on the same day that her son was gay and had AIDS. She reacted to this with hostility and openly maintained a prayer vigil outside the intensive care unit, praying that her son would die because of the shame he had caused her. The patient could hear his mother praying. One hour later the patient died, much to the surprise of his physician, since he did not appear to be terminal.

What do these reports have in common? Not the diagnosis or the setting or time in which they occurred. Some would say all of these patients had characteristics suggesting they were hexed, voodooed, hoodooed, or cursed.

It has been frequently noted that a person's belief that he has been subjected to sorcery and is condemned to death will result in his death. Well-known behavioral and medical researchers such as Cannon (13) have pointed out that both slowly developing fatal illnesses and sudden death attributed to emotional or stressful factors can be found throughout recorded history. Although illness and death have been described in current literature as occurring without any clear-cut physiopathology,

95

psychosocial and emotional factors are suspected as playing a role in the etiology rather than the power of a sorcerer or the wrath of a vengeful deity.

VOODOO

So-called voodoo or hex death is a classic example of a biopsychosocial interaction. It is a dramatic demise that occurs when a person feels cursed by another believed powerful enough to kill or powerful enough to create a feeling of hopelessness. The victim has to believe that the hex works and that he cannot control it. The role of the community and family is crucial. If a hexed person resists his fate, the community, including the family, withdraws support. The hexed feels cast out, isolated, alone. He sees death as the only escape from an intolerable loneliness. Only when he accepts the inevitability of death does the community return and act in various ritual ways suggesting death positively.

There are all kinds of counterparts of so-called voodoo death, hexing-like phenomena, and faith healing in modern society. It is more pervasive in our pluralistic culture than supposed. This includes people of all social classes, diverse ethnic backgrounds, and various religious groups.

One reason for highlighting voodoo in this chapter is the Haitian link in the AIDS epidemiological chain. I hope it will rapidly become apparent that the reference to voodoo has little to do with either the formal religion or a mystical or divine explanation for the AIDS epidemic.

AIDS IN HAITI: VOODOO OR VIRUS

The incidence of AIDS among Haitians, including recent immigrants to the United States, provides some important demographic variables in understanding the epidemiology of AIDS rather than suggesting more exotic explanations rooted in religion or witchcraft. The Haitian data are an especially important example of how the illness can spread in a heterosexual community.

When AIDS started to claim Haitians, especially those in the United States who were recent immigrants, the juxtaposition of a mystifying disease with an exotic culture created much attention and speculation.

It was suggested by some that the disease might be transmitted through some spiritual or voodoo ritual. The fact that this was raised publicly in the 20th century may be a function of the threat of a strange disease associated with and possibly spread by an alien group as the feared source (12).

Some of the earliest cases reported from Haiti suggest many of the points that will be reviewed.

One case noted by Leibovich (36) was that of Sister Y, a Sister of Charity. She performed admirably during her long years on the island. Toward the end of her apostolate, she abandoned her veil in order to devote herself to the spiritual welfare of the prostitutes in Port-au-Prince. She fell sick and was hospitalized in Montreal.

She confided to her doctors before dying that she had a single intimate contact with a Haitian man 4 years before falling ill. She assumed her illness was punishment from God for succumbing to the pleasures of the flesh and deserting her vows.

Her Canadian physicians confirmed that she had AIDS, but Sister Y believed she was a victim of her own human fall from grace. Her doctors believed it was caused by the transmission of the virus during intercourse or possibly that she was a victim of the local paramedical tradition of self-administered injections of vitamin C, B_{12}, or other drugs.

There might even be a direct link between voodoo and AIDS in Haiti, but not as a result of hexes. The country swarms with voodoo priests (one for every 100 inhabitants). Puncture and injection is a common procedure in some religious healing rituals. It is possible that unsterilized syringes might have been involved in the spread of AIDS (36).

There are some principles of voodoo death or hexing that may have implications in influencing the psychological states of persons from many social and cultural groups. These attitudes and beliefs, which are so essential to hexing and faith healing, may be present in somewhat different form in many cultures and account for the fears and social reactions we encounter. Further, the victim of a voodoo spell may have psychobiological reactions that are similar to those of groups at risk for AIDS.

Some current health problems are briefly considered in which the biopsychosocial interactions seem to be similar to those operating in voodoo or hexing. Of particular importance are the possible biological mechanisms that are set off by a state of hopelessness and despair.

Table 1 organizes some of the major elements found in most systems of voodoo, hexing, evil eye, and cursing. This table will be a guide in the analysis of other similar phenomena.

HEALTH AREAS WITH COMPONENTS OF HEXING

Oppressive Socioeconomic Conditions

A startling correlation was reported between stressful socioenvironmental factors and excessive mortality rates in an epidemiological study involving an inner-city catchment area. The mortality rate from a wide variety of illnesses was so high that the catchment area was called a death zone (32). The studies suggested that the high mortality rate may be related to an accumulation of serious and adverse psychosocial circumstances.

Other catchment areas had deficient resources, faring as badly in many socioeconomic indices, but there was a sense in many of these inner-city persons that they were trapped and helpless to do anything about their condition.

One hypothesis was that mortality, and perhaps morbidity, may be increased in stressful social settings in which hopelessness, loss of a feeling of mastery and

TABLE 1. *Factors in voodoo death*

Voodoo elements	Primitive hexing
Communication from external world or social structure	Message from an authority, a chief or a shaman, e.g., by "pointing the bone," announcing the victim's doom, the curse, the hex, or the prophecy; the victim must be aware of the message
Personal belief system	Belief in power of hex and hexer
Perception of own power	Sense of loss of control, the inevitability of the fate and of being hopelessly trapped
Behavior of victim	Goes off by self; may refuse food and drink
Community/family behavior	Withdrawal of interest and contact, fearful curse could affect them; family encourages acceptance by patients of their fate; lack of social support; ritualized social contact if inevitability of death is accepted
Psychological reaction of victim	"Give up," feels hopeless, helpless; death only escape from intolerable loneliness
Biological reaction	Death from unknown sources

control of one's environment, despair, and a sense of futility are created. A possible consequence of such a psychological state created by environmental and social conditions may be an increased biological vulnerability.

Culture shock may have similar impact on physical health as oppressive social conditions. Marshall (40) described the plight of the Hmong, many of whom escaped to refugee camps in Thailand and from there emigrated to the United States. Recently a strange illness has been occurring in healthy young Hmong men that kills them in their sleep, leaving no physical traces. It was speculated that the Hmong have been dying of fright, homesickness, and grief. The culture shock of relocating from the mountain jungles of Laos to the high rises of American cities may be overwhelming. The stresses of modern American society may lead to feelings of impotence, of oppression by an environment over which the Hmong can gain no mastery. Such feelings are similar to those found in victims of voodoo death.

Hexing the Persons with an Incurable Illness

Let us now consider how a health care team and a patient's family may "hex" a patient with an illness believed to be incurable. We all have difficulty facing one of the natural consequences of life, the death process. We adapt by not focusing on it. When confronted with this natural but frightening occurrence in another person, we often "cast him out." Through our behavior and attitude, we create a state of hopelessness, a feeling of inevitability, a loss of the sense of mastery of life. It may be that this psychological state of hopelessness makes the individual more vulnerable to biological problems and possibly hastens death.

The similarities are striking between the attitudes of the primitive community toward the hexed person and modern attitudes toward the patient diagnosed as having an incurable illness, especially if it is believed that the patient may be terminal. Like the primitive community, the surviving family and sometimes the health care staff in modern society often withdraw interest from the dying patient as a vital participant in day-to-day family affairs. Family members often carry out, especially in the hospital setting, certain preparatory rituals such as drawing the shades, lowering voices, and behaving unnaturally toward the dying patient (64). These gestures of complete capitulation and abandonment, amounting almost to a premortem burial, are strikingly similar to the behavior in the community of a hexed person, where death is presented as the only acceptable solution.

When the illness is cancer, for example, the patient sometimes dies too quickly for the malignancy to have had time to kill. Such a death resembles the death produced by "pointing the bone" among primitives; the physician, in effect, points the bone at the patient when he makes the diagnosis of cancer, which is considered terminal by most people.

Loss, Separation, and Loneliness

If hopelessness can speed the death of a patient with terminal illness, what about its effect on those who are not sick? A number of reports have singled out real or threatened loss as being associated with the onset of cancer, thyrotoxicosis, asthma, tuberculosis, ulcerative colitis, obesity, leukemia, rheumatoid arthritis, congestive heart failure, lupus disease, and diabetes (34,39,51,52,55).

The concept of "separation, loss, and depression" advanced by Schmale (51) and Engel (21,22) does not establish the cause of disease but rather the setting or one of the possible necessary conditions that allow disease to appear when it does. More specifically, it has been suggested that the psychic state of helplessness or hopelessness may be related to increased biological vulnerability. There are innumerable clinical case reports of sudden death (2,3,14,16,20,22,26,31,49,63) as well as the incidence of more lingering, debilitating illnesses that suggest the influence of psychosocially induced emotional states acting through the brain, autonomic nervous system, and neuroendocrine system.

THE HEXING OF HOMOSEXUALS WITH AIDS

Feeling isolated, helpless, and alienated, together with being viewed as a pariah, may have similar effects on the AIDS patients as having the "bone pointed" or being socially shunned or lacking social support so that death is felt to be their only resource.

The phenomena may result from the AIDS patient's reactions to family's response, social and religious beliefs, and the response of the health care team, employees, and lovers.

The problems created by these factors may be worsened by CNS infection from HTLV-III or CNS infections associated with opportunistic infections, e.g., cryptococcus or toxoplasmosis, which results in decreased cognitive abilities and a lessening of the patient's ability to cope with the life events.

The last vestige of hope is often removed when the patient is confronted by the tragic refusal of health care staff and families to provide care and support. Many patients perceive or sense other people (family, health care staff, society) as wishing that the patient would disappear or die and not endanger them. This is clearly suggested by the suggestions to quarantine AIDS patients, i.e., to remove them from society so they will not damn the rest of the community.

The sense of loss and abandonment generated by family rejection can be profound. Some gays are so fearful of rejection that they never disclose their life-style or diagnosis to their family.

One urban family, notified by their son with AIDS of his plan to visit, said "You can visit but must stay in a hotel; we have read that gays carry AIDS germs, and your mother and I do not wish the risk of contracting it."

The realities of the illness and the response of others to them lead many patients to feel they have lost any measure of control of their lives and that they are at the mercy of a community that wants them dead. The loss of mastery of their lives, the isolation, the stigmatization leads to a sense of helplessness, despair, and hopelessness as tragic and as devastating as that produced by oppressive social conditions, the diagnosis of other terminal diseases, loss of loved ones, or the rupture of cultural and social bonds.

There have been a large number of articles and reports in the professional literature, numerous publications, and the public media. Table 2 reviews some of these in the categories used to analyze the components of hexing and related phenomena.

UPDATING THE STRESS CONCEPT:
BIOPSYCHOSOCIAL SPECIFICITY

Has the major point been to impress you that stress is an important factor in dealing with the AIDS problem? The answer is yes, but with qualifications. There is a need to revise stress concepts. It has become increasingly apparent that stress is not a specific unitary entity. It is a convenient code word that subsumes a large variety of internal and external forces acting on the organism.

Early stress researchers looked primarily at stress responses from a biological perspective (54), although it was noted repeatedly that stress responses were influenced by psychosocial as well as biological and physical factors. Even when it was finally accepted or at least considered possible that life stress, psychological reactions, emotions, thoughts, and behavior might be legitimate factors influencing or influenced by body functions, this did not lead to relinquishing of the mind–body

TABLE 2. *Voodoo factors in AIDS*

Factor	AIDS
Communication from external world or society	Message from medical authority of fatal disease. Told they are a threat to family, friends, co-workers. Told they are unclean, loathsome, and sinful—reinforced by lack of physical contact and isolation. Fearful of being isolated, deprived of medical and social support. Message that they are unwanted, no longer acceptable in society, and doomed to die.
Personal belief system	Belief in validity of scientific knowledge of doctor. Need support from loved ones. Share cultural value system in community—homophobic. Believe they have violated social, religious, and family taboos. Disease is punishment for life-style.
Perception of own power	Unable to control course or severity of disease or of own life. Fearful of loss of body functions and inevitability of death.
Behavior of victim	Withdrawal from family and friends, uncommunicative. May not notify family. Some react to uncertainty with anger at health care staff, overly demanding, which leads to negative feedback. Give up any self-supporting behavior, totally helpless, suicidal.
Community and family behavior	Fearful may catch disease. Fearful of social ostracism. Encourage victim to adopt isolation; quarantine and mass screening for marker of evil. Expulsion from military, occupation, school, family. Victim seen as unclean, a pariah, a sinner, cursed by an angry God. Fearful God's wrath will be visited on family, community. Health care staff turn away. Viewed as lavender plague—suggestion wear lavender stars. Dread of homosexuality. Disease called nature's revenge. Viewed as depraved.
Psychological reaction of victim	Guilt, shame, remorse, depression, despair; fear of being abandoned, isolated, alienated, despised as threat to society and family. Loss of hope in the future. Profound sense of loss of all support.
Biological reaction	CNS and neuroendocrine changes associated with hopelessness, with possible worsening of immune dysfunction, possible role as cofactor in activating virus. Increased rate of biological deterioration. Depressed, seropositive, asymptomatic patients may be more vulnerable to onset of active infection.

dichotomy or a biomedical causality model, i.e., a specific cause leading to a specific effect. The inclusion of psychosocial factors as potential influences on the body seems to have required the adoption of the stress model in which stress now achieved the status as a causative agent like bacteria, poisons, tumors, etc. However, the stress model was, at best, a pseudo systems model.

The notion of specific biological patterns associated with definable psychosocial events and emotional signals that mobilize a specific behavioral response now seems a more useful framework than to group all psychosocial and environmental demands as stress.

THE BIOLOGY OF HOPELESSNESS

Rather than talking about an overall category of stimuli called stressors as potentially significant influences on biological functions, my focus is on a specific type of emotional response, namely, hopelessness, despair, and depression.

The animal observations that are most pertinent are those in which loss, separation, or the inability to master or control the environment is experienced. Experiments have shown that animals exposed to conditions they cannot master or control may be vulnerable to premature death as well as to a variety of biological changes (33). There are also a number of reports of animals dying suddenly of unknown causes in situations such as captivity or on being transferred from a familiar to an unfamiliar locale. Deaths have occurred after the demise of mates, and sudden death has been observed in primates separated from mothers or experiencing what appear to be meaningful losses (21).

In most animal studies, when sudden death occurs, the animal has been exposed to conditions similar to human psychosocial stresses, e.g., a threatening situation. The death seems related to ventricular arrhythmias associated with sympathetic nervous system overstimulation (19,38). In a few studies, cardiac slowing and arrest associated with massive vagal discharge has been reported (7,15,15a,45).

Other studies have reported that psychosocial, environmental, and mechanical stressors produce increases in plasma adrenal corticoids and other hormones through well-known neuroendocrine pathways (46). These hormonal changes are often accompanied by alterations in immune functions that lead to vulnerability to the action of latent oncologic viruses and other insipient pathological processes normally held in check by an intact immunologic apparatus.

In some experiments, animals were exposed to unpredictable shock and hence were unable to avoid or escape the shock. The response of these animals, which is called learned helplessness, is felt by some investigators to be an excellent animal model for human depression (53). These helpless animals have shown decreased T-cell number and function (35). It was noted that the experimental conditions suppressed the stimulation of lymphocytes in adrenalectomized animals. Hence, stress-related adrenal secretion of corticosteroids or catecholamines is not required for stress-induced suppression of lymphocyte stimulation by T-cell mitogen in the rat (35,61).

In studies of learned helplessness, Post (43) indicates that the ability to cope with a noxious stimulus can determine the change in brain norepinephrine. If an animal is subjected to shock from which it can escape by appropriate mechanisms, it will not evince depletion in brain or plasma norepinephrine. By contrast, a yoked control animal receiving a shock of equal intensity and duration will show depletion in norepinephrine when its behavior is inconsequential to removal of the painful stimulus. Placing the animal back in the environment in which it was originally shocked is sufficient to reproduce some of the original biochemical depletion (1).

Stein (50,61) studied in humans the effect of conjugal bereavement in men whose wives had advanced cancer and found that the ability of their lymphocytes to respond to an activating agent declined significantly in a month or two after their wives' death. Suppression of mitogen-induced lymphocyte stimulation appeared to be a direct consequence of bereavement.

Since depression is one consequence of bereavement, Stein examined the lymphocyte responses in patients hospitalized with severe depression and found these also to be suppressed. Lymphocyte stimulation by PHA, con A, and PWM were significantly lower for hospitalized depressed patients. T and B cells were also lower. Functional activity of the lymphocyte and the number of immune competent cells are decreased in clinically depressed patients.

Evidence for anatomic and chemical connections between CNS and immune system has been accumulating. Work by Stein (62) and others in animals has shown that lesions of the anterior but not the posterior hypothalamus reduce cellular and antibody-mediated immune responses to antigenic substances. Life events causing psychological distress may produce immune suppression through a number of pathways; e.g., CRF may trigger release of ACTH, which stimulates the release of corticosterone, which may suppress immune function. Increased HPA activity is characteristic of major depressive disorder. Corticosterones suppress the number of lymphocytes and the mitogen response. Pert et al. (42,48) have reported that subjects who are made to feel helpless show macrophages that move more sluggishly than usual, probably because of changes in neuropeptides. This may be a reason why patients who feel hopeless do worse than those who remain optimistic. Pert has suggested that neuropeptides may be a key biochemical unit of emotion, since they appear in such high concentrations in the limbic system.

The CNS and immune system may communicate directly through specific nerve connections. Bullock (11) has reported ANS fibers that go directly to the thymus, where T cells mature.

Recent work has also suggested that right and left neocortices have different effects on the immune system (44). The left cortex seems to be involved in regulating activity of the immune system, especially the activities of T cells, with lesions of left cortex resulting in some T-cell dysfunction. In humans it is possible that right brain dominance may be similar to decreasing left brain function. The right hemisphere may be involved in the processing of negative emotions, especially depression. The point to be made is that altering the function of an area of the central nervous system can change the responsivity of the immune system, which in turn can influence resistance to infection or growth of cancer cells.

Not only can the nervous system influence immune responses; more recent work shows immune responses can alter nerve cell activities. The cells of the immune system may function in a sensory capacity, relaying signals to the brain about stimuli such as invading pathogens (5,6,56). The immune system can communicate back to the hypothalamus and the autonomic and endocrine systems via substances produced by immune cells, which Hall has termed immunotransmitters (30).

POSSIBLE SPECIFIC BIOPSYCHOSOCIAL INFLUENCES ON AIDS

The CNS, endocrine, and ANS changes associated with states of depression and hopelessness could influence the activation of and the course of AIDS. After transmission, HIV can exist in a latent, nonreplicating form. Activation is related to a *tat* gene, which is responsible for transacting transcriptional activation (24,57). AIDS becomes a clinical problem when viral genes are activated and new virus particles are formed, which then infect fresh T4 cells, one of HTLV-III's primary targets.

A key question is what activates viral genes. A widely held notion is that further challenges to the immune system by another infection are responsible, for example, intestinal parasites, cytomegalovirus, EBV, or coexisting venereal diseases such as syphilis, GC, or chancroid. Other possible cofactors that have been mentioned are the medical use of steroids, the use of antineoplastic agents, nutritional deficiency states, age, alcohol, ionizing radiation, and exposure to chemicals (18,23,57).

Therefore, it is possible that the disease may proceed more rapidly in a person whose immune system is already impaired by drugs or infection. Is it possible that changes associated with endocrine and CNS activity triggered by life events and emotional reactions could also impair the immune system or operate as a cofactor? This is not such an outlandish question, since a frequently reported finding in psychoimmunological studies has been the decreased T-helper cell function, which has been noted to increase the risk for other viral infections. It is possible that endogenous substances released in reaction to specific psychological states might influence the cells so that the entrance of the virus into the cell is facilitated, or specific psychobiological states might influence the virus that is already in the cell so that it changes from a dormant to an active state.

Are there host susceptibility factors that increase the risk of AIDS or are responsible for activating the virus that has lived in an inactive state in the lymphocytes (and possibly the brain)? It is also not understood why some persons with active infections deteriorate rapidly and die while others have a less rapid and deteriorating course. Are there influences that make some persons more susceptible? In particular, is there some reason that some AIDS-infected persons die far more rapidly than would be clinically expected? What will be the effect on persons as they become aware of becoming seropositive? Will a knowledge that they carry the virus produce in some persons a psychological state that could set in motion biological changes that might activate the virus? Solomon and Temoshok (60) report that the differences in outcome they noted in AIDS patients (with PCP) were consistent with the literature on helplessness and hopelessness. Patients dying more quickly had a lower score on a control scale, suggesting that they tend to feel powerless in the face of overwhelming forces. Further, the unfavorable outcome group utilized less problem-solving help.

THE BIOLOGY OF HOPE

If future studies provide data that hopelessness and depression produce changes that may worsen the risk of AIDS, then the question would have to be asked, is it possible that the opposite state, hope, could decrease the risk? Dramatic reversals of chronic, even terminal, hopeless states have been described not only by patients who have seen faith healers but by patients sent to special clinics with international reputations if they have experienced a feeling that there is still hope. As soon as the patient feels that something can be done and that people have not given up, their attitude and psychological state change, and a slowing of the physical disease process has been described. Cousins (17,17a) has vividly and dramatically described the healing effects of hope, humor, and a sense of mastery on his own serious illness. His publications remind us that positive emotions as well as a message of hopefulness from an authoritative, benevolent, helping figure, regardless of whether it is a doctor, a healer, a shaman, or a family member, may not only create a sense of well-being but may set in motion reparative biological processes.

The sick person's expectant faith in his or her ultimate recovery is further increased by the conviction that he or she shares with the healer and the community a set of assumptions about the cause of the illness and the appropriate treatment. The therapeutic ritual may provide a plan of action for the patient, family, and community that gives them all a sense of purpose and mastery.

A central feature of folk healing involves elements that increase the participants' self-esteem. The involvement of members of the afflicted person's community is viewed as evidence of community support and strengthens the supplicants' self-esteem, sense of worthiness, and acceptability. The feeling of being wanted as part of the living community can reverse what, at times, appears to be an inevitable death.

A few years ago this might have seemed "way out." More recently clinicians and scientists have begun to examine improvements in clinical states associated with faith, hope, meditation, and psychotherapy. Relief of pain and a feeling of euphoria are some features of "shamanic" healing that have also been identified as the effects of endorphins. The therapeutic or protective effect of "shamanic" practices has often been ascribed to a "placebo" effect. It is interesting that more recently endorphins have been suggested as the biological mediator of the placebo effect (37).

Benson (4) has suggested that the relaxation response in yoga, meditation, and prayer may have its healing source in an integrated hypothalamic response resulting in a generalized decrease in sympathetic nervous system activity.

Rossi (47) has presented a psychophysiological rationale for understanding how psychological factors can foster healing. He feels that state-dependent memory, learning, and behavior are the missing links in previous theories of mind–body relationships. This phenomenon, he feels, is the common denominator between traditional western medicine and all the holistic, shamanistic, and spiritualistic approaches to healing.

There are cancer patients who survive much longer than expected. Others die more quickly than predicted. The long survivors have been noted by some to be less anxious and depressed and to show faith and inner confidence (8–10). These are often people who state from the onset they will fight the disease. Persons who die sooner than expected have been described as seeming helpless and full of despair.

Cancer patients utilizing relaxation and mental imagery have been observed by Hall to show increases in their thymosin levels and lymphocyte counts (28,30) together with an attenuation of their cancer (27). Hall and Goldstein (29) have shown that thymosin can stimulate the maturation of immune cells and, in addition, that thymosin acts in the brain and may influence behavior. There is some evidence that mice treated with thymosins become more active and aggressive and are better able to learn simple tasks. Patients treated with thymosins to bolster their immune system indicate that they feel better and some have shown improvement in depressed states.

Solomon (58,60) has wondered if happiness, security, a sense of control, relaxation, and other positive emotions are accompanied by immune enhancement. He has described a patient with ARC who was treated psychiatrically for a depression. The patient's ARC symptoms decreased in association with diminished depression and increased assertiveness. In spite of a worsening helper/suppressor T-cell ratio, the patient had renewed vigor and resumed working full time. Solomon feels that the patient's superb attitude, determination, fighting spirit, and social support played a significant role in his improvement. Solomon, Temoshok, and their colleagues are currently engaged in an intensive immunologic and psychologic study of factors associated with long-term survival of AIDS patients.

Most patients with AIDS have elevated levels of thymosin α-1, and Hall and Goldstein (29) have shown that this substance localizes in circumventricular areas of the brain involved in neuroendocrine regulation. Further, Hall and Goldstein (30) proposed that thymosin peptides function as immunotransmitters to modulate the functioning of the immune system. Solomon wonders if the elevation of thymosin α-1 in AIDS is a compensatory effort at immune stimulation.

The studies that have been mentioned suggest that a feeling of hope associated with either an increased sense that one can cope (or be helped by others to cope) with the problems with which he is confronted (illness, social, or interpersonal) may be accompanied by biological changes that enhance physical as well as mental health.

CONCLUDING STATEMENT

Research employing a biopsychosocial rather than a biomedical model must be taken seriously in AIDS research. The heavy emphasis on defining the pathophysiological mechanisms and the search for vaccines and chemical interventions often tend to push this area of study into the background.

Medical research has always tended to delay studies in what appears to be soft research or humanistic concerns at a time when the research community embarks on the enticing search for the magic bullet.

There is no intention to suggest that there should be any decrease in studies such as the development and use of antiviral drugs or vaccines. Rather, if our research were guided by an integrative model, then studies of drug agents would automatically incorporate into their design studies of psychosocial and CNS factors that might influence the response to these drugs.

The profound effect of AIDS virus on the brain, the panic that the emergence of the illness has engendered, the attitudinal biases related to high-risk groups, the mode of transmission, conflict over potential infectivity, and the terrible sense of hopelessness created by the illness all suggest that this area of study must be adequately supported and integrated into the overall research and program planning.

A biopsychosocial perspective is certainly necessary to develop a humane and comprehensive approach to patient care. This humanistic reason would be sufficient to adopt this model. However, there are additional compelling reasons to consider a broad multisystems approach; e.g., prevention requires influencing health-related behavior, and prevention requires explication of etiology. This may require identifying potential cofactors, some of which may involve the influence of psychosocial factors and emotional reactions on biological systems.

The goal of this chapter was not to highlight a mental–spiritualistic view of the etiology and cure of AIDS. Further, it is not necessary to preach on mind–brain as a potent influence on biological functions. There has been great awareness of and sensitivity to the influence of prejudicial social factors affecting the adequacy of preventive, therapeutic, and rehabilitation efforts. Clinical researchers have suggested the impact of the diagnosis on patients, health care staff, and family and the need to consider this in developing clinical programs. In spite of this awareness, the psychosocial component of the biopsychosocial model of illness has not been thoroughly integrated into the conceptual models guiding the research in spite of the recent flurry of psychoimmunological investigations in which the T cell, one of the prime targets of the HTLV-III, is affected by states of depression and hopelessness. The failure to replace the biomedical with the biopsychosocial conceptual model guiding AIDS research is also noteworthy now that the predilection of the virus for brain cells has been established.

Solomon (59) has pointed out that it is amazing how easily we forget the impact that nonphysical environmental signals can have on CNS functions, especially if those signals are psychologically meaningful ones. Loud noise, bright lights, odors, and changes in atmospheric pressure and temperature are all acceptable subjects for biological stress studies, but signs or sounds that cause fear, hopelessness, love, and hope are often dismissed as significant influences on biological functions. It may be a familiar and even comfortable idiosyncratic human need to keep science away from the unique mind and soul of the human. However, it appears that we can no longer afford this luxury of preserving our soul's immortality by dissociating it from the body. This effort to maintain man's spiritual likeness to God may have to be relinquished so that we can develop a true biopsychosocial approach in our effort to comprehend and treat AIDS.

REFERENCES

1. Anisman, H. (1986): Vulnerability to depression: Contribution of stress. In: *Neurobiology of Mood Disorders*, edited by R. Post and J. C. Bullough, pp. 407–431. Williams & Wilkins, Baltimore.
2. Barber, T. (1985): Death by suggestion. *Psychosom. Med.*, 23:153–158.
3. Bauer, J. (1957): Sudden unexpected death. *Postgrad. Med.*, 22:311.
4. Benson, H. (1983): The relaxation response and norepinephrine. *Integ. Psychiatry*, 1:15–18.
5. Besedovsky, H., del Rey, A., Sorkin, E., DaPrada, M., Burri, R., and Honegger, C. (1983): The immune response evokes changes in brain noradrenergic neurons. *Science*, 221:564–566.
6. Besedovsky, H., and Sorkin, B. (1981): Immunologic–neuroendocrine circuits. In: *Psychoneuroimmunology*, edited by R. Adler, pp. 545–574. Academic Press, New York.
7. Binik, Y. (1977): Sudden death in the laboratory rat. *Psychosom. Med.*, 39:82–93.
8. Blumberg, E. M., Nest, P. M., and Ellis, F. N. (1954): A possible relationship between psychological factors and human cancer. *Psychosom. Med.*, 16:276.
9. Borysenko, J. (1982): Behavioral–physiologic factors in the development and management of cancer. *Gen. Hosp. Psychiatry*, 4:69–74.
10. Borysenko, M., and Borysenko, J. (1982): Stress, behavior and immunity. *Gen. Hosp. Psychiatry*, 4:59–67.
11. Bullock, K. (1985): Neuroanatomy of lymphoid tissue. In: *Neural Modulation of Immunity*, edited by R. Guillemin, M. Cohn, and T. Melnechuk, pp. 111–141. Raven Press, New York.
12. Cahill, K., editor (1983): *The AIDS Epidemic*. St. Martins Press, New York.
13. Cannon, W. B. (1934): *Bodily Changes in Pain, Hunger, Fear and Rage*. Appleton-Century, New York.
14. Comfort, P. (1981): Sorcery and sudden death. *J. R. Soc. Med.*, 74:332–333.
15. Corley, K. C. (1975): Cardiac responses associated with "yoked chair" shock avoidance in squirrel monkeys. *Psychophysiology*, 12:439–444.
15a. Corley, K. C. (1977): Myocardial degeneration and cardiac arrest in squirrel monkeys. *Psychophysiology*, 14:322–328.
16. Cottington, E. M. (1980): Environmental events preceding sudden death in women. *Psychosom. Med.*, 42:567–574.
17. Cousins, N. (1979): *Anatomy of an Illness*. W. W. Norton, New York.
17a. Cousins, N. (1983): *The Healing Heart*. W. W. Norton, New York.
18. Curran, J. W., et al. (1985): The epidemiology of AIDS: Current status and future prospects. *Science*, 229:605–617.
19. DeSilva, R. (1982): Central nervous system risk factors for sudden cardiac death. In: *Sudden Cardiac Death*, edited by H. M. Greenberg and E. M. Dwyer, pp. 143–161. New York Academy of Sciences, New York.
20. Dimsdale, S. C. (1977): Emotional causes of sudden death. *Am. J. Psychiatry*, 134:1361–1366.
21. Engel, G. L. (1971): Sudden and rapid death during psychological stress: Folklore or folkwisdom. *Ann. Intern. Med.*, 74:771–782.
22. Engel, G. L. (1980): The clinical application of the biopsychosocial model. *Am. J. Psychiatry*, 137:535–544.
23. Fauci, A. S., Macher, A. M., and Longo, D. L. (1983): Acquired immunodeficiency syndrome: Epidemiologic, clinical, immunologic and therapeutic considerations. *Ann. Intern. Med.*, 100:92–106.
24. Folks, T., Posell, D. M., Lightfoote, M. M., Benn, S., Martin, H. A., and Fauci, A. S. (1985): Induction of HTLV/LAV from a non-virus-producing T-cell line. *Science*, 231:600–602.
25. Godwin, J. (1976): *Unsolved: The World of the Unknown*. Doubleday, Garden City, NY.
26. Goodfriend, M., and Wolpert, E. (1976): Death from fright. *Psychosom. Med.*, 38:348–355.
27. Hall, H. H. (1983): Hypnosis and the immune system. *Am. J. Clin. Hypnosis*, 25:92–103.
28. Spangelo, B., Hall, N., and Goldstein, A. L. (1987): Biology and chemistry of thymosine peptides-modulation of immunity and neuroendocrine circuits. *Ann. N.Y. Acad. Sci.*, 496:196–204.
29. Hall, N. R., and Goldstein, A. L. (1983): The thymus–brain connection: Interactions between thymosin and the neuroendocrine system. *Lymphokine Res.*, 2:1–6.
30. Hall, N. R., McGillis, J., Spangelo, B., and Goldstein, A. L. (1985): Evidence that thymosin and other biologic response modifiers can function as neuroactive immunotransmitters. *J. Immunol.*, 135(2):806S–811S.

31. Howie, D. (1968): Scared to death. *J. Florida Med. Assoc.*, 55:150–151.
32. Jenkins, C. D., et al. (1973): Zones of excess mortality in Massachusetts. *N. Engl. J. Med.*, 296:1354–1356.
33. Kaufman, I., and Rosenbaum, L. A. (1975): The reaction to separation in infant monkeys. *Psychosom. Med.*, 29:648–675.
34. Kirkpatrick, R. (1981): Witchcraft and lupus erythematosus. *J.A.M.A.*, 245:1937–1938.
35. Laudenslager, M., Ryan, S. M., Drugan, R. C., Hyson, R. L., and Maier, S. F. (1983): Coping and immunosuppression: Inescapable but not escapable shock suppresses lymphocyte proliferation. *Science*, 221:568–570.
36. Leibovitch, J. (1985): *A Strange Virus of Unknown Origin.* Ballantine Books, New York.
37. Levine, J., Gordon, N., and Fields, H. (1978): The mechanism of placebo analgesia. *Lancet*, 2:654–657.
38. Lown, B. (1980): Psychophysiologic factors in sudden cardiac death. *Am. J. Psychiatry*, 137:1325–1335.
39. Lynch, J. (1977): *The Broken Heart.* Basic Books, New York.
40. Marshall, E. (1981): The Hmong: Dying of culture shock. *Science*, 212:1008.
41. Mathis, J. L. (1964): A sophisticated version of voodoo death. *Psychosom. Med.*, 26:104–106.
42. Pert, C., Ruff, M., Weber, R., and Herkenham, M. (1985): Neuropeptides and their receptors: A psychosomatic network. *J. Immunol.*, 135(2):820S–826S.
43. Post, R. (1985): Potential of neuroscience research. In: *The Integration of Neuroscience and Psychiatry*, edited by A. A. Pincus and A. Purdiev, pp. 22–38. APA Press, Washington.
44. Renoux, G., and Biziere, K. (1986): Brain neocortex lateralized control of immune regulation. *Integ. Psychiatry*, 4:32–36.
45. Richter, C. P. (1957): On the phenomena of sudden death in animals and man. *Psychosom. Med.*, 19:191–198.
46. Riley, V., Fitzmaurice, M., and Spackman, D. H. (1981): Psychoneuroimmunologic factors in neoplasia. In: *Psychoneuroimmunology*, edited by R. Ader, pp. 31–102. Academic Press, New York.
47. Rossi, E. L. (1986): *The Psychobiology of Mind–Brain Healing.* W. W. Norton, New York.
48. Ruff, M. R., and Pert, C. B. (1984): Small cell carcinoma of the lung: Macrophage specific antigens suggest hemopoietic stem cell origin. *Science*, 225:1034–1086.
49. Saul, L. J. (1966): Sudden death at impasse. *Psychoanal. Forum*, 1:88–89.
50. Schleifer, S. J., Keller, S. E., and Stein, M. (1985): Stress effects of immunity. *Psychiatr. J. Univ. Ottawa*, 10(3):125–131.
51. Schmale, A. H. (1958): Relationship of separation to disease. *Psychosom. Med.*, 20:4.
52. Schmale, A. H., and Iker, H. (1966): The psychological setting of uterine cervical cancer. *Ann. N.Y. Acad. Sci.*, 125:807–813.
53. Seligman, M. (1976): *Helplessness.* W. H. Freeman, San Francisco.
54. Selye, H. (1976): *The Stress of Life.* McGraw-Hill, New York.
55. Shekelle, R. B. (1981): Psychological depression and 17-year risk of death from cancer. *Psychosom. Med.*, 43:2.
56. Smith, E. M., Meyer, W. J., and Blalock, J. E. (1982): Virus-induced corticosterone in hypophysectomized mice: A possible lymphoid adrenal axis. *Science*, 218:1311–1312.
57. Sodorski, J. G., Rosen, C. A., and Haseltine, W. R. (1984): Transaction, transcription of the long terminal repeat of human T-lymphocyte viruses in infected cells. *Science*, 225:381–382.
58. Solomon, G. (1985): The emerging field of psychoneuroimmunology. *Advances*, 2(1):6–19.
59. Solomon, G., Amkraut, A. A., and Kaspan, P. (1974): Immunity, emotions and stress. *Psychother. Psychosom.*, 23:209.
60. Solomon, G., and Temoshok, L. (1987): A psychoneuroimmunologic perspective on AIDS research. *J. Appl. Soc. Psychol.*, 17:286–308.
61. Stein, M. (1981): A biopsychosocial approach to immune function and medical disorders. *Psychiatr. Clin. North Am.*, 4:203–221.
62. Stein, M., Schleifer, S., and Keller, S. (1981): Hypothalamic influence on immune responses. In: *Psychoneuroimmunology*, edited by R. Ader, pp. 429–448. Academic Press, New York.
63. Weiss, S. (1940): Instantaneous physiologic death. *N. Engl. J. Med.*, 223:793–797.
64. Weissman, P. D., and Hackett, T. (1961): Predilection to death. *Psychosom. Med.*, 23:232–256.

Psychological, Neuropsychiatric, and Substance Abuse Aspects of AIDS, edited by T. Peter Bridge et al. Raven Press, New York © 1988.

Neuropsychiatric Impairment in Patients with AIDS

*David R. Rubinow, *Russell T. Joffe, †Pim Brouwers, †Kathleen Squillace, ‡H. Clifford Lane, and †Allan F. Mirsky

Biological Psychiatry Branch, †Laboratory of Psychology and Psychopathology, Intramural Research Program, National Institute of Mental Health, ‡Laboratory of Immunoregulation, National Institute of Allergy and Infectious Disease, National Institutes of Health, Bethesda, Maryland 20892

A variety of behavioral responses and psychiatric syndromes have been described in relation to AIDS. First, given the uniformly grim prognosis that accompanies AIDS, the frequent experience by AIDS patients of symptoms such as anxiety, sadness, and regret is surprising to no one. Second, formal psychiatric syndromes, major depressive disorder and generalized anxiety disorder, may appear and require therapeutic intervention. Third, organic mental syndromes have been reported both in association with CNS lymphoma and opportunistic infections and as part of an HIV-induced subacute encephalitis (25). The discovery of HIV DNA (24) and HIV-infected giant cells (15) in the brains of patients with AIDS, the culture of HIV from the CSF and brains of AIDS patients (13,16), the intra-blood–brain-barrier synthesis of HIV-specific IgG (21), and the identification of HTLV-III viral receptors in brain (18) suggest that the brain might be directly affected by HTLV-III infection and not merely experience an "innocent bystander reaction" to AIDS-related opportunistic infections.

As part of an attempt to describe the neuropsychiatric concomitants of AIDS, we performed structured psychiatric interviews and neuropsychological testing in patients with AIDS ($n = 13$) who had no clinical or laboratory evidence of systemic infection or neurological involvement and in a group of age-, sex- (male), and education-matched homosexual controls ($n = 10$) (14). All patients were admitted to the NIAID for participation in experimental protocols, and all gave written and oral informed consent to participate in this study. Controls were recruited from the local community through the NIH volunteer office and had demonstrated the absence of medical illness by chemical and laboratory screening. Psychiatric assessment was performed by means of a modified Schedule for Affective Disorders and Schizophrenia—Lifetime interview (SADS-L) (26) and two self-rating instruments, the Beck Depression Inventory (3) and the SCL-90 (a 90-item questionnaire that yields eight factor scores) (8). Neuropsychological assessment surveyed both general and specific (abstraction and categorization, visuospatial organization, visuo-motor performance, and attention and concentration) cognitive function. These tests included:

1. Wechsler Adult Intelligence Scale—Revised (WAIS-R) (31).
2. Halstead Category Test (10).
3. Trail-Making Test (1).
4. Rey Osterreith Complex Figure Test (17).
5. Cancellation Test (28).
6. Wisconsin Card Sort (4).
7. Wechsler Memory Scale (30).
8. Test of Selected Reminding and Restricted Reminding (Buschke) (7).
9. Stroop Color–Word Test (27).
10. Continuous Performance Task (CPT) (22).
11. Raven's Progressive Matrices (20).
12. Babcock Story Recall Test (2).
13. Harris Hand Dominance Test (11).

In addition a personality profile was obtained with the Minnesota Multiphasic Personality Inventory (MMPI) (12).

RESULTS

Psychiatric

As reported elsewhere (14), no difference was observed in the prevalence of current psychiatric disorders between patients (two adjustment disorders and one substance abuse disorder) and controls (three adjustment disorders). A trend was observed for an increased prevalence of past history of major depressive disorder in the patients ($n = 5$) compared with the controls ($n = 1$) ($p = 0.06$, Fisher's exact test) and of adjustment disorder in the controls ($n = 5$) compared with the patients ($n = 1$) ($p = 0.06$, Fisher's exact test). Patients had significantly higher scores on the Beck Depression Inventory ($p < 0.02$) and a trend toward elevated scores on the depression subscale of the SCL-90 ($p < 0.1$). Only the two patients with the adjustment disorder with depressed mood scored in the depressed range (greater than 15) (3) on the Beck Depression Inventory.

Neuropsychological

Significantly decreased performance in the patients compared with the controls was noted on the following tests: WAIS full-scale IQ ($p < 0.05$), verbal IQ ($p < 0.05$), WAIS vocabulary subtest ($p < 0.01$), similarities subtest ($p < 0.05$), Digit–Symbol subtest ($p < 0.05$), Halstead Category Test ($p < 0.05$), Trail–Making Tests Trial B ($p < 0.05$), and the number completed and number correct on all three sections of the Cancellation Task ($p < 0.05$ to 0.01). Additionally, patients scored significantly higher on the hysteria ($p < 0.01$) and hypochondriasis ($p < 0.05$) subscales of the MMPI. Patients scored significantly higher on the copying component of the Rey Osterreith Complex Figure Test ($p < 0.05$).

DISCUSSION

Our data suggest that patients with AIDS show decreased general cognitive function as well as a potential focal dysfunction in the absence of evidence of overt CNS involvement. Additionally, AIDS patients appear somewhat more likely to have had a past history of depression. These data are consistent with those of Tross et al. (29), which similarly demonstrated cognitive impairment in AIDS patients without overt CNS involvement, although our data differ in our failure to demonstrate a memory deficit as indicated by scores on the Weschler, Buschke, and Babcock tests.

Several methodologic points deserve comment. First, our findings may represent the product of chronic or terminal illness, preoccupation with somatic functioning, or disturbances of mood rather than a specific concomitant of AIDS viral infection. One therefore requires several different control groups in order to ascertain the significance of the relative cognitive impairment observed in the AIDS patients. Second, the tests that we employed are screening tests and do not permit much in the way of conclusive statements about the specificity of deficits and may be insensitive to fairly selective alterations in cognition. Third, our data suggest that there may be a two-factor component to the neuropsychological impairment observed. Whereas findings of deterioration on "hold" functions such as verbal IQ may be consistent with focal and specifically limbic pathology, the reduced performance on self-paced timed tasks (Trail-Making, Digit–Symbol, and Cancellation tests) suggests that motivation alterations, perhaps resulting from depressed mood and preoccupation with illness, might have contributed to test results. Fourth, longitudinal testing is required in order to determine the constancy and clinical relevance of cognitive dysfunction and, additionally, to reveal other factors (e.g., labile mood) that may affect performance or suggest focal involvement.

These problems notwithstanding, our data suggest the relevance of neuropsychiatric compromise to patients with AIDS as well as the relevance of AIDS to the neuroscientist. Recent evidence has increasingly demonstrated the mutual regulatory interactions of the immune, neuroendocrine, and central nervous systems (5,6,9,19,23). These three systems are stimulus–response systems that display signal recognition and memory and that transmit information to one another as part of an integrated homeostatic response. Thus, further attempts to define the mechanism of AIDS-related neuropsychological deficits may tell us not only about the pathogenesis, course, and significance of these deficits but may as well inform us about immune–central nervous systems interactions. The clinical relevance of these interactions is suggested by recent demonstration of interleukin-2-induced neuropsychiatric toxicity in cancer patients (K. Denicoff et al., *unpublished data*) as well as by the report of α-interferon-induced organic affective and mental syndromes in patients with chronic active hepatitis (P. Renault et al., *unpublished data*). Finally, continuing study of neuropsychologic function in patients with HIV viral infections may provide important clues to those vulnerability factors that affect disease acquisition as well as the illness-related behavioral factors that may influence immune functions and/or course of illness.

REFERENCES

1. Army Individual Test (1944): *Manual of Directions and Scoring.* War Department, Adjutant General's Office, Washington.
2. Babcock, H., and Levy, L. (1940): *Revision of the Babcock Examination for Measuring Efficiency of Mental Functioning.* C. H. Stoelting, Chicago.
3. Beck, A. T., Ward, C. H., and Mendelson, M. (1961): An inventory for measuring depression. *Arch. Gen. Psychiatry,* 41:561–571.
4. Berg, E. A. (1948): A simple objective technique for measuring flexibility in thinking. *J. Gen. Psychol.,* 39:15–22.
5. Besedovsky, H. O., de Rey, A. E., and Sorkin, E. (1985): Immune–neuroendocrine interactions. *J. Immunol.,* 135(2):750S–754S.
6. Blalock, J. E., Harbour-McMenamin, D., and Smith, E. M. (1985): Peptide hormones shared by the neuroendocrine and immunologic systems. *J. Immunol.,* 135(2):858S–861S.
7. Buschke, H., and Fuld, P. A. (1974): Evaluating storage, retention and retrieval in disordered memory and learning. *Neurology (Minneap.),* 11:1019–1025.
8. Derogatis, L. R. (1984): *SCL-90-R Manual.* Clinical Psychometric Research, Towson, MD.
9. Hall, N. R., McGillis, J. P., Spangelo, B. L., and Goldstein, A. L. (1985): Evidence that thymosins and other biologic response modifiers can function as neuroactive immunotransmitters. *J. Immunol.,* 135(2):806S–811S.
10. Halstead, W. C. (1947): *Brain and Intelligence.* University of Chicago Press, Chicago.
11. Harris, A. J. (1954): *Harris Test of Lateral Dominance.* The Psychological Corporation, New York.
12. Hathaway, S. R., and McKinley, J. C. (1951): *The Minnesota Multiphasic Personality Inventory Manual (Revised).* Psychological Corporation, New York.
13. Ho, D. D., Rota, T. R., Schooley, R. T., Kaplan, J. C., Allan, J. D., Groopman, J. E., Resnick, L., Felsenstein, D., Andrews, C. A., and Hirsch, M. S. (1985): Isolation of HTLV-III from cerebrospinal fluid and neural tissues of patients with neurologic syndromes related to the acquired immunodeficiency syndrome. *N. Engl. J. Med.,* 313:1493.
14. Joffe, R. T., Rubinow, D. R., Squillace, K., Lane, C. H., Duncan, C. C., and Fauci, A. S. (1986): Neuropsychiatric manifestations of acquired immune deficiency syndrome (AIDS). *Psychopharmacol. Bull.,* 22:684–688.
15. Koenig, S., Gendelman, H. E., Orenstein, J. M., Dal Canto, M. C., Pezeshkpour, G. H., Yungbluth, M., Janotta, F., Aksamit, A., Martin, M. A., and Fauci, A. S. (1986): Detection of AIDS virus in macrophages in brain tissue from AIDS patients with encephalopathy. *Science,* 233:1089–1093.
16. Levy, J. A., Shimabururo, J., Hollander, H., Mills, J., and Kaminsky, L. (1985): Isolation of AIDS-associated retroviruses from cerebrospinal fluid and brain of patients with neurological symptoms. *Lancet,* 1:586–588.
17. Osterreith, R. A. (1944): Le test de copie d'une figure complexe. *Arch. Psychol.,* 30:206–256.
18. Pert, C. B., Hill, J. M., Farrar, W. L., and Ruscetti, R. W. (1985): Autoradiographical distribution of the AIDS virus receptor (entry protein) in primate brain. In: *Annual Meeting of the American College of Neuropsychopharmacology, Maui, Hawaii, December 9–13,* p. 30.
19. Pert, C. B., Russ, M. R., Weber, R. J., and Herkenham, M. (1985): Neuropeptides and their receptors: A psychosomatic network. *J. Immunol.,* 135(2):820S–826S.
20. Raven, J. C. (1958): *Standard Progressive Matrices.* H. K. Lewis, London.
21. Resnick, L., Di Marzo-Veronese, F., Schupbach, J., Tourtellotee, W. W., Ho, D. D., Muller, F., Shapshak, P., Vogt, M., Groopman, J. E., Markham, P. D., and Gallo, R. C. (1985): Intra-

blood–brain barrier synthesis of HTLV-III-specific IgG in patients with neurologic symptoms associated with AIDS or AIDS-related complex. *N. Engl. J. Med.,* 313:1498.

22. Rosvold, H. E., Mirsky, A. F., Sarason, I., Bransone, E. D., Jr., and Beck, L. H. (1956): A continuous performance test of brain damage. *J. Consult. Psychol.,* 20:343–350.
23. Roszman, T. L., Jackson, J. C., Corss, R. J., Titus, M. J., Markesbery, W. R., and Brooks, W. H. (1985): Neuroanatomic and neurotransmitter influences on immune function. *J. Immunol.,* 135(2):769S–772S.
24. Shaw, G. M., Harper, M. E., Hahn, B. H., Epstein, L. G., Gajdusek, D. C., Price, R. W., Navia, B. A., Petito, C. K., O'Hara, C. J., Groopman, J. E., Cho, E. S., Oleske, J. M., Wong-Stall, F., and Gallo, R. C. (1985): HTLV-III infection in brains of children and adults with AIDS encephalopathy. *Science,* 227:177–181.
25. Snider, W. D., Simpson, D. M., Nielsen, S., Gold, J. W. M., Metroka, C. E., and Posner, J. B. (1983): Neurological complications of acquired immune deficiency syndrome: Analysis of 50 patients. *Ann. Neurol.,* 14:403–418.
26. Spitzer, R. L., and Endicott, J. (1978): *Schedule for Affective Disorders and Schizophrenia— Lifetime Versions (SADS-L),* 3rd ed. Psychiatric Institute, New York.
27. Stroop, J. R. (1935): Studies of interference in serial verbal reactions. *J. Exp. Psychol.,* 18:643–662.
28. Talland, G. A. (1965): *Deranged Memory.* Academic Press, New York.
29. Tross, S., Price, R., Sidtis, J., Hollan, J., Wolfe, L., and Navia, B. (1987): Neuropsychological complications of AIDS. *Psychopharmacol. Bull. (in press).*
30. Wechsler, D. A. (1945): A standardized memory scale for clinical use. *J. Consult. Psychol.,* 19:87–95.
31. Wechsler, D. (1981): *Wechsler Adult Intelligence Scale—Revised.* The Psychological Corporation, New York.

Psychological, Neuropsychiatric, and Substance Abuse Aspects of AIDS, edited by T. Peter Bridge et al. Raven Press, New York © 1988.

Neuropsychological Manifestations and Predictors of HIV Disease in Vulnerable Persons

Allan F. Mirsky

Laboratory of Psychology and Psychopathology, Intramural Research Program, National Institute of Mental Health, National Institutes of Health, Bethesda, Maryland 20892

In the other chapters of this volume and in the previous presentations or publications of the contributors, a number of neuropsychological findings have emerged with some regularity: in patients suffering from AIDS, changes occur in such cognitive functions as problem solving, language, memory, vigilance, and visuomotor–spatial abilities and in motor efficiency (9,17; D. R. Rubinow et al., *this volume*). Aside from these changes, findings have also been reported indicating alterations in mood or affect, usually of a dysphoric nature (13; D. G. Ostrow, *this volume*). In one report, the dysphoric changes also presented as a previous history of major affective disorder (9).

I wish to make four general points with respect to those neuropsychological findings:

1. There is a reasonably good fit between the dense AIDS virus receptor clusters in the brain using the animal model developed by Pert and colleagues (15; C. B. Pert et al., *this volume*) and some of the neuropsychological results. Specifically, mood changes and memory losses could well be related to destruction of hippocampal and amygdala tissue. The findings of Price in the neuropathological studies of the brains of patients dying from AIDS fit somewhat better with the reported deficits in attention, concentration, and vigilance.
2. The occurrence of dysphoria/depression in the AIDS cases is difficult to interpret.
3. The cognitive changes present some opportunities for research studies and, at the same time, dangers for the patients themselves and for those with the responsibility of dealing with them or for planning their care.
4. Future studies aimed at predicting development of active HIV disease in persons at risk may well take advantage of certain sensitive methods used in the study of other putative central nervous system disorders, methods that are based on

cognitive psychophysiology/electrophysiology. These could conceivably enhance the predictive power of the test battery.

With respect to the neuropsychological/neuroanatomical fit, the following correlations may be pointed out. The reported changes in speed of response may be related to the basal ganglia effects described by Pert et al. (15). Both the caudate and putamen have a major role in the modulation of motor output. In addition, recent clinical observations by Healton et al. (7) and by Heilman et al. (8) have suggested that these structures are involved in attention as well, possibly through their anatomic connections to the prefrontal cortex. The confluence of effects produced by lesions in the caudate, putamen, and cingulate gyrus are certainly compatible with the deficits reported in motor control and in vigilance/attention/concentration described by the Tross, Ostrow, and Joffee groups (9,13,17). The correlations are even stronger when one adds the lesions in the subcortical gray nuclei reported by Price. Figure 1 shows some of the portions of an attention system

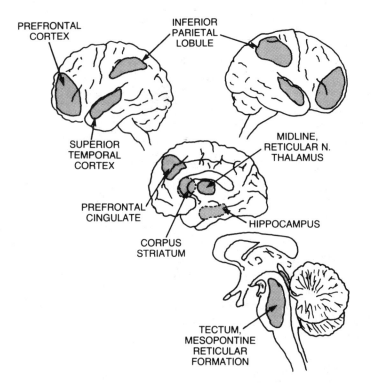

FIG. 1. A hypothetical system within the human brain specialized for the behavioral functions referred to as "attention." The components of the system are inferred primarily from clinical research on patients suffering from brain injuries and/or epilepsy as well as from neuropsychological studies with nonhuman primates.

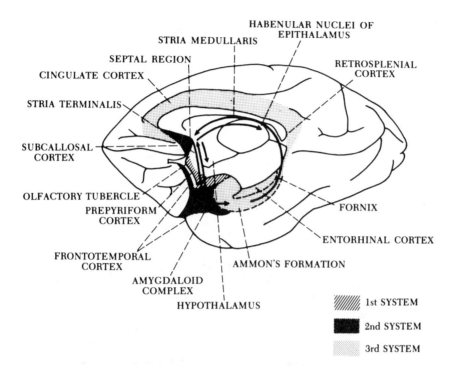

FIG. 2. The components of the limbic system or "olfactory brain" as described by Pribram and Kruger; according to their 1954 formulation, there are three olfactory brain subsystems, each of which plays a specialized and differentiated role with respect to the support of emotion. Ammon's formation is another term for hippocampal formation. (Reproduced with permission from Pribram and Kruger, ref. 16.)

that the virus could be attacking; the caudate and putamen are indicated in phantom on this figure.

Concerning the affective/dysphoric changes, if these are clearly related to brain lesions, as opposed to being a reactive (and appropriate) depression, then the tissue destruction seen in the cingulate, septum, and amygdala could provide a substrate for this disturbance. These structures are part of the well-known limbic system, the anatomical support system for the expression of emotion first described by Broca (2), rediscovered by Papez (14), and then brought up to date so magnificently by MacLean (10) and Pribram and Kruger (16). Figure 2, reproduced from Pribram and Kruger, helps to illustrate this point.

On the question of dysphoria/depression in AIDS cases, several comments are in order. Some of the reported neuropsychological deficits could be caused by depression per se. There are a number of reports in the literature indicating that affective disturbances can have deleterious effects on cognitive processes. To separate these two effects would require correlational studies and/or comparison of cases with and without significant depression (assuming that there are AIDS cases without significant depression). In any event, this variable is potentially significant as a source of confounding in these data.

It needs to be established whether there are concurrent changes in both attention and memory. Attentional losses could very well be primary. We need better definition and assessment of recent versus remote memory effects in these patients, since a comparison of the two classes of memory loss could help clarify the role of attention.

The cognitive changes seen in AIDS present the opportunity to develop a battery of neuropsychological tests that could well predict the onset of active disease before the physical symptoms become manifest. At some point in the future, these test scores may be critical data in the event an effective treatment has been developed; we presume that such therapy must be administered early in the history of the disorder in order to be most efficacious. We may need all the advance notice possible, and the data from psychological tests may provide some of the earliest prodromal signs.

Those charged with the responsibility of modifying the sexual practices of AIDS-vulnerable people must recognize the following facts. We are asking persons with AIDS to modify behavior in major ways. However, the brain, the source and support of all behaviors, has been seriously compromised by the disease. This emphasizes the necessity of developing support systems, whether they be individuals, groups, or other networks, to help guide and supplement the potentially faulty cognitive apparatus of the AIDS patient. The situation is strikingly similar to that of Alzheimer's disease.

Since attention/vigilance/concentration seems to be almost universally reported as impaired in AIDS patients, it would seem essential to employ the most sensitive techniques available for the purpose of assessing early changes in these behaviors. It would also be of considerable interest to try to ascertain the type of attentional

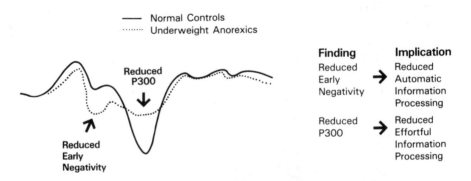

FIG. 3. Schematic view of event-related potential results obtained by Duncan et al. (3) in their study of patients with anorexia nervosa. In the result depicted, underweight anorexic subjects showed both reduced early negativity, which is correlated with the mismatch negativity of Naatanen et al. (12), and reduced P300. The implications of these findings for information processing are represented on the figure.

loss that is taking place. Event-related brain potentials (ERP) would seem to be an extremely good approach toward this end. Since these measures of speed and efficiency of cognitive processing are based on brainwave activity, they are one step closer to the dysfunctional brain structures than the overt behaviors themselves. They can provide clues to the locus of the interference in the neuropsychological information-processing system.

Of the several ERP components that have been linked to information processing, two (among several) are perhaps of special interest. The mismatch negativity (MMN) is an early, preattentive measure, apparently indexing what the cognitive psychologists refer to as automatic information processing (12). The second or P300 component is firmly linked to attention, expectancy, and memorability (5), or effortful or controlled information processing in the lexicon of the cognitive psychologists. The P300 may be of special interest for the present discussion since there are data to support the view that this ERP component is in part generated in the hippocampus (6). If hippocampal cell loss is an early manifestation of AIDS, the P300 could be an index of the central pathophysiology in this disease. Figure 3 shows the ERP, recorded from the scalp, elicited by an attention-demanding stimulus in a special psychological test paradigm. These data were gathered in a study of patients suffering from severe anorexia nervosa. The average ERPs from a group of such cases are compared with that from a group of normal control women (3).

The MMN appears between 50 and 200 msec post-stimulus (given the appropriate task); the P300 appears between 250 and 400 msec (under appropriate task

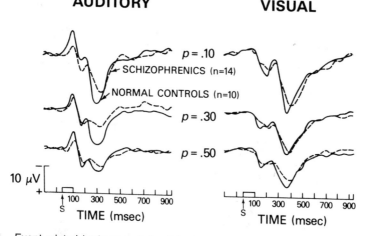

FIG. 4. Event-related brain potentials elicited in the course of a discrimination reaction time task by auditory and visual target stimuli of varying probabilities: $p = 0.10$ refers to 10% probability of a target as compared to a nontarget stimulus; $p = 0.30$ refers to 30% probability; etc. The P300 is the positive-going waveform seen at about 300 msec following stimulus (S) onset. Schizophrenic patients show reduced P300 component amplitudes in auditory visual tasks; this is especially pronounced at low stimulus probabilities ($p = 0.10, 0.30$).

conditions). The P300 is better known and is established to be significantly reduced in amplitude in various clinical states in which attention impairment is a key symptom (i.e., schizophrenia, eating disorders, dyslexia). In this study both MMN and P300 were reduced, suggesting a deficit in both automatic and controlled information processing in this group. In contrast, Fig. 4 presents the results of a recent ERP study in schizophrenia (4); here the deficit shown is restricted to P300, presumably reflecting the well-known attention disturbance in this disorder. This finding, which has been replicated frequently in schizophrenia research, is of particular relevance for this discussion, since there are data suggesting that some persons who are vulnerable to schizophrenia (on genetic grounds) may also show reduced P300 waves (11). There have been reports, as well, of P300 alterations in persons genetically vulnerable to alcoholism (1). The possibility thus exists that this metric might provide a measure of vulnerability to AIDS.

These electrophysiological methods could provide the basis for an assessment or assay that, in conjunction with an appropriate neuropsychological test battery, could be repeated on a systematic basis. This could be considered as part of a regular health checkup in AIDS-vulnerable patients. It seems likely that such procedures could enhance significantly our ability to detect central nervous system manifestations early and, it is hoped, to institute effective therapies when they are developed.

REFERENCES

1. Begleiter, H., Porjesz, B., Bihari, B., and Kissin, B. (1984): Event-related brain potentials in boys at risk for alcoholism. *Science*, 225:1493–1496.
2. Broca, P., editor (1888): *Mémoires sur le Cerveau de l'Homme*. C. Reinwald, Paris.
3. Duncan, C. C., Kaye, W. H., Perlstein, W. M., Jimerson, D. C., and Mirsky, A. F. (1985): Cognitive processing in eating disorders: An ERP analysis. *Psychophysiology*, 22:588.
4. Duncan, C. C., Perlstein, W. M., and Morihisa, J. M. (1987): Probability and modality effects on brain potentials in schizophrenia: Preliminary findings. In: *Proceedings of the Eighth International Symposium on Current Research in Event-Related Brain Potentials. Electroencephalography and Clinical Neurophysiology*, edited by J. W. Rohrbaugh, R. Johnson, Jr., and R. Parasuraman (*in press*).
5. Duncan-Johnson, C., and Donchin, E. (1982): The P300 component of the event-related brain potential as an index of information processing. *Biol. Psychol.*, 14:1–52.
6. Halgren, E., Squires, N. K., Wilson, C. L., Rohrbaugh, J. W., Babb, T. L., and Crandall, P. H. (1980): Endogenous potentials generated in the human hippocampal formation and amygdala by infrequent events. *Science*, 210:803–805.
7. Healton, E. B., Navarro, C., Bressman, S., and Brust, J. C. M. (1982): Subcortical neglect. *Neurology* (N.Y.), 32:776–778.
8. Heilman, K. M., Watson, R. T., Valenstein, E., and Damasio, A. R. (1983): Localization of lesions in neglect. In: *Localization in Neuropsychology*, edited by A. Kertesz, pp. 471–492. Academic Press, New York.
9. Joffe, R. T., Rubinow, D. R., Squillace, K., Lane, C. H., Duncan, C. C., Fauci, A. C., and Mirsky, A. F. (1985): Neuropsychiatric manifestations of acquired immune deficiency syndrome. Paper presented at 24th Annual Meeting of the American College of Neuropsychopharmacology.
10. MacLean, P. D. (1949): Psychosomatic disease and the "visceral brain." *Psychosom. Med.*, 11:338–353.
11. Mirsky, A. F., and Duncan, C. C. (1986): Etiology and expression of schizophrenia: Neurobiological and psychosocial factors. *Annu. Rev. Psychol.*, 37:291–319.

12. Naatanen, R., Sams, M., and Alho, K. (1986): The mismatch negativity: The ERP sign of a cerebral mismatch process. In: *Cerebral Psychophysiology: Studies in Event-Related Potentials. Electroencephalography and Clinical Neurophysiology,* Suppl. 38, edited by C. W. McCallum, R. Zappoli, and F. Denoth, 172–178.
13. Ostrow, D. G., Joseph, J., Monjan, A., Phair, J., Polk, F., Rinaldo, C., Detels, R., and Kaslow, R. (1985): Psychological correlates of AIDS risk and HTLV-III exposure. Paper presented at 24th Annual Meeting of the American College of Neuropsychopharmacology.
14. Papez, J. W. (1937): A proposed mechanism of emotion. *Arch. Neurol. Psychiatry,* 38:725–743.
15. Pert, C. B., Hill, J. M., Farrar, W. L., and Ruscetti, F. W. (1985): Autoradiographical distribution of the AIDS virus receptor (entry protein) in primate brain. Paper presented at 24th Annual Meeting of the American College of Neuropsychopharmacology.
16. Pribram, K. H., and Kruger, L. (1954): Functions of the "olfactory brain." *Ann. N.Y. Acad. Sci.,* 58:109–138.
17. Tross, S., Price, R., Sidtis, J., Holland, J., Wolf, L., and Navia, B. (1985): Neuropsychological complications of AIDS. Paper presented at 24th Annual Meeting of the American College of Neuropsychopharmacology.

Psychological, Neuropsychiatric, and
Substance Abuse Aspects of AIDS,
edited by T. Peter Bridge et al.
Raven Press, New York © 1988.

Drugs of Abuse and Virus Susceptibility

Herman Friedman, Thomas Klein, Steven Specter, Susan Pross,
Catherine Newton, D. K. Blanchard, and Raymond Widen

*Department of Medical Microbiology and Immunology, University of South Florida
College of Medicine, Tampa, Florida 33612*

It is widely accepted that retroviruses cause malignancy as well as immunodeficiency not only in lower animal species, such as rodents, cats, dogs, cattle, as well as birds, but also in man. The recent discovery of the human immunodeficiency virus (HIV) as the etiologic agent of acquired immunodeficiency syndrome (AIDS) in man indicates that retroviruses, at least of the lentivirus group, can also cause a devastating collapse of the immune response in humans (5). The HIV infection not only causes increased susceptibility to malignancies such as Kaposi's sarcoma and lymphomas and leukemias but also increases susceptibility to opportunistic bacterial, fungal, and viral infections. However, it is widely recognized that only about 10 to 30% or so of those individuals who have evidence of being exposed to or infected with this virus (i.e., high-risk group showing evidence of antibody to the virus or virus antigens) have to date developed overt AIDS. Thus, it is felt that there must be cofactors involved along with the virus for full development of the syndrome, including collapse of the immune system.

Retrovirus infection of mice is controlled by a variety of factors including genetic susceptibility to the virus but also the type of virus, the host's condition, route of exposure to the virus, etc. (1). It is also known that resistance to viruses depends on functioning host defense mechanisms involving nonspecific and immune cells as well as humoral and subcellular factors. Numerous studies over the past few decades have shown that tumor viruses in particular, as well as many other viruses, may alter a wide variety of immune responses, both humoral and cellular (1). For example, virus infection may interfere temporarily or permanently with normal immune function as well as function of cells such as macrophages either involved in phagocytosis or as regulators of other immune cells. These lymphoreticular cells also produce a variety of soluble mediators including interleukins, interferons, and pharmacologically active molecules that affect the function of other cells. Recently some studies on possible cofactors important in virus infection, especially substances or agents that increase the susceptibility to viruses and their effects, have focused attention on drugs considered "drugs of abuse" used for "recreational" purposes in this country and elsewhere. Among these substances are marijuana and cocaine.

In regard to marijuana, a number of studies over the last decade or so have focused attention on various components of this complex plant material, including purified cannabinoids such as Δ^9-tetrahydrocannabinol (THC) and its less psychoactive metabolic product 11-OH THC. Studies in this laboratory have confirmed and extended the observations that THC may have marked suppressive effects on various components of the immune system, both cellular and humoral. As shown in the present study, these cannabinoids at nontoxic doses can depress *in vitro* the functional activity of T and B lymphocytes as well as macrophages. The drugs also affect the ability of these cells to produce soluble mediators of immunity, including interleukins and interferons, which are important in various immune responses and also in resistance to viral infections, including those caused by retroviruses. Thus, it appears from these studies that cannabinoids, widely used by individuals who are considered at high risk for AIDS, have the ability to serve as cofactors in altering the immune status of the host and thus contributing to the increased susceptibility to retrovirus infection and eventual development of AIDS.

MATERIALS AND METHODS

For these studies the purified cannabinoid components THC and 11-OH THC were used. These components were obtained from the National Institute on Drug Abuse, Rockville, MD. The compounds were dissolved in either dimethyl sulfoxide (DMSO) or ethanol. Stock preparations were prepared in the appropriate vehicle and used immediately. For *in vitro* studies, spleen cells were obtained from normal BALB/c mice and dispersed cell suspensions prepared for lymphoproliferation studies in sterile RPMI 1640 medium containing 10% fetal calf serum (FCS) and antibiotics as described (4). Peritoneal macrophage preparations were obtained from normal mice. The ability of the macrophages to spread on glass surfaces or to phagocytize yeast particles was determined in the presence or absence of THC or 11-OH THC exactly as described (6). For human studies, peripheral blood lymphocytes were obtained from whole blood collected by venapuncture by centrifugation on Ficoll–Hypaque. Human volunteers were used only if they denied a history of use of drugs of abuse during the previous 3 months.

The ability of spleen cells to produce antibody when challenged *in vitro* with sheep erythrocytes was determined by the localized antibody plaque cell assay (PFC) as described previously (10). In brief, 10×10^6 dispersed viable spleen cells in individual wells of culture plates were immunized with 2×10^6 SRBC, and the cultures were incubated for 5 days at 37°C in an atmosphere of 5% CO_2 and air. The number of PFCs was then determined by the localized plaque assay exactly as described (10). The effects of THC or 11-OH THC were determined in these cultures treated at the time of culture initiation and immunization.

Allogeneic mixed cell cultures were prepared exactly as described previously, and the effect of cannabinoids on this response was determined by the thymidine uptake assay (3). The effect of these drugs on lymphoid cell ability to produce interleukins (IL-1 or IL-2) and interferon was determined exactly as described previously: culture supernatants of spleen cells, after stimulation with bacterial LPS, were assayed for IL-1 activity with thymocytes from C_3H/HeJ mice (7) or for interferon activity by the ability of graded quantities of supernatants to protect L929 cells from the cytopathogenic effects of vesicular stomatitis virus (2). The effect of cannabinoids on natural killer cell activity was determined as described (9).

RESULTS

Tetrahydrocannabinol was found to inhibit markedly the ability of mouse macrophages to spread *in vitro*, an indicator of macrophage activity, as well as to phagocytize yeast particles (Tables 1–3). A dose as low as 0.1 μg THC had an inhibitory effect on macrophage spreading. A concentration of 1 to 5 μg THC had the ability to inhibit markedly the phagocytic activity of the macrophages. Cell viability was inhibited only with doses greater than 15 or 20 μg THC. Thus, it was apparent that these two functional activities of macrophages, i.e., spreading *in vitro* and phagocytosis of yeast particles, could be markedly inhibited at doses of THC that had no effect on the viability of the cells.

Treatment of spleen cells with THC as well as 11-OH THC also modulated antibody responsiveness to sheep erythrocytes (Table 4). Addition of 5 to 10 μg THC to mouse spleen cell cultures *in vitro* immunized for 5 days with sheep erythrocytes resulted in a marked inhibition of the antibody response as compared to control cultures not treated with the cannabinoids. It is of interest, however, that a 10-fold lower dose of THC resulted in somewhat enhanced antibody responsiveness (Table 4). The possibility that low doses of cannabinoids can enhance immune function is currently under investigation.

TABLE 1. *Effect of Δ^9-THC on spreading of mouse adherent peritoneal cells on glass surfaces*

Addition (μg/ml)[a]	Days of exposure to THC[b]		
	1	3	6
20.0	26 ± 4	32 ± 6	67 ± 9
10.0	36 ± 7	37 ± 6	64 ± 11
5.0	38 ± 9	41 ± 5	84 ± 7
1.0	42 ± 6	47 ± 6	73 ± 8
0.1	62 ± 9	77 ± 8	87 ± 6
0.05	71 ± 4	91 ± 6	98 ± 5
0.01	106 ± 11	102 ± 7	110 ± 11

[a]Dose of THC added to cultures of normal mouse peritoneal cells.
[b]Mean percentage of spread cells ± SEM; three to five determinations per data point. Medium containing 0.1% DMSO only used as control for 100% spreading value.

TABLE 2. *Effect of Δ⁹-THC on yeast particle phagocytosis by peritoneal or splenic adherent cells after 24 hr culture*

THC dose (μg/ml)[a]	Peritoneal cells[b]		Spleen cells[b]	
	cpm ± SE	Percentage of control	cpm ± SE	Percentage of control
Medium only	37,081 ± 2,915	—	39,830 ± 2,702	—
THC				
0.1	42,185 ± 4,096	113.8	37,881 ± 3,132	95.1
1.0	40,384 ± 4,813	108.9	31,836 ± 1,567	79.9
5.0	23,193 ± 768	62.5	25,420 ± 2,305	63.4
10.0	27,245 ± 2,218	73.5	22,081 ± 1,757	55.4

[a]Indicated dose of THC added to cultures of adherent cells from peritoneum or spleen for 24 hr at 37°C before testing for yeast phagocytosis by radioactive assay.
[b]Average cpm ± SE for six cultures tested for phagocytosis 24 hr after culture initiation and treatment with indicated dose of THC.

TABLE 3. *Effect of Δ⁹-THC on yeast phagocytosis by adherent spleen cells at varying times after incubation*

THC dose (μg/ml)[a]	Phagocytosis assay by radiolabel test on day[b]		
	+1	+2	+4
0.05	112 ± 17	128 ± 12	112 ± 18
0.1	97 ± 8	112 ± 13	109 ± 12
5.0	47 ± 9	68 ± 11	87 ± 22
10.0	33 ± 17	54 ± 10	72 ± 12

[a]Indicated dose of THC added to cultures of adherent spleen cells for indicated number of days before assay for phagocytosis of yeast by radioactive test.
[b]Average percentage of yeast uptake for six cultures per group, in triplicate, as percentage uptake by splenic adherent cells in control medium only (100%).

Both THC and 11-OH THC were also found to inhibit markedly the blastogenic responsiveness of murine spleen cells *in vitro*. Treatment of the cells with 5 to 10 μg of these drugs markedly inhibited the ability of the cells to be stimulated to undergo blastogenesis when activated *in vitro* with the T-cell mitogens concanavalin A (Con A) or phytohemagglutinin (PHA). The responsiveness to the B-cell mitogen bacterial LPS was even more suppressed in the presence of these cannabinoids (4). Thymocytes stimulated with the plant mitogens were even more inhibited than spleen or lymph node cells when graded doses of THC or 11-OH THC were incubated with the cell cultures at the time of culture stimulation (Table 5). Thymic cell populations contain a greater percentage of immature lymphocytes than the cell populations from peripheral lymphoid organs such as the lymph node or spleen.

The alloantigen response of mouse lymphocytes was also markedly reduced by the presence of the cannabinoids. As indicated in Table 6, responses of normal

TABLE 4. *Influence of THC on antibody-forming capacity of mouse splenocyte cultures*

Group[a]	PFC ± SD[b]	
	Experiment 1	Experiment 2
Control	32 ± 26	136 ± 33
SRBC[c] only	794 ± 316	2,175 ± 915
SRBC plus		
DMSO	452 ± 151	3,094 ± 934
THC, 1.0 μg/ml	1,951 ± 1,357	2,706 ± 653
5.0 μg/ml	979 ± 528	2,273 ± 224
10.0 μg/ml	432 ± 276	755 ± 381

[a]Mouse splenocytes cultured for 5 days without SRBC, with SRBC, or with SRBC plus vehicle or THC. The splenocytes were subsequently harvested and antibody-forming capacity of the various groups determined by localized hemolysis in gel.
[b]Plaque-forming cell response ± standard deviation.
[c]SRBC, sheep red blood cell antigen.

TABLE 5. *Differential susceptibility of spleen, lymph node, and thymus cells to suppression by THC and 11-hydroxy THC*

Cannabinoid dose (μg/ml)	Percentage of control response[a]		
	Spleen	Lymph node	Thymus
THC			
1	100	100	65
3	100	94	61
5	100	96	68
10	62	78	43
11-OH THC			
1	96	100	100
3	96	100	100
5	83	100	100
7	97	100	48
10	73	84	28

[a]Cells from various organs were exposed in culture to either THC or 11-hydroxy THC and stimulated with the mitogen Con A. The extent of ^{3}H-thymidine incorporation was subsequently determined as the percentage of vehicle (DMSO or ethyl alcohol)-treated cells.

mouse spleen cells cultured with mitomycin-C-treated stimulator cells from an allogeneic donor mouse strain were markedly inhibited in the presence of THC, indicating that this parameter of the immune response, i.e., cell-mediated target cell killing presumably by T cells, could be readily inhibited by cannabinoids *in vitro*.

Natural killer (NK) cells are considered important in resistance to a wide variety of tumors as well as to intracellular pathogens such as viruses, bacteria, fungi, etc. As seen in Table 7, THC injection into mice had a strong inhibitory effect on the

TABLE 6. *Effect of THC on the proliferation response of murine splenocytes stimulated by an allogeneic challenge*

Group[a]	CPM $\times$ 10^{-3} at responder-to-stimulator ratio		
	4	2	1
Medium control	17.5	10.4	4.6
DMSO (0.05%)	23.5	10.3	2.9
THC 5.0 μg/ml	4.8	2.3	1.1
7.5 μg/ml	2.9	0.8	0.1
10 μg/ml	0.3	0.2	0.0

[a]Splenocytes from BALB/c (responders) mixed with mitomycin-C-treated C3H/HeJ (stimulators) and incubated in medium alone, DMSO (0.05%), or THC at 5 to 10 μg/ml concentrations and assayed for proliferative activity after 4 days by addition of ^{3}H-thymidine.

TABLE 7. *Suppression of murine natural killer cell activity following acute administration of THC[a]*

Treatment	Days after injection	Percentage cytotoxicity	
		E : T 10	E : T 100
Control		14.5 $\pm$ 1.5[b]	34.2 $\pm$ 2
DMSO (0.1%)	1	12.5 $\pm$ 2.8	26.7 $\pm$ 4.9
	3	12.8 $\pm$ 2.8	29.2 $\pm$ 2.8
THC (50 mg/kg)	1	7.8 $\pm$ 1.5	23.8 $\pm$ 3.7
	3	7.5 $\pm$ 2.4	15.8 $\pm$ 3.7

[a]Mice were given a single intraperitoneal injection of either DMSO or THC (50 mg/kg), and either 1 or 3 days later spleens were removed and NK activity determined.
[b]Mean percentage cytotoxicity $\pm$ standard error mean; $n = 6$.

NK activity. Similar results were obtained with human NK cell preparations cultured with varying concentrations of THC (Table 8). In addition, the ability of human peripheral blood leukocytes to undergo blastogenesis when stimulated with the T-cell mitogens Con A or PHA was also markedly inhibited by 5 to 10 μg THC as well as 11-OH THC (data not shown).

The ability of murine spleen cell cultures to be stimulated to produce interleukins or interferon was also markedly suppressed when THC was added to the cell cultures at the time of stimulation with the cytokine inducer. There was a 50 to 80% suppression of the ability of the lymphoid cells to produce IL-1 or IL-2 and interferon in the presence of 5 μg THC added at the time of culture initiation (Tables 9–12). THC inhibited interferon production by both adherent and nonadherent cell cultures (Table 13) and also suppressed interferon-forming capacity of splenocytes

TABLE 8. *Suppression of human natural killer cell activity by THC as function of time of exposure*[a]

Treatment	Percentage cytotoxicity					
	0[b]	1	2	3	4	18
Control	54[c]	48	57	32	43	31
DMSO (0.1%)	40	46	47	33	41	36
THC						
1 μg/ml	50	45	52	36	42	—
10 μg/ml	47	29	26	9	16	1
20 μg/ml	55	4	4	1	1	—

[a]PBLs incubated with medium only, DMSO, or THC for various times, washed twice to remove THC, and assayed for NK activity.
[b]Hours of exposure to THC.
[c]Mean percentage cytotoxicity for a representative experiment.

TABLE 9. *Reduced interleukin 1 production by splenic macrophages exposed in culture to THC*

Group[a]	IL-1 activity (cpm $\times$ 10^{-3})	Percentage of control
Control (culture medium only)	20.4	—
DMSO	18.9	93
THC 5.0 μg/ml	17.7	87
7.5 μg/ml	14.3	70
10.0 μg/ml	4.0	20

[a]Splenocytes enriched for macrophages following 20 hr culture and rinsing. Adherent cells cultured for an additional 24 hr with IL-1-inducing antigen mixture and various test substances. Supernatant fluids from cultures harvested and tested for IL-1 activity (^{3}H-thymidine incorporation into thymocytes).

TABLE 10. *Reduced interleukin 1 production by peritoneal macrophages from mice chronically injected with THC*

Group[a]	IL-1 activity (cpm $\times$ 10^{-3})				
	16[b]	26	36	46	56
Hank's solution	—	27.3	36.7	36.8	59.2
DMSO (0.05%)	—	23.0	22.0	30.9	85.7
THC (50 mg/kg)	31.2	1.6	18.9	11.5	39.0

[a]Mice injected with Hank's, DMSO, or THC for various periods of time and peritoneal cells harvested. Cells were stimulated for 48 hr in culture with an IL-1-inducing antigen mixture. Supernatant fluids from the cultures were harvested and added to thymocyte cultures for determination of IL-1 activity.
[b]Days of THC treatment.

TABLE 11. *Suppression of interleukin 2 production by THC in cultures of mouse splenocytes*

Group[a]	IL-2 (units/ml)	Percentage reduction
Medium	6.7	—
DMSO (0.05%)	5.7	15
THC		
5.0 μg/ml	4.6	31
7.5 μg/ml	1.9	72
10.0 μg/ml	1.0	85

[a]Splenocytes cultured in presence of medium only, DMSO, or THC and stimulated with Con A for 24 hr. Supernatant fluids from these cultures were harvested and cultured in varying dilutions with the IL-2-dependent cell line CTLL.

TABLE 12. *Effect of THC on IFN production by normal splenocytes*

	IFN (units/ml)		
Treatment[a]	PHA (2 μg/ml)	LPS (μg/ml)	Legionella (10^8 cells/ml)
None[b]	100	100	90
DMSO (0.05%)[c]	100	100	88
THC			
5.0 μg/ml	56	76	38
7.5 μg/ml	20	53	22
10.0 μg/ml	15	65	15

[a]Splenocytes incubated for 24 hr with various mitogens and either THC or DMSO; supernatants harvested and assayed for IFN activity.
[b]Mitogens only.
[c]Equivalent to amount of DMSO in THC preparation at 10 μg/ml.

when chronically injected into mice (Table 14). In addition, exogenous IL-2 was able to overcome the depression of human NK function by 5 to 10 μg THC (data not shown). Regarding the association of THC and altered immunity in retrovirus infection, preliminary studies indicate that a concentration of 1 μg/ml THC can suppress lymphocyte blastogenesis of Friend leukemia virus-infected mice although this concentration did not affect normal spleen cells.

DISCUSSION AND CONCLUSIONS

The results of this study support the view that purified components of marijuana such as THC and the less psychoactive metabolite 11-OH THC may have modulatory effects on both cellular and humoral components of the immune response sys-

TABLE 13. *Effect of THC or DMSO control on induction of IFN by LPS in various spleen cell populations*

	IFN (units/ml) induced by LPS in		
Substance tested[a]	Spleen cells	Adherent[b] cells	Nonadherent[c] cells
None (control)	100	100	100
DMSO			
0.05%	100	53	65
0.025%	100	53	65
THC			
5 μg/ml	65	24	30
10 μg/ml	56	17	24

[a]Test substances added at indicated concentration to indicated cultures with 5 μg LPS and supernatants collected 24 hr later for IFN assay.
[b]Adherent spleen cells prepared by adhering whole spleen cultures to plastic wells for 2 hr, washing with warm RPMI + 10% FCS, and adding 1 ml fresh medium.
[c]Nonadherent cells recovered from washed cultures, centrifuged, and cultured separately at concentration corresponding to original culture.

tem. The possible immunosuppressive properties of cannabinoids have been considered controversial, especially during the last decade or so, when studies of this type were performed with lymphoid cells from individuals who smoked marijuana cigarettes (8). It should be noted that marijuana has at least 50 components, many of which are psychoactive, and some of which are immunomodulatory. The immune system itself is quite complex and consists of several distinct cell types and many different soluble factors involved in immune responses, both humoral and cellular. The use of different techniques to examine components of the immune system in man and animals may also have contributed to the disparate results reported by others.

In the present studies it was found unequivocally that graded concentrations of THC or 11-OH THC markedly affected the functional activity of distinct cell classes cultured *in vitro* and examined for specific capabilities. The same reactions that were examined in this study are widely acknowledged to be important in antimicrobial immunity, including immune responses to a wide variety of viruses, some of which are known to be tumorogenic and immunomodulatory, including the retroviruses. It is widely accepted that macrophages, for example, are important as immunoregulatory cells that produce soluble factors important in immune responses but also are phagocytic and considered the first line of defense against a wide variety of microbial pathogens, including viruses. Retroviruses are now known to replicate in macrophages and may actually be disseminated by these cells or may be controlled and eliminated by functional macrophages.

In the present study, THC, even in extremely small doses, was found to inhibit

TABLE 14. *Effect of chronic in vivo exposure of mice to THC on induction of IFN in whole spleen cell cultures*

Treatment of mice[a]	In vivo stimulant	Day after treatment spleen cell cultures tested				
		+16	+26	+36	+46	+56
THC	Con A	200[b] (50)	234 (78)	167 (56)	30 (30)	106 (53)
	LPS		58 (89)	10 (15)	10 (15)	34 (32)
	Legionella		17 (32)	20 (20)	10 (19)	10 (20)
DMSO	Con A	200 (100)	300 (100)	200 (67)	100 (100)	234 (117)
	LPS		65 (65)	65 (100)	53 (82)	130 (123)
	Legionella		53 (100)	100 (100)	20 (38)	48 (100)
Medium control	Con A	200	300	300	100	200
	LPS		100	65	65	106
	Legionella		53	100	53	48

[a]Mice injected intraperitoneally on day 0 and at 5-day intervals with THC at concentration of 1 mg/mouse, control medium, or DMSO in medium only.

[b]Average units of IFN for three mouse spleen cultures per group on day indicated after initial treatment.

murine macrophages in their most fundamental activities, i.e., spreading on smooth surfaces as well as phagocytizing a microbial particle, i.e., yeast. The ability of macrophages to produce interleukin 1 is widely known as an important function of these cells. THC was found in the present study to suppress IL-1 production in the spleen cell cultures as well as in peritoneal exudate cell cultures (*unpublished data*). Thus, it appears that soluble mediator production by these cells on stimulation with a known IL-1 inducer is compromised by THC.

The ability of spleen cells to produce antibody on challenge with a T-cell-dependent antigen such as sheep erythrocytes was also found in the present study to be markedly inhibited by prior incubation with cannabinoids. Antibody is a known constituent of antimicrobial immunity, but its role in controlling infection by retroviruses in man or experimental animals is uncertain. Nevertheless, the suppressive effect of cannabinoids on production of antibody, at least by relatively large doses *in vitro*, suggests that antibodies that are important in protection against some viruses may be suppressed by cannabinoids, and this could contribute to altered susceptibility to infection after exposure to these drugs.

It is widely accepted that interferons play an important role in antiviral defenses. Results of the present study also showed that interferon production by lymphoid cells was markedly compromised by treatment of the cells with THC. Furthermore, interferon production *in vivo* was also markedly suppressed by chronic administration of this cannabinoid.

The ability of lymphoid cells to recognize antigens and undergo proliferation is considered a correlate of cell-mediated immunity. Thus, it was of interest that THC as well as 11-OH THC suppressed the ability of murine spleen cells to undergo blastogenesis when stimulated with the T-cell mitogens Con A and PHA as well as the B-cell mitogen LPS. Furthermore, the suppression of the ability of lymphoid cells to undergo an allogeneic reaction against histoincompatible target cells provided evidence that cannabinoids interfere with this T-cell function *in vitro*, and if similar suppression occurs *in vivo*, this may contribute to heightened susceptibility of an individual to a virus such as HIV, which is known to infect T cells preferentially and undoubtedly is controlled by T-cell activity, especially effector killer T cells (11).

Natural killer cells are thought to be related to T cells. These T cells are important in natural resistance against not only tumor cells but also viruses and other intracellular microorganisms. As shown in the present study, THC had marked suppressive effects on NK activity for murine and human cells *in vitro*. The NK activity was also found to be markedly suppressed in animals given acute injections of THC. Thus, an important cell type was compromised by exposure to THC.

Although the mechanisms whereby cannabinoids diminish the activity of macrophages and lymphocytes as well as NK cells is not clear, nor is the mechanism whereby humoral factors secreted by these cells, such as antibody, interleukins, and interferons, are depressed is not known, it is likely that such impairment is not related to cell death because cannabinoid suppression is uniformly reversible. Also, doses of THC found to suppress cellular and humoral immune parameters were quite low, i.e., in the range of 5 μg per 10^6 cells. This is severalfold less than the doses that resulted in increased loss of viability of the cells in culture.

Compounds such as THC and 11-OH THC are known to be lipophilic molecules and may alter the lipid membranes of cells, including lymphoid cells. Normal immune functions are thought to depend in part on the integrity of membrane components of lymphoid cells, including T and B lymphocytes or macrophages. It is conceivable that perturbation of the lipid-containing membranes of relevant lymphoid cells in the presence of cannabinoids may contribute either partially or fully to the immune impairment induced by these compounds. Although it is unlikely that one or even a few exposures to THC *in vivo* results in marked suppression of immune competence, continued effects on immunity by repeated exposure to even small doses of cannabinoids may be sufficient in the presence of other immunomodulating factors, including opportunistic microorganisms such as viruses and bacteria, to make an individual much more susceptible to immunological perturbations induced by a retrovirus such as HIV. Further studies concerning the immunomodulatory effects of marijuana and its components may be of value in examining these drugs as possible cofactors in development of AIDS in man.

SUMMARY

It is widely recognized that various microorganisms including viruses have immunomodulatory effects and, under appropriate circumstances, may markedly suppress the immune response mechanisms. Cannabinoids present in marijuana also have immunomodulatory effects. In the present studies THC as well as its metabolic product 11-OH THC were studied in regard to their effects *in vivo* and *in vitro* on selected parameters of the immune response system known to be important in antiviral resistance, including immunity to retroviruses. Cannabinoids markedly suppressed the ability of murine macrophages to spread on glass (an important functional marker of macrophages) as well as to phagocytize yeast particles.

Splenic macrophage cultures treated with the cannabinoids also were deficient in their ability to produce interleukin 1 on appropriate stimulation with bacterial LPS. Spleen cells capable of producing antibody to sheep erythrocytes when stimulated with this antigen *in vitro* were markedly affected when treated with graded doses of THC or 11-OH THC. Furthermore, the blastogenic responsiveness of normal mouse splenocytes to the T-cell mitogens Con A and PHA as well as the B-cell mitogen *E. coli* LPS was markedly suppressed by graded concentrations of the cannabinoids in doses that did not affect the viability of the cells. Natural killer cell activity of normal mouse spleen cells was also markedly inhibited by THC and 11-OH THC. Similarly, these cannabinoids suppressed the blastogenic responsiveness and NK activity of human peripheral blood leukocytes from normal individuals. The ability of mouse spleen cells to produce interferon on *in vitro* stimulation was also suppressed by THC. In addition, injection of THC into mice suppressed blastogenic responsiveness of spleen cells, NK activity, and the production of interferon by lymphoid cells. Thus, it was apparent that these cannabinoids had immuno-modulatory effects, both *in vivo* and *in vitro,* at noncytotoxic small doses and impaired the ability of the lymphoid cells to express immune function necessary for antiviral resistance.

REFERENCES

1. Bendinelli, M., Matteucci, D., and Friedman, H. (1985): Retrovirus-induced acquired immunodeficiencies. *Adv. Cancer Res.,* 45:125–181.
2. Blanchard, D. K., Klein, T. W., Friedman, H., and Stewart, W. E. (1985): Kinetics and characterization of interferon production by murine spleen cells stimulated with *Legionella pneumophila* antigens. *Infect. Immun.,* 49:719–723.
3. Bradley, L. M. (1980): Mixed lymphocyte responses. In: *Selected Methods in Cellular Immunology,* edited by B. B. Mishell and S. M. Shiigi, pp. 162–164. W. H. Freeman, San Francisco.
4. Klein, T. W., Newton, C. A., Widen, R., and Friedman, H. (1985): The effect of delta-9-tetrahydrocannabinol and 11-hydroxy-delta-9-tetrahydrocannabinol on T-lymphocyte and B-lymphocyte mitogen responses. *J. Immunopharmacol.,* 7:451–466.
5. Lane, H. C., and Fauci, A. S. (1985): Immunologic abnormalities in the acquired immunodeficiency syndrome. *Annu. Rev. Immunol.,* 3:477–500.
6. Lopez-Cepero, M., Friedman, M., Klein, T., and Friedman, H. (1986): Tetrahydrocannabinol-induced suppression of macrophage spreading and phagocytic activity *in vitro. J. Leukocyte Biol.,* 39:679–686.
7. Mizel, S. B., Oppenheim, J. J., and Rosenstreich, D. L. (1978): Characterization of lymphocyte-activating factor (LAF) produced by the macrophage cell line, P388D₁. *J. Immunol.,* 120:1497–1503.
8. Nahas, G. G., Morishima, A., and Desoize, B. (1977): Effects of cannabinoids on macromolecular synthesis and replication of cultured lymphocytes. *Fed. Proc.,* 39:1748–1752.
9. Specter, S. C., Klein, T. W., Newton, C., Mondragon, M., Widen, R., and Friedman, H. (1986): Marijuana effects on immunity: Suppression of human natural killer cell activity by delta-9-tetrahydrocannabinol. *Int. J. Immunopharmacol.,* 8:741–745.
10. Vogel, F. R., Klein, T. W., Stewart, W. E., Igarashi, T., and Friedman, H. (1985): Immune suppression and induction of gamma interferon by pertussis toxin. *Infect. Immun.,* 49:90–97.
11. Walker, C. M., Moody, D. J., Stites, D. P., and Levy, J. A. (1986): CD8⁺ lymphocytes can control HIV infection *in vitro* by suppressing virus replication. *Science,* 234:1563–1566.

Psychological, Neuropsychiatric, and
Substance Abuse Aspects of AIDS,
edited by T. Peter Bridge et al.
Raven Press, New York © 1988.

Suppression of Human and Mouse Lymphocyte Proliferation by Cocaine

Thomas W. Klein, Catherine A. Newton, and Herman Friedman

*Department of Medical Microbiology and Immunology, University of South Florida
College of Medicine, Tampa, Florida 33612*

The increasing use of cocaine in recent years has prompted questions concerning the public health risk of abusing this drug. Indeed, recent reports document that large doses of cocaine can be very toxic and even lethal (8). To address the question of a possible negative impact of cocaine on biological systems, we examined the influence of this drug on lymphocyte function. We felt this model to be appropriate because several reports have suggested an influence of cocaine on immune function (9,11,12) and also because the extensive literature that exists on lymphocyte function supports the use of these cells as a model system of cell biology. In the present chapter, we demonstrate that cocaine HCl added to cultures of either human peripheral blood lymphocytes or mouse splenic lymphocytes suppresses the response of these cells to T-cell mitogens at doses that do not result in cell damage sufficient to cause the nonspecific uptake of vital dyes. The response to B-cell mitogens appears to be less affected by cocaine treatment.

MATERIALS AND METHODS

Single-cell suspensions (2×10^6 cells/ml) of splenocytes from BALB/c mice (Jackson Laboratories, Bar Harbor, ME) were prepared as previously described (6). Splenocytes were cultured in medium RPMI-1640 (Gibco, Grand Island, NY) containing 10% fetal calf serum (Hyclone Laboratories, Logan, UT) and antibiotics. The cells were cultured for 48 hr in 96-well culture plates (Costar, Cambridge, MA) with various combinations of the mitogens concanavalin A (Con A; Sigma Chemical, St. Louis, MO), phytohemagglutinin (PHA; Burroughs Wellcome, Greenville, NC), *E. coli* lipopolysaccharide (LPS; Sigma) or cocaine HCl (Sigma). Subsequently, the cultures were pulsed for 18 hr with 0.5 μCi of ^{3}H-thymidine (ICN, Irvine, CA) and harvested by a cell harvester, and the extent of thymidine incorporation was determined by scintillation counting.

Heparinized venous blood was obtained from healthy volunteers, and the mononuclear cell fraction was isolated as previously described (2). Briefly, the whole blood was diluted (1 : 1) with saline and layered on Ficoll–Paque (Pharmacia, Piscataway, NY). Following centrifugation, the mononuclear cell layer was washed two to three times, and the resultant cells were cultured exactly as described for mouse splenocytes.

The count-per-minute data from the replicate experiments were normalized by calculating a percentage of control wherein:

$$\% \text{ of control} = \frac{\text{cpm (mitogen + cocaine)}}{\text{cpm (mitogen only)}} \times 100$$

Triplicate wells are performed in each experiment, and the data represent the means of four separate experiments in the human studies and eight experiments in the mouse studies.

RESULTS AND DISCUSSION

To our knowledge no reports have appeared analyzing the influence of cocaine on cultured lymphocytes. Therefore, initially we designed a dose–response study using cocaine concentrations previously reported to influence cell function in culture (10). Table 1 demonstrates a suppression of mouse lymphocyte proliferation in response to the T-cell mitogen Con A with increasing concentration of cocaine. At a dose of 200 μg/ml the drug reduced the response 75%. On the other hand, mouse splenocytes responsive to the B-cell mitogen lipopolysaccharide were generally unaffected in the dose range examined.

In order to determine whether the suppression of proliferation to T-cell mitogens at high doses of cocaine reflected an effect on cell viability, splenocytes were cul-

TABLE 1. Effect of cocaine on mouse splenic
lymphocyte proliferation in response
to T cell and B cell mitogens

Cocaine (μg/ml)	Lymphocyte proliferation[a]	
	Con A	LPS
25	94.7 ± 7	88.0 ± 8
50	82.4 ± 8	89.8 ± 6
100	74.0 ± 11	93.9 ± 7
200	26.9 ± 6	87.9 ± 7

[a]Cocaine and mitogens were added to splenocytes at the start of culture. Data are expressed as mean % control ± SEM of eight experiments. The activity ranges for Con A (5 μg/ml) and LPS (10 μg/ml) were 125–280 × 10^3 cpm and 46–106 × 10^3 cpm, respectively.

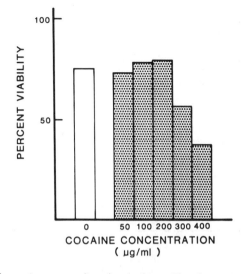

FIG. 1. Murine splenocytes were cultured as in the proliferation assay, and portions of the cells were subsequently mixed with an equal volume of trypan blue. Dye exclusion was determined microscopically, and the percentage viability determined.

tured in the presence of varying doses of cocaine exactly as in the proliferation assay and were analyzed for trypan blue dye exclusion (7). Leukocytes that are no longer viable will not exclude the dye and therefore appear blue when examined microscopically. Figure 1 demonstrates that the mouse splenocytes treated with cocaine at concentrations as high as 200 μg/ml maintain viability as well as nontreated splenocytes. However, increasing the concentration to 300 or 400 μg/ml resulted in a loss of cell viability. These results suggest that the depression of the Con A response at 100 and 200 μg of cocaine did not reflect diminished cell viability in response to the drug.

Based on the results obtained with mouse lymphocyte cultures, we next determined whether a similar suppressive effect of cocaine occurred on the T-cell proliferation response of human lymphocytes. Cultures of peripheral blood leukocytes obtained from four different human donors were stimulated with the T-cell mitogens Con A and PHA, and the effects of varying doses of cocaine were determined. Figure 2 demonstrates that, as with mouse lymphocyte proliferation, human T-lymphocyte proliferation in response to mitogens is suppressed at doses of 200 μg/ml. At lower doses, the PHA response appears to be more complex, and additional studies in this dose range are currently in progress.

To our knowledge, the results reported here are the first to demonstrate an effect of cocaine on cultured mouse and human lymphocytes. Although preliminary, our results suggest that cocaine is relatively nontoxic for these cells and that T-cell responses are more sensitive to drug effects than B-cell responses. Cocaine, when administered to the whole animal, is known to affect adrenergic mechanisms (1).

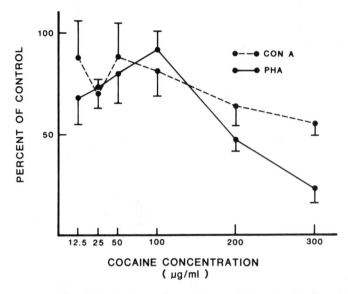

FIG. 2. Human peripheral blood mononuclear cells were isolated and cultured with mitogens and cocaine. Data are expressed as mean percentage of control ± SEM of four experiments. The activity ranges for Con A (5 μg/ml) and PHA (2.5 μg/ml) were 40–60 × 10^3 cpm and 70–90 × 10^3 cpm, respectively.

In culture, it appears to have local anesthetic effects on ion permeability (5,10). Lymphocyte proliferation is known to be regulated by adrenergic receptors (4) and to be controlled by membrane events such as Ca^{2+} flux (3). These and other mechanisms are currently under investigation to account for the cocaine-induced modification of cultured T-lymphocyte proliferation.

REFERENCES

1. Banerjee, S. P., Sharma, V. K., Kung-Cheung, L. S., Chanda, S. K., and Riggi, S. J. (1979): Cocaine and D-amphetamine induce changes in central beta-adrenoceptor sensitivity: effects of acute and chronic drug treatment. *Brain Res.*, 175:119–130.
2. Boyum, A. (1968): Isolation of mononuclear cells and granulocytes from human blood. *Scand. J. Lab. Clin. Invest.*, 21(Suppl. 97):77–89.
3. Cahalan, M. D., Chandy, K. G., DeCoursey, T. E., and Gupta, S. (1985): A voltage-gated potassium channel in human T lymphocytes. *J. Physiol. (Lond.)*, 358:197–237.
4. Coffey, R. G., and Hadden, J. W. (1985): Neurotransmitters, hormones, and cyclic nucleotides in lymphocyte regulation. *Fed. Proc.*, 44:112–117.
5. Just, W. W., and Hoyer, J. (1977): The local anesthetic potency of norcocaine, a metabolite of cocaine. *Experientia*, 33:70–71.
6. Klein, T. W., Newton, C. A., Widen, R., and Friedman, H. (1985): The effect of delta-9-tetrahydrocannabinol and 11-hydroxy-delta-9-tetrahydrocannabinol on T-lymphocyte and B-lymphocyte mitogen responses. *J. Immunopharmacol.*, 7:451–466.
7. Mishell, B. B., Shiigi, S. M., Henry, C., et al. (1980): Preparation of mouse cell suspensions. In: *Selected Methods in Cellular Immunology*, edited by B. B. Mishell and S. M. Shiigi, pp. 3–27. W. H. Freeman, San Francisco.

8. Sander, R., Ryser, M. A., Lamoreaux, T. C., and Raleigh, K. (1985): An epidemic of cocaine associated deaths in Utah. *J. Forensic Sci.*, 30:478–484.
9. Savona, S., Nordi, M. A., Lennette, E. T., and Karpatkin, S. (1985): Thrombocytopenia purpura in narcotic addicts. *Ann. Intern. Med.*, 102:737–741.
10. Togna, G., Tempesta, E., Togna, A. R., Dolci, N., Cebo, B., and Caprino, L. (1985): Platelet responsiveness and biosynthesis of thromboxane and prostacyclin in response to *in vitro* cocaine treatment. *Haemostasis*, 15:100–107.
11. Van Dyke, C., Stesin, A., Jones, R., Chuntharapai, A., and Seaman, W. (1986): Cocaine increases natural killer cell activity. *J. Clin. Invest.*, 77:1387–1390.
12. Watson, E. S., Murphy, J. C., ElSohly, H. N., ElSohly, M. A., and Turner, C. E. (1983): Effects of the administration of coca alkaloids on the primary immune responses of mice: interaction with delta-9-tetrahydrocannabinol and ethanol. *Toxicol. Appl. Pharmacol.*, 71:1–13.

Psychological, Neuropsychiatric, and
Substance Abuse Aspects of AIDS,
edited by T. Peter Bridge et al.
Raven Press, New York © 1988.

Neuroimmunomodulation by Opiates and Other Drugs of Abuse: Relationship to HIV Infection and AIDS

*R. M. Donahoe and †A. Falek

*Laboratory of Psychoimmunology and †Human and Behavioral Genetics Laboratory,
*†Department of Psychiatry, Emory University School of Medicine, and the Georgia
Mental Health Institute, Atlanta, Georgia 30306

Since the earliest documentation of the AIDS epidemic (16,29,42), intravenous (i.v.) drug abusers have constituted approximately 17% of AIDS cases in the United States (4,21). Also, from 8 to 10% of AIDS cases associated with homosexuality and bisexuality share drug abuse as a cofactor (4,21). Furthermore, drug abusers are often the source for transmission of heterosexual and pediatric AIDS (4,21,39). The relative ease with which AIDS has spread throughout the world is attributable in large measure to the insidious nature of the etiologic agent of AIDS, the human immunodeficiency virus (HIV-1) (14,26,35). This is a particular problem with addicts because their typically pathological, self-destructive, compulsive behaviors create an ideal circumstance for the spread of infectious agents, especially those that are transmitted as chronically latent viruses (8). Thus, even though there is evidence that some addicts can reduce their risks for AIDS through self-motivated behavioral changes (6), the relationship between drug addiction and AIDS remains a high-priority public health concern.

Although needle sharing is unquestionably a major factor in the spread of AIDS by addicts, the fact that various abused drugs are themselves immunomodulatory (28,32,37,45–47,49) and immunocompromising (17,41,44,46) has led to the suggestion (9,11,12) that such drugs, in particular opiates, may directly alter susceptibility to HIV-1 and exacerbate the complications of AIDS. In the present chapter, we review information linking drug abuse with altered immunity and discuss the possible causes for this effect and its relevance to the spread as well as the treatment and prevention of AIDS.

145

EVIDENCE THAT DRUG ABUSERS ARE IMMUNOSUPPRESSED

From as early as 1907 (1,43), evidence has accumulated that opiate addiction leads to depressed immune function. In the late 1960s and 1970s, the observations that opiate addicts often suffered from opportunistic infection (8,18,27,41) and cancer (18,20,40,41) were construed as indicating that they were experiencing immunosuppression. Contemporary with these observations, Brown et al. (3) showed that heroin addicts had depressed lymphocyte mitogenic responsiveness and elevated levels of immunoglobulin production. In 1980, McDonough et al. (32) from our laboratory showed that opiate addicts had depressed levels of total T cells as determined by the ability of T cells to form E-rosettes with sheep erythrocytes (E). This information corroborated the earlier findings of Wybran et al. (49) that morphine depressed formation of active T-cell E-rosettes *in vitro*. Because Wybran et al. (49) and McDonough et al. (32) found that the morphine effects they observed were reversible by naloxone, they conjectured that these effects were mediated through opiate receptors. Indeed, the presence of opiate receptors on lymphocytes has been confirmed by several investigators using radioligand competition assays (19,34), including a recent study from our laboratory employing tritiated naloxone as ligand and highly enriched T-cell preparations (29).

Experimentation with animal models has also demonstrated the immunoregulatory and immunocompromising (17,44) potential of morphine. In addition, endogenous opioids, enkephalin (38,49) and endorphin (15,31), as well as morphine also affect various aspects of immune function (48). Therefore, despite the fact that much work remains to characterize fully the role of opioids in immunoregulatory phenomena, particularly *in vivo,* the inference is clear that such effects may well influence host susceptibility to opportunistic disease. Because of this circumstance, there is intense interest in learning how opiates influence the susceptibility of addicts to HIV infection and AIDS.

Our laboratory has made several observations of relevance to the possible role of opiates in AIDS. Most importantly, we (9,12,32) have shown, as have others (6,25), that opiate addicts exhibit signs of immunodepression even in the absence, or apparent absence, of HIV infection (6,9,12). In fact, our findings that T-cell E-rosette formation is depressed in heroin addicts (12,32) must be construed as evidence of immunodepression because the data of Kerman et al. (22,23) have established that depression of this T-cell parameter correlates with poor immunoresponsiveness. Recently, we showed (9), as illustrated by the data in Table 1, that opiate addicts free of AIDS had depressed levels of the ratio between their T-helper/inducer (Th) and T-suppressor/cytotoxic (Ts) cells (Th/Ts), which also is an indication of immunodepression in addicts. This latter observation is in agreement with the findings of Layon et al. (25) and have been corroborated by a much larger study of HIV-negative addicts by Des Jarlais et al. (6).

Unfortunately, information documenting immunodepression in HIV-negative opiate addicts does not prove that such addicts are actually immunocompromised or even that this state is induced by opiates. In fact, these types of information are

TABLE 1. *Effects of heroin addiction on expression of lymphocyte antigenic surface markers*

| Test group | Mean percent of leukocytes (±SD) reactive with | | Mean Th/Ts (%) | Number Th/Ts (%) ratios within, above, or below 1 or 2 SD from mean control value | | | |
	OKT-4 (Th)	OKT-8 (Ts)		1 SD above	Within 1 SD	1 SD below	2 SD below
Addicts (n = 21)	38 (±11) [8.2 ± 2.8][a]	25 (±8) [5.2 ± 2.4]	1.7 (±0.6) (p > 0.06)	0 (0%)	12 (57%)	4 (19%)	5[b] (24%)
Control (n = 12)	44 (±15) [10.6 ± 4.2]	21 (±8) [4.9 ± 0.7]	2.2 (±0.6)	3 (25%)	6 (50%)	3 (25%)	0 (0%)

[a]Bracketed figures are mean absolute numbers ±SD (× 10^6) of the respective T-cell subset in Ficoll/Hypaque-separated leukocytes from 20 ml of whole blood.

[b]These five addicts were long-term chronic heroin abusers of at least 10 years duration (mean = 13.1 years) and are referred to in the text as showing severely depressed ratios, i.e., Th/Ts < 1.0.

Adapted from Donahoe et al. (9).

TABLE 2. *Case report on the demographics of drug abuse and the immunological status of a Chicago heroin addict*[a]

Drug history	
Heroin abuse/addiction	18 years
Alcohol abuse	18 years
Marijuana abuse/addiction	18 years
Tobacco use	18 years
Cocaine abuse	4 years
Immunological status (depressed)	
Th/Ts	0.78
Total E-rosettes	52%

[a]Personal: Addict # J291; male; 30 years old.

essentially impossible to obtain by retrospective analyses of addiction because evidence of immunodepression obtained under such circumstances must be rectified against a number of other factors common to the addiction milieu, aside from the direct effects of opiates, that may also be of etiological relevance; these include (a) immune paralysis from antigenic overload, (b) prior or intercurrent infections or other pathologies, (c) individual genetic predisposition, (d) polydrug effects, (e) erratic addiction-withdrawal episodes, and (f) nutritional factors. Indeed, in all likelihood, a combination of any or all such factors contributes to the immunocompetency of a given addict at any given time.

The case report shown in Table 2 helps to illustrate the problem. Despite clear evidence of immunodepression in this HIV-negative addict as the result of E-rosette and Th/Ts analyses, the extremely chronic history of polydrug abuse that is also apparent makes it impossible to conclude that this immunodepression is actually opiate related; nor is it possible to say that the characterization of immunodepression used actually indicates a state of compromised immune capacity.

FURTHER EVIDENCE THAT OPIATE ADDICTION COULD AFFECT SUSCEPTIBILITY TO HIV

Despite the fact that the role of opiates in compromising the immune status of opiate addicts is presently conjectural, we (9) and D. C. Des Jarlais (*personal communication*) have shown that heroin addicts without depression of Th/Ts experience enhancement of the percentage of their circulating T4[+] Th cells as a function of the duration of their heroin abuse. This evidence (9), illustrated in Fig. 1, suggests an important way that opiate addiction could exacerbate susceptibility of addicts to HIV infection and AIDS because elevation of Th expression could result in addicts having more cell targets for HIV to infect since the receptor by which HIV gains entry to Th cells is the Th antigenic marker itself, the T4 molecule (5,24,33). These data are also interesting because, in analogy to the association between hypergam-

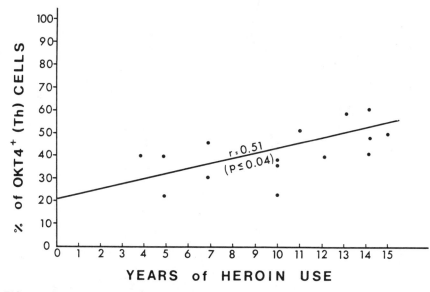

FIG. 1. Regression analyses and coefficient of correlation derived from a comparison of the duration of heroin use by the study addicts and the percentage of OKT4$^+$ (Th) cells in their peripheral blood. (Adapted from Donahoe et al., ref. 9.)

maglobulinemia and hyper-Th activity in autoimmune disorders, hyperexpression of Th might also account for elevated levels of immunoglobulins reported to occur in long-term heroin addicts (3).

SUBSTANTIATION OF THE ABILITY OF OPIATES TO MODIFY EXPRESSION OF T4

The evidence that Th cells were modulated in heroin addicts prompted us to develop assays to determine whether T4 molecules could be modulated by opiates *in vitro*. To this end, we generated cytofluorometric assays based on principles worked out in our laboratory for analyses of the effects of morphine on the kinetics of E-rosette formation (10,28). Detailed description of these assays is the topic for several manuscripts currently in preparation, although a preliminary description has already been published (9).

Briefly, the protocol design was (a) to incubate mononuclear leukocytes for 10 min at 37°C; (b) to expose these cells to 10^{-9} M morphine in buffered saline at 23°C (controls unexposed); (c) to chill cells on wet ice and saturably bind all 9.6 epitopes of the E receptors on the cell surface with anti-E-receptor (T11) monoclonal antibodies (MAb); (d) to cross link E-receptor/T11-MAb complexes with goat anti-mouse IgG; (e) to block uncommitted antigen-combining sites on the goat anti-mouse IgG with saturating levels of mouse IgG; (f) to incubate separate sets of cells

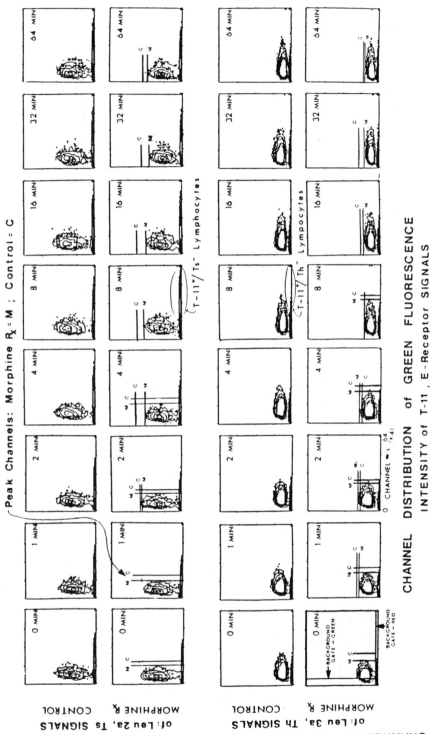

Peak Channels: Morphine R$_X$ = M ; Control = C

(T-11$^+$/Ts$^-$ Lymphocytes)

(T-11$^+$/Th$^-$ Lymphocytes)

O CHANNEL = (×4)

BACKGROUND GATE — GREEN

BACKGROUND GATE — RED

CHANNEL DISTRIBUTION of GREEN FLUORESCENCE
INTENSITY of T-11 , E-Receptor SIGNALS

CHANNEL DISTRIBUTION of RED FLUORESCENCE INTENSITY
of Leu 2a, Ts SIGNALS
of Leu 3a, Th SIGNALS

MORPHINE R$_X$ CONTROL
MORPHINE R$_X$ CONTROL

at 37°C to induce capping of cross-linked T11, E-receptor molecules; (g) to stop the capping reaction after variable periods of incubation at 37°C (0, 1, 4, 8, 32, and 64 min) by placing the cells in a wet ice bath; (h) to stain the chilled cells with one of two combinations of fluorescently conjugated MAbs [anti-T11 conjugated with fluorescein (FITC, fluoresces green) plus either anti-Th (Leu3a) or anti-Ts (Leu2a) MAbs conjugated with phycoerythrin (PE, fluoresces red)]; (i) to fix the stained cells in 0.1% paraformaldehyde; (j) to evaluate the cells cytofluorometrically by using a FACS-IV (Becton-Dickinson, Mountain View, CA) cytofluorometer employing an argon laser for excitation of UV light measured at a 488-nm line setting and operating at 200-mW power to excite both FITC and PE. With this assay we have been able to assess simultaneously the effects of morphine on both T11 and either Leu2a or Leu3a antigenic markers.

A representative result of the assay described above is illustrated in Fig. 2 as two-color FACS plots. These data graphically indicate that at varying times during the kinetic assessment opiates are inhibiting expression of all three antigenic markers studied. Initially, expression of the E-receptor marker is inhibited, whereas inhibition of Ts and Th occur later in the kinetic sequence. Interestingly, the effect of morphine on Th marker expression fluctuates over time between depression and enhancement, illustrating a difference in responsiveness to morphine of Th cells versus Ts cells. These data substantiate the possibility that alteration of the levels of circulating Th cells and Th/Ts ratios in heroin addicts as described above could be related to opiates themselves.

COMMONALITIES IN THE ACTIONS OF BEHAVIORALLY ACTIVE SUBSTANCES

The types of phenomena described thus far in this report suggest that opiates influence the behavior of T cells by modulating expression of surface membrane receptors/markers in a cooperative fashion. Notably, we have found that alcohol has similar effects. It enhances expression of E receptors *in vivo* and *in vitro* (28) and modulates expression of Th and Ts *in vivo* (11). Furthermore, we have shown (12), as illustrated in Fig. 3, that cocaine reverses, even to the point of enhancement, the depression of E-rosetting by heroin in polydrug abusers. Even more, alcohol ame-

---

FIG. 2. Two-color FACS plots of the channel distribution of fluorescence intensity of cells stained with FITC-conjugated T11 MAb (green signals) and either PE-conjugated Leu2a (**top two sets** of figures) or Leu3a (**bottom two sets**) MAbs. Cells were either exposed to 10^{-9} M morphine or untreated, as indicated. Cells were cross linked at the T11/anti-T11 complex by exposure to antimouse antibody and then incubated at 37°C for the indicated durations to induce capping of these cross-linked molecules. The capping process was stopped by placing cells on wet ice. The cells were then stained with the fluoresceinated MAb, fixed, and analyzed on the FACS. The farther right the channel intensities of green signals are, the greater the number of T11 markers present per cell. The closer to the top the channel intensities of red signals are, the greater the number of Th or Ts markers per cell. Where differences in channel intensities are visible between morphine-treated (M) and control (C) Th and Ts cells, lines are drawn for the respective peak channels of fluorescence intensity and labeled with M or C as appropriate. (Adapted from Donahoe et al., ref. 9.)

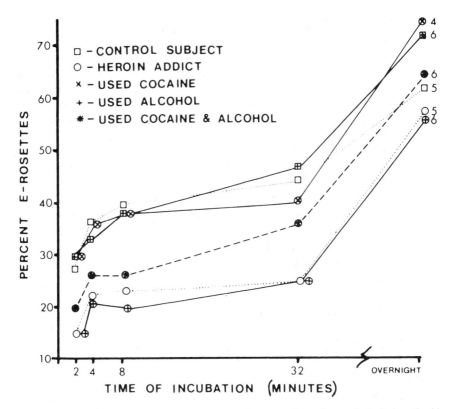

FIG. 3. The effects of simultaneous or independent use of cocaine and alcohol on the kinetics of E-rosette formation for T cells from heroin addicts as compared with those from control subjects who did or did not use alcohol. The number of subjects studied for each experimental group appears at the end of the plotted curves. Each point represents the mean percentage of duplicate samples. (Adapted from Donahoe et al., ref. 12.)

liorates the ability of cocaine to reverse the effects of opiates when all three drugs are being abused simultaneously (12). This is especially notable in view of the fact that alcohol use by heroin addicts not using cocaine has no significant effect on the E-rosette depressive effects of heroin. These immunomodulatory effects of alcohol and cocaine are not surprising because others have reported that these drugs are immunomodulatory (28,45–47) and also that the immunologic effects of alcohol and cocaine can be antagonistic (47). These observations suggest that all abused substances can be of consequence to the susceptibility of addicts to HIV and their subsequent vulnerability to development of AIDS. The importance of this issue is emphasized by the incidence of polydrug abuse among heroin addicts (from Chicago, the rate presently is over 90%; *unpublished data*) not to mention also the pervasive problem of drug abuse in our society today, regardless of types of drugs being considered or the combinations in which they are used.

BASIC IMPLICATIONS OF THE IMMUNOMODULATORY EFFECTS OF ABUSED DRUGS

As described previously, alcohol (28) and cocaine (12) enhance rosette formation, and opiates (12,32,46) depress this T-cell functional parameter. However, under certain conditions, morphine can also enhance parameters of T-cell function (*unpublished data*), whereas alcohol can have depressive effects (46). Thus, immunological effects of abused drugs cannot inerrantly be described solely as enhancing or depressing. Furthermore, dichotomous immunological responses are not even inimical to normal immunological function. Regulation of an immune response by various immunomodulators is often of a reciprocal nature, depending on the time a regulator is introduced into the immune response process, on the dose used, and on the type of response being measured. For example, such effects have been recorded for interferon, an endogenous immunomodulator (36), and endotoxin, an exogenous one (13).

Our findings and conclusions regarding the mechanisms involved in drug-induced changes in T-cell function are relevant for explaining why drugs of abuse and their endogenous counterparts have the potential to influence dichotomously various immune parameters. Thus, the immunomodulatory effects of behaviorally active substances probably relate, at least in part, to their common ability to modulate expression of T-cell membrane surface receptor proteins (9,10). According to this thesis, behaviorally active substances either enhance or inhibit expression of selected T-cell receptors by influencing a process termed receptor microdisplacement. This process, described originally by Bernard et al. (2), is one whereby receptors lying dormant at the cell surface become ligand receptive through alteration of their molecular configuration. An important feature of the microdisplacement concept demonstrated by our *in vitro* studies of the phenomenon (9,10) is that this process is cyclically connected with a series of sequentially dependent receptor-modulating processes, as outlined in Fig. 4. According to this conceptualization, once ligand and receptor interact, the ligand–receptor complex is either processed directly through endocytosis or through an indirect endocytic pathway that initially involves receptor–ligand patching and capping. Then, through endocytic recycling, receptors are reprocessed and reinserted into the cell surface membrane, where they remain dormant until up-regulated to a ligand-receptive state via microdisplacement. At this stage, the receptors are capable of perpetuating the cycle as long as ligands are available to them, and the receptor supply does not become exhausted.

This conceptualization leads to the conclusion that enhancement and inhibition of microdisplacement are rate-limiting factors in controlling the interaction of ligand with receptor. Presumably, when the receptor systems being controlled in this way are of immunological relevance, the ultimate effect will be pertinent to immunoresponsiveness. Indeed, such control over B-cell antigen recognition and processing has already been well defined (7). Moreover, when these conceptualizations are generalized, receptor microdisplacement can be envisioned as an essential regulatory process in the adaptive response of a host to all manner of changes in its

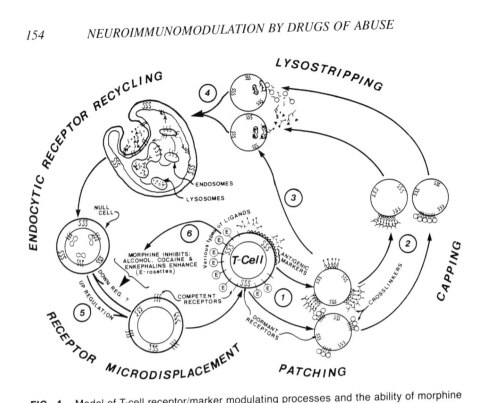

FIG. 4. Model of T-cell receptor/marker modulating processes and the ability of morphine and other behaviorally addicting drugs to intervene. Depending on receptor density and configuration, ligand concentration, thermal conditions, and the physiological state of the cell, a ligand-receptive T cell in the center has two options in responding to ligand-induced receptor activation. **Pathway 1:** It may coalesce receptor–ligand complexes into patches. **Pathway 6:** It may directly activate cell membrane microdisplacement processes to up-regulate receptors lying dormant within the cell. If, after patching, the nature and concentration of the ligand allow for cross linking of receptor–ligand complexes, then capping processes (**pathway 2**) may be activated, which eventually lead to lysostripping and shedding of ligand and receptors and, finally, to their endocytosis. Where cross linking does not occur because of insufficient ligands and/or cross linkers and/or inadequate thermal conditions, the patched receptor–ligand complexes may be endocytosed as in **pathway 3**. Endocytosed receptor–ligand complexes will be processed in endosomes and lysosomes (if temperatures are adequate), and receptors will be recycled in endosomes back to the cell surface (**pathway 4**). Recycled receptors will be inserted into the cell surface membrane, assuming a dormant and later a ligand-receptive, competent configuration relative to their microdisplacement status (**pathway 5**). When sufficient receptors of ligand-receptive form are available on the T cell, a new series in the cycle of receptor modulation can be initiated by ligand binding. Behaviorally addictive drugs appear to intervene in this cycle through depression (morphine) or enhancement (alcohol, cocaine) of receptor microdisplacement. Ligand concentrations, thermal conditions, and the physiological state of the cell are the major factors involved in receptor modulation through these various reaction pathways. (Adapted from Donahoe et al., ref. 9.)

environment, including those mediated through psychological as well as immuno-logical and other types of stimuli.

A particularly interesting feature of the concepts discussed here is that, regardless of whether receptor microdisplacement is enhanced or inhibited, the ultimate outcome in terms of responsivity may be the same because the processes controlled by microdisplacement are cyclical. Thus, if microdisplacement is inhibited as the result of receptor–ligand interaction, nonresponsiveness should result because the ability of the receptor to bind ligand will be inhibited. In turn, if circumstances dictate that microdisplacement is enhanced, and this enhancement is chronic enough, nonresponsiveness should also result because the supply of dormant receptors available to undergo microdisplacement and become ligand receptive will be exhausted. This perspective on the regulatory potential of microdisplacement processes is useful for explaining how drugs that have seemingly opposing cellular biological effects, such as opiates (32) and alcohol (28) and opiates and cocaine (12), in respect to their influence over E-rosette formation are ultimately able to precipitate the same kind of systemic effect on a recipient organism, i.e., depression of behavioral responsivity.

However, this is not to say that drugs with opposing cellular effects cannot have opposing systemic effects. An example of this latter situation is evident with substances that enhance E-rosetting, such as endogenous opioids (49), that also can be beneficial to host immunocompetency (38), as compared with the effects of exogenous opiates (heroin and morphine), which inhibit E-rosetting (12,32,49) and have proven capacity to induce immunodepression (44). Perhaps in circumstances in which endogenous opioids enhance immunity, they do not cause dormant receptor supplies to be exhausted. Indeed, in the situation in which the immunoenhancing peptide enkephalin is administered exogenously (38), it is very likely that the chronicity of exposure of immune cells to the peptide is insufficient to exhaust dormant receptors via enhancement of microdisplacement because enkephalins are so readily degraded by circulating and cell-bound proteases.

Regardless of the mechanisms involved, it is notable that the influence of drugs over microdisplacement processes can ultimately lead to beneficial as well as deleterious effects at the systemic level. A major problem in the past in assessing the immunological consequences of drug addiction has been that results often seemed in conflict with one another. Considering the cyclical nature of microdisplacement processes, dichotomous effects of addictive drugs on immune function are not surprising.

In conclusion, the findings and concepts discussed here open new perspectives on ways to investigate the immunological effects of drugs of abuse that should be useful in determining the immunocompromising potential of such drugs as well as the basic mechanisms related to their cellular and systemic effects. Furthermore, such findings and concepts are particularly relevant to the AIDS issue because they provide a working hypothesis from which to investigate the association between drugs of abuse and the outcome of exposure to infection with HIV and secondary opportunistic infections commonly associated with AIDS.

ACKNOWLEDGMENTS

This work was supported in part by the National Institute on Drug Abuse (grant DA-01451) and by the State of Georgia, Department of Human Resources.

REFERENCES

1. Atchard, C., Benard, H., and Gagneux, C. (1909): Action de la morphine sur les proprietes leukococytaires; leuka-diagnastic du morphinisme. *Bull. Mem. Soc. Med. Hosp. Paris*, 28:958–966.
2. Bernard, A., Gelin, C., Raynal, B., Pham, D., Gosse, C., and Boumsell, L. (1982): Phenomenon of human T cells rosetting with monoclonal antibodies. "Modulation" of a partially hidden epitope determining the conditions of interaction between T cells and erythrocytes. *J. Exp. Med.*, 155:1317–1333.
3. Brown, S. W., Stimmel, B., Taub, R. N., Kochwa, S., and Rosenfield, R. E. (1974): Immunological dysfunction in heroin addicts. *Arch. Intern. Med.*, 134:1001–1006.
4. Curran, J. W., Morgan, W. M., Hardy, A. M., Jaffe, H. W., Darrow, W. W., and Dowdle, W. R. (1985): The epidemiology of AIDS: Current status and future prospects. *Science*, 229:1352–1357.
5. Dalgleish, A. G., Beverley, P. C. L., Clapham, P. R., Crawford, D. H., Greaves, M. F., and Weiss, R. A. (1984): The CDA (T4) antigen is an essential component of the receptor for AIDS retrovirus. *Nature*, 312:763–767.
6. Des Jarlais, D. C., Friedman, S. R., and Hopkins, W. (1985): Risk reduction for the acquired immunodeficiency disease syndrome among intravenous drug users. *Ann. Intern. Med.*, 103:755–759.
7. Dintzis, R. A., Vogelstein, B., and Dintzis, H. M. (1982): Specific cellular stimulation in the primary immune response: Experimental test of a quantized model. *Proc. Natl. Acad. Sci. U.S.A.*, 79:884–888.
8. Dismukes, W. E., Karchmer, A. W., Johnson, R. F., and Dougherty, W. J. (1968): Viral hepatitis associated with illicit parenteral use of drugs. *J.A.M.A.*, 206:1048–1052.
9. Donahoe, R. M., Bueso-Ramos, C., Donahoe, F., Madden, J. J., Falek, A., Nicholson, J. K. A., and Bokos, P. (1987): Mechanistic implications of the findings that opiates and other drugs of abuse moderate T-cell surface receptors and antigenic markers. *Ann. N.Y. Acad. Sci.*, 496:711–721.
10. Donahoe, R. M., Madden, J. J., Hollingsworth, F., Shafer, D., and Falek, A. (1985): Morphine depression of T cell E-rosetting: Definition of the process. *Fed. Proc.*, 44:95–99.
11. Donahoe, R. M., Madden, J. J., Hollingsworth, F., Shafer, D. A., Falek, A., Nicholson, J. K. A., and Bokos, P. (1985): Immunomodulation by behaviorally active drugs provides a paradigm for connecting AIDS-like processes and psychoneuroimmunology. In: *Neuroimmunomodulation: Proceedings of the First International Workshop on Neuroimmunomodulation*, edited by N. H. Spector, pp. 201–204. International Working Group on Neuroimmunomodulation, Bethesda.
12. Donahoe, R. M., Nicholson, J. K. A., Madden, J. J., Donahoe, F., Shafer, D. A., Gordon, D., Bokos, P., and Falek, A. (1986): Coordinate and independent effects of heroin, cocaine and alcohol abuse on T-cell E-rosette and antigenic marker expression. *Clin. Immunol. Immunopathol.*, 41:254–264.
13. Donahoe, R. M., and Peters, R. L. (1979): Limulus amebocyte lysate assay used in evaluating immunoregulatory effects of endotoxin in type-C RNA virus reagents. In: *Biomedical Application of the Horseshoe Crab (Limulidae)*, edited by E. Cohen, pp. 473–483. Alan R. Liss, New York.
14. Gallo, R. C., Salahuddin, S. Z., Popovic, M., Shearer, G. M., Kaplan, M., Haynes, B. F., Palker, T. J., Redfield, R., Oleske, J., and Safai, B. (1984): Frequent detection and isolation of cytopathic retroviruses (HTLV-III) from patients with AIDS and at risk for AIDS. *Science*, 224:500–503.
15. Gilman, S. C., Schwartz, J. M., Milner, R. J., Bloom, F. E., and Feldman, J. D. (1982): β-

Endorphin enhances lymphocyte proliferative responses. *Proc. Natl. Acad. Sci. U.S.A.,* 79:4226–4230.

16. Gottlieb, M. S., Schroff, R., Schanker, H. M., Weisman, J. D., Fan, P. T., Wolf, R. A., and Saxon, A. (1981): *Pneumocystis carinii* pneumonia and mucosal candidiasis in previously healthy homosexual men: evidence of a newly acquired cellular immunodeficiency. *N. Engl. J. Med.,* 305:1425–1431.

17. Gungor, M., Cenc, E., Sagduyu, H., Eroglu, L., and Koyuncloglu, H. (1980): Effect of chronic administration of morphine on primary immune response in mice. *Experientia,* 36:1309–1310.

18. Harris, P. D., and Garret, R. (1972): Susceptibility of addicts to infection and neoplasia. *N. Engl. J. Med.,* 287:310.

19. Hazum, E., Chang, K. J., and Cuatrecasas, P. (1979): Specific non-opiate receptors for β-endorphin. *Science,* 205:1033–1035.

20. Hewer, T., Rose, E., Ghadirian, P., Castegnaro, M., Bartsch, H., Malaneile, C., and Day, N. (1978): Ingested mutagens from opium and tobacco pyrolysis and cancer of the esophagus. *Lancet,* 2:494–495.

21. Jaffe, H. W., Bregman, D. J., and Selik, R. M. (1983): Acquired immune deficiency syndrome in the United States: The first 1,000 cases. *J. Infect. Dis.,* 148:339–345.

22. Kerman, R. H., and Geis, W. P. (1976): Total and active T-cell dynamics in renal allograph recipients. *Surgery,* 79:398–407.

23. Kerman, R. H., Floyd, M., Van Buren, C. T., and Kahan, B. D. (1980): Improved allograph survival of strong immune responder–high risk recipients with adjuvant antithymocyte globulin therapy. *Transplantation,* 30:450–454.

24. Klatzman, D., Champagne, E., Chamarets, S., Greust, J., Guetard, D., Hercend, T., Gluckmon, J.-C., and Montagnier, L. (1986): T-lymphocyte T4 molecule behaves as the receptor for human retrovirus LAV. *Nature,* 312:767–768.

25. Layon, J., Idris, A., Warzynski, M., Shere, R., Brauner, D., Patch, O., McCulley, D., and Orris, P. (1984): Altered T-lymphocyte subsets in hospitalized intravenous drug abusers. *Arch. Intern. Med.,* 133:1376–1380.

26. Levy, J. A., Hoffman, A. D., Kramer, S. M., Landis, J. A., Shimabukuro, J. M., and Oshiro, L. S. (1984): Isolation of lymphocytopathic retroviruses from San Francisco patients with AIDS. *Science,* 225:840–842.

27. Louria, D. B. (1974): Infectious complications of nonalcoholic drug abuse. *Annu. Rev. Med.,* 25:219–231.

28. Madden, J. J., Donahoe, R. M., Smith, I. E., Martinson, D. E., Moss-Wells, S., Klein, L., and Falek, A. (1984): Increased rate of E-rosette formation by T-lymphocytes of pregnant women who drink alcohol. *Clin. Immunol. Immunopathol.,* 36:67–79.

29. Madden, J. J., Donahoe, R. M., Zwemer-Collins, J., Shafer, D. A., and Falek, A. (1987): The binding of naloxone to human T-lymphocytes. *Biochem. Pharmacol.,* 36:4103–4109.

30. Masur, H., Michelis, M. A., Greene, J. B., Onorato, I., Vande Stouwe, R. A., Holzman, R. S., Wormser, G., Brettman, L., Lange, M., Murray, H. W., and Cunningham-Rundles, S. (1981): An outbreak of community-acquired *Pneumocystis carinii* pneumonia: initial manifestation of cellular immune dysfunction. *N. Engl. J. Med.,* 305:1431–1438.

31. Mathews, P. M., Froelich, C. J., Sibitt, W. L., Jr., and Bankhurst, A. D. (1983): Enhancement of natural cytoxocity by β-endorphin. *J. Immunol.,* 130:1658–1662.

32. McDonough, R. J., Madden, J. J., Falek, A., Shafer, D. A., Pline, M., Gordon, D., Bokos, P., Kuehnle, J. C., and Mendelson, J. (1980): Alteration of T and null lymphocyte frequencies in the peripheral blood of human opiate addicts: *in vivo* evidence of opiate receptor sites on T lymphocytes. *J. Immunol.,* 125:2539–2543.

33. McDougal, J. S., Kennedy, M. S., Sligh, J. M., Cort, S. P., Mawle, A., and Nicholson, J. K. A. (1986): Binding of HTLV-III/LAV to T4+ T cells by a complex of the 110K viral protein and the T4 molecule. *Science,* 231:382–385.

34. Mehrishi, J. N., and Mills, I. H. (1983): Opiate receptors on lymphocytes and platelets in man. *Clin. Immunol. Immunopathol.,* 27:240–249.

35. Montagnier, L., Chermann, J. C., Barre-Sinoussi, F., Chamaret, S., Gruest, J., Nugeyre, M. T., Rey, F., Dauguet, C., Axler-Blin, C., Vezinet-Brun, F., Rouzioux, C., Saimot, G.-A., Rozenbaum, W., Gluckman, J. C., Klatzmann, D., Vilmer, E., Griscelli, C., Foyer-Gazengel, C., and Brunet, J. B. (1984): A new human T-lymphotropic retrovirus; characterization and possible role in lymphadenopathy and acquired immune deficiency syndromes. In: *Human T-*

   Cell Leukemia/Lymphoma Viruses, edited by R. C. Gallo, M. Essex, and L. Gross, pp. 363–379. Cold Spring Harbor Laboratories, New York.

36. Moore, M. (1983): Interferon and the immune system 2: Effect of IFN on the immune system. In: *Interferons: From Molecular Biology to Clinical Application,* edited by D. C. Burke and A. G. Morris, pp. 181–209. Cambridge University Press, New York.

37. Nahas, G. G., Suica-Foca, N., Armand, J. P., and Monishima, A. (1974): Inhibition of cellular mediated immunity in marihuana smokers. *Science,* 183:419–420.

38. Plotnikoff, N. P., Murgo, A. J., Miller, G. C., Corder, C. N., and Faith, R. E. (1985): Enkephalins: Immunomodulators. *Fed. Proc.,* 44:118–122.

39. Rubinstein, A., Sicklick, M., Gupta, A., Bernstein, L., Klein, N., Rubinstein, E., Spigland, I., Fruchter, L., Litman, N., Lee, H., and Hollander, M. (1983): Acquired immunodeficiency with reversed T4/T8 ratios in infants born to promiscuous and drug-addicted mothers. *J.A.M.A.,* 249:2350–2356.

40. Sadeghi, A., Behmard, S., and Vasselinovitch, S. D. (1979): Opium: A potential urinary bladder carcinogen in man. *Cancer,* 43:2315–2321.

41. Sapira, J. D. (1968): The narcotic addict as a medical patient. *Am. J. Med.,* 45:555–588.

42. Siegal, F. P., Lopez, C., Hammer, G. S., Brown, A. E., Kornfeld, S. J., Gold, J., Hassett, J., Hirschman, S. L., Cunningham-Rundles, C., Adelsberg, B. R., Parham, D. M., Siegal, M., Cunningham-Rundles, S., and Armstrong, D. (1981): Severe acquired immunodeficiency in male homosexuals, manifested by chronic perianal ulcerative herpes simplex lesions. *N. Engl. J. Med.,* 305:1439–1444.

43. Terry, C. E., and Pellens, M. (1928): *The Opium Problem.* Bureau of Social Hygiene, New York.

44. Tubaro, E., Borelli, G., Croce, C., Cavallo, G., and Santiangeli, G. (1983): Effect of morphine on resistance to infection. *J. Infect. Dis.,* 148:656–666.

45. Van Dyke, C., Stein, A., Jones, R., Chuntharapai, A., and Seaman, W. (1986): Cocaine increases natural killer cell activity. *J. Clin. Invest.,* 77:1387–1390.

46. Wands, J. R. (1979): Ethanol and the immune response. In: *Biochemistry and Pharmacology of Ethanol,* edited by E. Majchrowicz and E. P. Noble, pp. 641–658. Plenum Press, New York.

47. Watson, E. S., Murphy, J. C., El Sohly, M. A., El Sohly, M. R., and Turner, C. E. (1983): Effects of administration of coca alkaloids on the primary immune response of mice: Interaction with delta-9-tetrahydrocannabinol and ethanol. *Toxicol. Appl. Pharmacol.,* 71:1–13.

48. Weber, R. J., and Pert, C. B. (1984): Opiatergic modulation of the immune system. In: *Central and Peripheral Endorphins: Basic and Clinical Aspects,* edited by E. E. Muller and A. R. Genezzani, pp. 35–42. Raven Press, New York.

49. Wybran, J., Appelboom, T., Famaey, J. P., and Govaerts, A. (1979): Suggestive evidence for receptors for morphine and methionine-enkephalin on normal human blood T lymphocytes. *J. Immunol.,* 123:1068–1070.

Psychological, Neuropsychiatric, and
Substance Abuse Aspects of AIDS,
edited by T. Peter Bridge et al.
Raven Press, New York © 1988.

Gender Differences in Response
to HIV Infection*

*Don C. Des Jarlais and †Samuel R. Friedman

*New York State Division of Substance Abuse Services, New York, New York 10047; and
†Narcotic and Drug Research, Inc., New York, New York 10027

There are many factors that affect the functioning of the immune system, including drugs, diet, stress, and Pavlovian conditioning. Discovery of cofactors that influence the effect of HIV on the immune system might lead to increased understanding of the pathogenic mechanisms of the virus as well as possible means for reducing the high fatality rate of HIV infection. Among gay men, the largest group to have developed AIDS in the United States, there is little evidence to date of any cofactors that influence the outcomes of HIV infection (1,2). In this chapter we review a variety of data indicating the existence of a gender-related cofactor in responses to HIV infection among intravenous drug users, the second largest group to have developed AIDS in the United States.

MALE–FEMALE DIFFERENCES IN HIV INFECTION

Over 93% of the cases of AIDS in the United States have occurred in males, with homosexual/bisexual men comprising the largest group at increased risk for the disease (Centers for Disease Control, *personal communication*). Consequently, there have been relatively few investigations of possible gender differences in HIV infection. Studies of intravenous drug users in New York, however, do show consistent evidence for male–female differences in the response to HIV infection. Females are substantially underrepresented among cases of AIDS among i.v. drug users in the city.

Data from persons entering treatment for heroin abuse provide the best basis for estimating the sex and ethnic distribution of i.v. drug users in New York City. (The

---

*Points of view or opinions in this chapter do not necessarily represent the official position or policies of Narcotic and Drug Research, Inc., the New York State Division of Substance Abuse Services, or the United States Government.

only major assumption required in using the treatment data is that there is a similar ratio of i.v. drug users entering treatment to total i.v. drug users in each of the sex and ethnic groups.) Females accounted for 27% of the heroin admissions to state-funded treatment programs in the years from 1980 through 1985 (3). Yet only 20% of the 2,634 heterosexual i.v. drug users who have developed AIDS in New York City have been females (4).

The underrepresentation of female i.v. drug users among the AIDS cases in New York City does not appear to be a result of less exposure to HIV among female i.v. drug users in New York. Our initial New York seroprevalence study found a higher seroprevalence rate among females (58%) than among males (48%) (5). A slightly higher rate was also found in the study by Weiss et al. (6) of i.v. drug users in treatment in New Jersey. (The sex differences in seroprevalence in these studies did not retain statistical significance after controlling for drug injection behavior.) More recent studies in the New York area have shown similar slightly higher seroprevalence rates among females (B. Primm, *personal communication*) or no sex differences (7). There are no studies showing significantly higher seroprevalence rates among male i.v. drug users in any sample from the New York City area.

In addition to the underrepresentation of female i.v. drug users in AIDS cases, sex differences in the clinical manifestations of AIDS have been observed. In the early stages of the AIDS epidemic in New York, Kaposi's sarcoma accounted for 12% of the cases in female i.v. drug users and only 4% of the cases in heterosexual male i.v. drug users (8). This sex difference is opposite in direction to the observed difference in non-AIDS Kaposi's sarcoma, which is predominantly a disease of males (9).

There are even sex differences in pediatric cases of AIDS. Among cases of maternally transmitted AIDS in New York City, male children with surveillance-definition AIDS have a higher cumulative mortality than female children—73% compared to 59%. This difference, however, is comparable to the mortality differences for all causes observed in children under 2 years of age in the City (10).

The differences in outcomes of HIV infection among i.v. drug users may begin well before the development of clinical AIDS. In a longitudinal study of HIV seropositive i.v. drug users without AIDS or ARC, we found a tendency for males to lose T4 cells at a rate faster than females. After controlling for continued drug injection, males lost an average of 118 T4 cells/mm^3 more than females over a 9-month follow-up ($p < 0.10$) (11).

DISCUSSION

All of the above gender differences in response to HIV infection suggest that females have less severe outcomes than males among i.v. drug users in New York City. They are underrepresented among i.v. drug users with AIDS; among heterosexual i.v. drug users with AIDS, females are more likely to develop KS, a less rapidly fatal form of AIDS; and female i.v. drug users may lose T4 cells at a lower rate after initial HIV infection. The consistency of the female–male differences across these different data sets is at least strongly indicative of a gender-related cofactor in response to HIV infection. The potential importance of this gender-related cofactor can be estimated by considering the underrepresentation of females among the heterosexual cases of AIDS among i.v. drug users in New York City. As noted above, females comprise only 20% of the cases of AIDS among heterosexual i.v. drug users in New York City, whereas they comprise 27% of the admissions to treatment for heroin abuse. Assuming equal rates of exposure to HIV, this under-representation corresponds to a 35% reduction in the number of female i.v. drug users who "should" have developed AIDS.

The existence of gender differences in the response to HIV infection should not be considered too surprising. Gender differences favoring females have also been observed in the response to hepatitis B infection, which has a similar epidemiology to AIDS and which may involve extensive involvement of the immune system as part of the disease process. Females infected with hepatitis B are less likely to remain in a carrier state (12) and are less likely to develop hepatic cancer as an outcome of the infection (13). The mechanisms for these differences in response to hepatitis B infection are not presently understood.

There are many possible mechanisms that might lead to male–female differences in response to HIV infection, and there may be multiple mechanisms related to the results noted above. These might include differences in sexual behavior or drug use behavior as well as hormonal differences. A subgroup of female i.v. drug users obtain drugs through sexual activity, whether through ongoing relationships with males who provide drugs, direct bartering of sex for drugs, or engaging in prosti-tution. Women who are sexually active with numerous partners are at great risk for exposure to a wide variety of sexually transmitted diseases, some of which may act as cofactors influencing HIV infection. For example, female i.v. drug users are more likely to have been exposed to cytomegalovirus than male i.v. drug users (14). Although one would ordinarily expect exposure to other infectious agents to in-crease severity of HIV immunosuppression (15), there may be specific infectious agents that reduce the severity of HIV immunosuppression. A sexually transmitted agent might be related to the increasing proportions of Kaposi's sarcoma in cases of AIDS among heterosexual male i.v. drug users, female i.v. drug users, gay i.v. drug users, and gay non-i.v. drug users (8).

Possible differences in drug use patterns between male and female i.v. drug users might also account for differences in response to HIV infection. The longitudinal study reported above, however, did control for both drug injection and noninjected drug use and still showed a tendency for HIV-seropositive male i.v. drug users to lose T4 cells more rapidly than seropositive female i.v. drug users.

Hormonal differences may be the "simplest" explanation of the sex differences in response to HIV infection, since they might encompass both the adult and pedi-atric findings. (One does, however, hesitate to call anything involving endocrine–immune system interaction "simple.") Croxson et al. (16) have shown some inter-action of prolactin with HIV infection. Research on hormonal interactions offers the opportunity to link the gender differences in HIV infection with gender differences in other immunologic responses and to contribute to greater understanding of the complex interactions between the endocrine and immune systems.

SUMMARY

There is strong epidemiologic evidence from studies of i.v. drug users in New York City for the existence of one or more gender-related cofactors in response to HIV infection. The strength of the evidence comes from the variety of data sets that indicate a gender-related cofactor and from the consistency of the pattern found: in all of the data sets, females appear to have a more "favorable" response than do males. The extent of underrepresentation of females in the cases of AIDS in i.v. drug users—a possible 35% reduction in the development of clinical AIDS—suggests that such a cofactor should be considered of practical importance. Identifying the mechanism(s) for a gender difference may lead to ways of deliberately affecting the course of the infection. Further research on the gender difference may also contribute to our understanding of interactions among the various components of the immune system and the interaction of the immune system with other behavioral and physiologic systems.

NOTE IN PROOF

Rothenberg and colleagues (17) have recently reported that females survive for shorter time after a diagnosis of AIDS than do males, controlling on a large number of variables including intravenous drug use. The mean difference in survival time (76 days) does not appear to be sufficient to outweigh the underrepresentation of females with AIDS among i.v. drug users. This new gender difference is in the opposite direction of the differences noted above and suggests differences in the time period from initial infection to the seeking of treatment as a possible unifying hypothesis for many of the observed gender differences.

ACKNOWLEDGMENTS

This research was supported in part by grant DA 03574 from the National Institute on Drug Abuse.

REFERENCES

1. Polk, B. F., Fox, R., Brookmeyer, R., Kanchanaraksa, S., Kaslow, R., Visscher, B., Renaldo, C., and Thair, J. (1987): Predictors of the acquired immunodeficiency syndrome developing in a cohort of seropositive homosexual men. *N. Engl. J. Med.*, 316(2):61–66.
2. Goedert, J. J., Biggar, R., Weiss, S., et al. (1985): Three year incidence of AIDS among HTLV-III-infected risk group members: A comparison of five cohorts. *Science*, 231:992–995.

3. New York State Division of Substance Abuse Services (1987): Current census and waiting lists for treatment programs. Management Information Systems.
4. New York City Department of Health (1986): *AIDS Surveillance*. Department of Health, New York.
5. Cohen, H., Marmor, M., Des Jarlais, D. C., et al. (1985): Behavioral risk factors for HTLV-III/LAV seropositivity among intravenous drug abusers. Presented at the 1st International Conference on the Acquired Immune Deficiency Syndrome, Atlanta, GA.
6. Weiss, S. H., Ginzburg, H. M., Goedert, J. J., et al. (1985): Risk for HTLV-III exposure and AIDS among parenteral drug abusers in New Jersey. Presented at the 1st International Conference on the Acquired Immunodeficiency Syndrome, Atlanta, GA.
7. Schoenbaum, E. E., Selwyn, P. A., Klein, R. S., et al. (1986): Prevalence of and risk factors associated with HTLV-III/LAV antibodies among intravenous drug users in methadone program in New York City. Presented at the 2nd International Conference on AIDS, Paris.
8. Des Jarlais, D. C., Marmor, M., Thomas, P., et al. (1984): Kaposi's sarcoma among four different AIDS risk groups. *N. Engl. J. Med.,* 310(17):1119.
9. Cutler, S. J., and Young, J. L. (1975): *Third National Cancer Survey: Incidence Data*. National Institutes of Health, Bethesda.
10. Thomas, P., Des Jarlais, D. C., O'Donnell, R., et al. (1986): The epidemiology of maternally transmitted AIDS in children in New York City. Presented at the Interscience Conference on Antibiotics and Antimicrobial Chemotherapies, New Orleans.
11. Des Jarlais, D. C., Friedman, S. R., Marmor, M., et al. (1987): Development of AIDS, HIV seroconversion, and co-factors for T4 cell loss in a cohort of intravenous drug users. *AIDS,* 1:105–111.
12. Szmunes, W., Harley, J., Ikram, H., et al. (1978): Sociodemographic aspects of the epidemiology of hepatitis B. In: *Viral Hepatitis: A Contemporary Assessment of Etiology, Epidemiology, Pathogenesis and Prevention,* pp. 297–320. The Franklin Institute Press, Philadelphia.
13. Peters, R. L. (1976): Pathology of hepatocellular carcinoma. In: *Hepatocellular Carcinoma,* edited by K. Okuda and R. L. Peters, pp. 107–114. John Wiley & Sons, New York.
14. Marmor, M., Des Jarlais, D. C., Spira, T., et al. (1985): AIDS and cytomegalovirus exposure in New York City drug abusers. Presented at the 1st International Conference on the Acquired Immunodeficiency Syndrome, Atlanta, GA.
15. Zagury, D., Bernard, J., Leonard, R., et al. (1986): Long-term cultures of HTLV-III-infected T cells: A model of cytopathology of T-cell depletion in AIDS. *Science,* 231:850–853.
16. Croxson, T. S., Rudolph, S., Chapman, W. E., et al. (1986): HTLV-III/LAV infection of the CNS with elevated serum prolactin. Presented at the 2nd International Conference on AIDS, Paris.
17. Rothenberg, R., Woelfel, M., Stoneburner, R., Milberg, J., Parker, R., and Truman, B. (1987): Survival with the acquired immunodeficiency syndrome. *N. Engl. J. Med.,* 317(21):1297–1302.

Psychological, Neuropsychiatric, and
Substance Abuse Aspects of AIDS,
edited by T. Peter Bridge et al.
Raven Press, New York © 1988.

Kaposi's Sarcoma and Nitrite Inhalants

Harry W. Haverkos

*Clinical Medicine Branch, Division of Clinical Research, National Institute on Drug
Abuse, Alcohol, Drug Abuse, and Mental Health Administration,
Rockville, Maryland 20857*

Kaposi's sarcoma (KS) is an important disease manifestation among patients with AIDS. It is the most common cancer reported among AIDS patients, and its sudden occurrence among homosexual men in New York and California was one of the earliest harbingers of the AIDS pandemic (4).

Kaposi's sarcoma is a neoplasm manifested by vascular nodules in the skin and other organs. The disease is generally multifocal, with a course ranging from indolent, with only skin lesions, to fulminant, with extensive visceral involvement (32). It was first described among elderly European men in 1872 and has subsequently been reported worldwide.

Nitrite inhalants were investigated as a possible cause of AIDS early in the epidemic, partly because of the preponderance of homosexual men who used nitrites among the early patients with AIDS. During pilot testing of questionnaires in 1981, Centers for Disease Control (CDC) investigators found that nitrites were used by nearly all homosexual men with AIDS. In addition, a 1981 survey of 420 men attending sexually transmitted diseases clinics showed that homosexual men reported the use of nitrites far more frequently than did heterosexual men and that the amount of use directly correlated with the number of different sexual partners (6). In 1982, Marmor et al. (23) reported significant associations between both use of amyl nitrite and sexual activity and the development of AIDS (all 20 patients in that study had KS) among homosexual men.

On the other hand, Marmor et al. reanalyzed their data by entering additional factors and using multivariate analysis; they found that still other variables appear to differentiate patients with AIDS from controls (22,24). Jaffe et al. (18) showed that nitrite inhalant use did not appear to be important in distinguishing patients with AIDS from controls. Measures of sexual activity were the best markers for the development of AIDS in that study. In addition, studies conducted by the National Institute for Occupational Safety and Health (CDC) showed no immunotoxic reactions in mice exposed to isobutyl nitrite vapors (20).

This chapter examines national surveillance data and a case comparison study to examine the role of nitrite inhalants, not as a cause of AIDS but as a cofactor in the development of KS in AIDS.

SURVEILLANCE

In 1981, CDC initiated surveillance in the United States for patients under age 60 with KS and opportunistic infections, including *Pneumocystis carinii* pneumonia (PCP), with no predisposing cause of immune deficiency. The initial CDC definition of AIDS did not require immunologic studies or testing for any possible viral causes, nor did it exclude patients with normal immunologic results (34).

Following the identification of human immunodeficiency virus (HIV) as the cause of AIDS, CDC changed the definition of AIDS to include HIV serology testing as part of the definition. AIDS patients with normal immunologic studies but not tested for HIV antibody could be included in the survey. In addition, KS patients over age 60 were included if the patient had a positive serologic or virologic test result for HIV (5).

Between June 1981 and February 9, 1987, 30,632 cases of AIDS in the United States were reported to the CDC; 6,484 (21.2%) patients had KS as one of their disease manifestations.

Kaposi's sarcoma associated with AIDS is unique (15). Unlike "classical" KS among elderly men or "endemic" KS in some patients of Africa, KS in AIDS is associated with HIV infection and cellular immune impairment (2,36). Furthermore, unlike the opportunistic infections associated with AIDS, KS occurs much more commonly among homosexual men than among AIDS patients of other risk

TABLE 1. *AIDS cases reported to the Centers for Disease Control through February 9, 1987 according to risk group, United States*

Group	Total no. of patients	Number of patients with KS	Percentage with KS
Homosexual/bisexual men	22,127	6,136	27.7
Intravenous drug users	5,128	155	3.0
Heterosexual contact			
Third world native	600	54	9.0
Other	547	13	2.4
Transfusion recipients	567	22	3.9
Hemophilia/coagulation disorder	254	5	2.0
Children[a]	444	12	2.7
Undetermined	965	87	9.0
Total	30,632	6,484	21.2

[a]Includes patients less than 13 years of age at time of diagnosis, including children with hemophilia/coagulation disorders and transfusion recipients.
From M. Morgan, Centers for Disease Control (*personal communication*).

TABLE 2. *AIDS cases reported to the Centers for Disease Control by year: February 9, 1987*[a]

Year	Total no. of patients	Number of patients with KS	Percentage with KS
1981	202	97	48.0
1982	741	247	33.3
1983	2,381	752	31.6
1984	4,375	1,096	25.1
1985	8,249	1,672	20.3
1986	13,055	2,334	17,9
1987	1,629	286	17.6
Total	30,632	6,484	21.2

[a]Data derived by using latest available *Weekly Surveillance Report* issued each year (1984–1986) by the Centers for Disease Control.

groups (Table 1) and is the only AIDS-defining illness in which the proportion of cases has declined (Table 2).

CASE COMPARISON STUDY

In order to pursue the unique epidemiology of KS in AIDS and to determine possible risk factors for its occurrence, we reanalyzed data from three epidemiologic studies conducted by the CDC (1,16,18). We compared patients by outcome of disease. Eighty-seven patients (47 with KS, 20 with PCP, and 20 with both) had participated in the earlier studies, and their interviews and laboratory results were available for analysis (17).

We found that patients with both KS and PCP resembled those with only KS much more closely than they did patients who developed only PCP. Those with KS or with both diseases reported more sexual partners [relative risk (RR) = 2.0], more receptive anal intercourse (RR = 4.4), more "recreational drug" use, and a higher incidence of non-B hepatitis (RR = 2.8) than patients with PCP only. The median number of sexual partners reported in the year prior to onset of illness was 125 by patients with KS only, 115 by those with both diseases, and 22.5 by those with PCP only. Statistically significant differences were also found for use of amphetamines (RR = 1.9), barbiturates (RR = 4.2), cocaine (RR = 1.8), ethyl chloride (RR = 6.0), LSD (RR = 2.5), marijuana (RR = 1.4), methaqualone (RR = 2.2), and nitrite inhalants (RR = 6.1). No statistically significant differences were found for sexually transmitted diseases (other than non-B hepatitis) or for any laboratory test performed (17).

Multivariate analysis suggests the relative importance of differences identified in univariate analysis. For the KS versus PCP and both KS and PCP versus PCP comparisons, total days of nitrite inhalant use differentiated between the disease groups better than any other variable available for analysis (17).

DISCUSSION

A multifactorial model can be postulated to explain the various manifestations of AIDS. We suggest that the natural history of AIDS begins with immune dysfunction resulting from HIV infection of T-helper lymphocytes. One or several cofactors, present in some but not necessarily all patients, then determine which, if any, malignancies or opportunistic infections the patient manifests. Our analysis suggests that a promoter or cofactor for KS is the use of large quantities of nitrite inhalants (17).

Two other epidemiologic studies have also found a strong association between KS and the use of large quantities of nitrite inhalants. One was conducted at Mount Sinai School of Medicine, New York (25), and the other was conducted in San Francisco (30). On the other hand, results of three epidemiologic studies presented at the International Conference in Paris, France, in June 1986 do not support the associations (8,11,31). However, in the three latter studies, investigators did not collect as detailed information about nitrite inhalants as in the former studies. For example, the earlier studies report quantitative lifetime nitrite exposure; the latter studies query nitrite use only in the 6 months or 2 years prior to interview. One of the latter studies does not quantitate nitrite use in its analysis (31).

Amyl nitrite has been used medically since 1897 as a treatment for angina pectoris and later as a diagnostic maneuver in cardiac auscultation (3). It is a clear, yellowish liquid that is packaged in a cloth-covered ampule and administered by inhalation. When the ampule is broken, it makes a snapping sound; thus the nicknames "snappers" or "poppers." In the 1960s sales of amyl nitrite rose sharply because of its abuse as an inhalant for getting "high" and as an aphrodisiac. This led to its reinstatement as a prescription drug by the Food and Drug Administration (FDA) in 1968 (29). Since 1968, other volatile nitrites containing isomers of amyl and butyl alcohol and butyl nitrite have been marketed as "room odorizers" and sold in bottles containing 10 to 30 ml of liquid for $5 to $15 each. Since their labels state that they are not to be inhaled, they are sold legally over the counter in bookstores, pornographic and "head" shops, and by mail order under such names as *Locker Room* and *Rush*. Until recently, male homosexuals indulged in these drugs more than did other groups (29,35). More recently, abuse among adolescents has been reported more (33).

At present, no federal agency regulates the sales or use of the volatile nitrites sold as room odorizers. The FDA has determined that butyl nitrite is not a drug and therefore not under the provisions of the Food, Drug, and Cosmetic Act. The National Institute on Drug Abuse (NIDA) has held symposia and published information on nitrite inhalants; however, NIDA has no authority to take regulatory action. The Consumer Product Safety Commission has applied restrictions on labeling but has not taken action against nitrites under the Federal Hazardous Substances Act. Recently, 11 states have passed laws regarding labeling, sales, and/or use of volatile nitrites.

There have been several hypotheses concerning the possible mechanism by which nitrites may promote the likelihood of KS in homosexual men infected with HIV. First, nitrite inhalants may act directly on the immune system (12). Second, nitrosamines, metabolites of nitrites, may be carcinogenic (19). Interactions of nitrites and mouse skin lipids have been shown to produce potentially carcinogenic substances (26). Third, the vasodilatory action of nitrite inhalants may, in some unknown way, promote KS, a malignancy of blood vessels (17). Finally, the use of nitrite inhalants may only be a marker for another cofactor, e.g., an "unidentified" virus.

In addition to the concerns about the inconsistencies of the epidemiologic studies, there have been other concerns raised by investigators about the significance and importance of the association of nitrite inhalant use and KS. Although nitrite use may be contributory to the development of KS among homosexual men, it is not likely to explain the KS seen in Africa and Haiti (27). Even though KS among homosexual men with AIDS and among Africans appears to be the same histologically, there may be a variety of different causes or pathways to the same histologic process. A contributing factor for KS associated with AIDS may not be necessary for the development of KS in endemic areas. It may also be difficult to determine the effects of increased surveillance for KS in developing countries engendered by the publicity associated with the AIDS pandemic and the increased awareness, identification, and reporting of endemic KS cases as AIDS related. Increased use of the HIV antibody test in Africa and Haiti should help distinguish between these two forms of KS. Although less likely, another explanation for endemic KS in developing countries may be nutritional or other environmental exposures to nitrites or nitrosamines in some other form.

If the use of nitrite inhalants is a necessary cofactor in the development of KS in AIDS, how does one explain the KS cases in the United States occurring in risk group members other than homosexual men? First, the CDC definition of AIDS is not 100% specific and includes some KS cases that are probably "classical" rather than AIDS related (7). The recent addition of cases over age 60 is likely to add more "classical" KS cases to the survey (5). Second, the pathologic diagnosis of KS is not uniform from pathologist to pathologist. A few of the KS cases reported to CDC have not been confirmed by more experienced investigators by review of skin biopsies from intravenous drug abusers (D. Mildvan, Beth Israel Medical Center, New York, *personal communication*) and from children (D. Porter, U.C.L.A. Medical Center, Los Angeles, *personal communication*). Finally, nitrite inhalant use is not limited to homosexual men but has been reported among adolescents (33) and intravenous drug abusers (R. Lange, Addiction Research Center, National Institute on Drug Abuse, Baltimore, *personal communication*). It would be helpful if physicians caring for patients with AIDS-associated KS would ask their patients about nitrite inhalant use.

Although there is no known animal model of KS, it may be interesting to challenge retrovirus-infected animals with large quantities of alkyl nitrites and look for skin changes consistent with KS. A few investigators, including those working with HIV-infected chimpanzees, have discussed such an experiment (28).

Interestingly, the proportion of AIDS patients with KS reported to CDC has dropped from approximately 50% in 1981 to approximately 20% in 1985 and 1986 (Table 2). Although there are many hypotheses to explain the declining trend of KS in AIDS, one possible explanation is a decrease in nitrite inhalant use.

Other potential cofactors have been hypothesized for KS. An association between cytomegalovirus (CMV) and KS was first noted by Giraldo et al. (13,14) in African patients with KS. More recently, Drew and colleagues (9) have reported a decreasing transmission of CMV among homosexual men that parallels the decreasing proportion of KS among homosexual men with AIDS. However, CMV is a common infection among heterosexuals, hemophiliacs, and blood transfusion recipients (10). If CMV is a cofactor in the development of KS, one would expect more KS in other risk group patients. Another explanation for the occurrence of KS early in the epidemic and its apparent decline is a change in the HIV itself over time or the existence of another "unidentified" virus acting as a cofactor (21,27).

In summary, the unique epidemiology of KS in AIDS suggests that a cofactor is needed in addition to HIV for its development and that the cofactor is highly associated with the homosexual lifestyle. Researchers who seek a cofactor for KS in AIDS would do well to design their studies and analyze their data in such a way as to consider that there may be separate causes or cofactors for the various forms of KS. Until more conclusive data are presented, persons at risk for exposure to HIV infection should refrain from using nitrite inhalants.

ACKNOWLEDGMENTS

I thank Drs. John Dougherty, Peter Hartsock, and Lynne M. Haverkos for reviewing the manuscript.

REFERENCES

1. Auerbach, D. M., Darrow, W. W., Jaffe, H. W., and Curran, J. W. (1984): Cluster of cases of the acquired immunodeficiency syndrome: Patients linked by sexual contact. *Am. J. Med.*, 76:487–492.
2. Biggar, R. J., Melbye, M., Kestems, L., et al. (1984): Kaposi's sarcoma in Zaire is not associated with HTLV-III infection. *N. Engl. J. Med.*, 311:1051–1052.
3. Brunton, T. (1897): *Lectures on the Actions of Medicines*, pp. 332–341. Macmillan, New York.
4. Centers for Disease Control (1981): Kaposi's sarcoma and *Pneumocystis* pneumonia among homosexual men—New York City and California. *Morbid. Mortal. Week. Rep.*, 30:305–308.
5. Centers for Disease Control (1985): Revision of the case definition of acquired immunodeficiency syndrome for national reporting—United States. *Morbid. Mortal. Week. Rep.*, 34:373–375.
6. Centers for Disease Control Task Force on Kaposi's Sarcoma and Opportunistic Infections (1982): Epidemiologic aspects of the current outbreak of Kaposi's sarcoma and opportunistic infections. *N. Engl. J. Med.*, 306:248–252.
7. Chamberland, M. E., Castro, K. G., Haverkos, H. W., et al. (1984): Acquired immunodeficiency syndrome in the United States: An analysis of cases outside high incidence groups. *Ann. Intern. Med.*, 101:617–623.
8. Darrow, W. W., Byers, R. H., Jaffe, H. W., et al. (1987): Cofactors in the development of AIDS and AIDS-related conditions. In: *International Conference on AIDS, Paris*, p. 99.

9. Drew, W. L., Mills, J., Hauer, L., and Miner, R. C. (1986): Declining prevalence of Kaposi's sarcoma in homosexual AIDS patients is paralleled by declining incidence of CMV infection. In: *26th Interscience Conference on Antimicrobial Agents and Chemotherapy.*
10. Drew, W. L., Mintz, L., Miner, R. C., et al. (1981): Prevalence of cytomegalovirus in homosexual men. *J. Infect. Dis.,* 143:188–192.
11. Goedert, J. J., Biggar, R. J., Melbye, M., et al. (1987): Effect of T4 count and cofactors on AIDS incidence in homosexual men infected with human immunodeficiency virus. *J.A.M.A.,* 257:331–334.
12. Goedert, J. J., Neuland, C. Y., Wallen, W., et al. (1982): Amyl nitrite may alter T lymphocytes in homosexual men. *Lancet,* 1:412–415.
13. Giraldo, G., Beth, E., and Haguenau, F. (1972): Herpes-type virus particles in tissue culture of Kaposi's sarcoma from different geographic regions. *J. Natl. Cancer Inst.,* 49:1509–1513.
14. Giraldo, G., Beth, E., and Huang, E. S. (1980): Kaposi's sarcoma and its relationship to cytomegalovirus (CMV). III. CMV DNA and CMV early antigens in Kaposi's sarcoma. *Int. J. Cancer,* 26:23–29.
15. Haverkos, H. W., Drotman, D. P., and Morgan, M. (1985): Prevalence of Kaposi's sarcoma among patients with AIDS [letter]. *N. Engl. J. Med.,* 312:1518.
16. Haverkos, H. W., Drotman, D. P., Pinsky, P. F., and Bregman, D. J. (1983): Case-control study of Kaposi's sarcoma and *Pneumocystis carinii* pneumonia in homosexual men residing outside New York City and California. In: *Program and Abstracts of the 23rd Interscience Conference on Antimicrobial Agents and Chemotherapy.* American Society for Microbiology, Washington.
17. Haverkos, H. W., Pinsky, P. F., Drotman, D. P., and Bregman, D. J. (1985): Disease manifestation among homosexual men with acquired immunodeficiency syndrome: A possible role of nitrites in Kaposi's sarcoma. *Sex. Transm. Dis.,* 12:203–208.
18. Jaffe, H. W., Choi, K., Thomas, P. A., et al. (1983): National case-control study of Kaposi's sarcoma and *Pneumocystis carinii* pneumonia in homosexual men. 1. Epidemiologic results. *Ann. Intern. Med.,* 99:145–151.
19. Jorgensen, K. A., and Lawesson, S.-O. (1982): Amyl nitrite and Kaposi's sarcoma in homosexual men [letter]. *N. Engl. J. Med.,* 307:893–894.
20. Lewis, D. M., Koller, W. A., Lynch, D. W., and Spira, T. J. (1985): Subchronic inhalation toxicity of isobutyl nitrite in Balb/c mice. II. Immunotoxicity studies. *J. Toxicol. Environ. Health,* 15:835–846.
21. Lo, S.-C. (1986): Isolation and identification of a novel virus from patients with AIDS. *Am. J. Trop. Med. Hyg.,* 35:675–676.
22. Marmor, M. (1984): Epidemic Kaposi's sarcoma and sexual practices among male homosexuals. In: *The Epidemic of Kaposi's Sarcoma and Opportunistic Infections,* edited by A. E. Friedman-Kien, pp. 291–296. Masson, New York.
23. Marmor, M., Friedman-Kien, A. E., Laubenstein, L., et al. (1982): Risk factors for Kaposi's sarcoma in homosexual men. *Lancet,* 1:1083–1087.
24. Marmor, M., Friedman-Kien, A. E., Zolla-Pazner, S., et al. (1984): Kaposi's sarcoma in homosexual men. A seroepidemiologic case-control study. *Ann. Intern. Med.,* 100:809–815.
25. Mathur-Wagh, U., Mildvan, D., and Senie, R. T. (1985): Follow-up at 4½ years on homosexual men with generalized lymphadenopathy [letter]. *N. Engl. J. Med.,* 313:1542–1543.
26. Mirvish, S. S., Babcock, D. M., Deshpande, A. D., and Nagel, D. L. (1980): Identification of cholesterol as a mouse skin lipid that reacts with nitrogen dioxide to yield a nitrosating agent (NSA), and of cholesteryl nitrite as the NSA produced in a chemical system from cholesterol. *Cancer Lett.,* 31:97–104.
27. Mortimer, P. P. (1987): Viral cause of Kaposi's sarcoma? *Lancet,* 1:280–281.
28. National Institute of Allergy and Infectious Diseases and Haverkos, H. W. (1987): Pathogenesis of AIDS, Associated Factors Workshop. *J. Infect. Dis.,* 156:251–257.
29. Newell, G. R., Mansell, P. W. A., Spitz, M. R., Reuben, J. M., and Hersh, E. M. (1985): Volatile nitrites: Use and adverse effects related to the current epidemic of the acquired immunodeficiency syndrome. *Am. J. Med.,* 78:811–815.
30. Osmond, D., Moss, A. R., Bachett, P., Volberding, P., Barre-Sinoussi, F., and Chermann, J.-C. (1985): A cases-control study of risk factors for AIDS in San Francisco. In: *International Conference on Acquired Immunodeficiency Syndrome (AIDS),* p. 24.
31. Polk, B. F., Fox, R., Brookmeyer, R., et al. (1987): Predictors of the acquired immunodeficiency syndrome developing in a cohort of seropositive homosexual men. *N. Engl. J. Med.,* 316:61–66.

32. Safai, B., and Good, R. A. (1981): Kaposi's sarcoma: A review and recent developments. *CA*, 31:2–12.
33. Schwartz, R. H., and Peary, P. (1986): Abuse of isobutyl nitrite inhalation (Rush) by adolescents. *Clin. Pediatr.*, 25:308–310.
34. Selik, R. M., Haverkos, H. W., and Curran, J. W. (1984): Acquired immunodeficiency syndrome (AIDS) trends in the United States, 1978–1982. *Am. J. Med.*, 76:493–500.
35. Sigell, L. T., Kapp, F. T., Fusaro, G. A., Nelson, E. D., and Falck, R. S. (1978): Popping and snorting volatile nitrites: A current fad for getting high. *Am. J. Psychiatry*, 135:1216–1218.
36. Stahl, R. E., Friedman-Kien, A., Dublin, R., Marmor, M., and Zolla-Pazner, S. (1982): Immunologic abnormalities in homosexual men. Relationship to Kaposi's sarcoma. *Am. J. Med.*, 73:171–178.
37. Tomasko, M. A., and Chudin, M. S. (1987): Kaposi's sarcoma in an elderly patient. *Ann. Intern. Med.*, 106:334–335.

Psychological, Neuropsychiatric, and
Substance Abuse Aspects of AIDS,
edited by T. Peter Bridge et al.
Raven Press, New York © 1988.

Ethanol-Associated Immunosuppression

*Thomas R. Jerrells, †Cheryl A. Marietta, ‡George Bone, †Forrest F. Weight, and ‡Michael J. Eckardt

Department of Pathology, University of Texas Medical Branch, Galveston, Texas 77550; †Laboratory of Physiologic and Pharmacologic Studies, National Institute on Alcohol Abuse and Alcoholism, Rockville, Maryland 20852; and ‡Laboratory of Clinical Studies, National Institute on Alcohol Abuse and Alcoholism, Bethesda, Maryland 20892

A number of investigators have suggested that prolonged and excessive consumption of ethanol (ETOH) results in alterations of host defense mechanisms manifested ultimately in increased susceptibility to infections from pathogenic and opportunistic organisms (11). Detrimental effects of ETOH on the ability to generate immune responses are thought to play a major role in this increased susceptibility to infection. Alterations in the immune system from the effects of ETOH also may be involved in other pathological aspects of alcoholism such as liver disease and autoimmunity.

A number of studies have shown that ETOH administration to experimental animals or ETOH abuse in humans has a profound effect on peripheral lymphoid organs as measured by a decrease in weights of the spleen and thymus (15,19). A loss of circulating leukocytes has been associated with ETOH intake or administration (2,12,16,17,20). Impairments in both humoral immune mechanisms, including antibody production (6,16,19), and aspects of cell-mediated immunity such as delayed-type hypersensitivity reactions (1,6,19) and lymphocyte proliferative responses to mitogens (14,20) also have been reported.

Although it is accepted that ETOH has an adverse effect on the immune system, neither the extent of this effect nor the mechanisms have been clearly elucidated. For instance, it has been suggested that impairments in immune responses do not occur in animals in the absence of hepatic disease (3); lymphocyte responses to mitogens were shown to be impaired in one study, but these impairments were not seen in the response to recall antigens (14); and human lymphocyte function was shown in one study not to be impaired (4) or only if the assay was performed in autologous plasma (20), suggesting the possibility of soluble suppressor factors. Because the model systems used in these studies were so different, it is difficult to define any general effects of ETOH on the immune system based on previous work.

To study some of these questions we have utilized a well-characterized model of ETOH dependency and withdrawal developed by Majchrowicz (13) to evaluate crit-

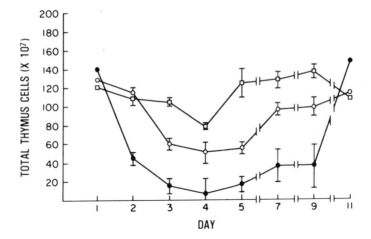

FIG. 1. Effects of ETOH administration on cell numbers in rat thymus. Male Sprague–Dawley rats were intubated with 8 to 11 g ETOH/kg body weight daily (●), one-half of this dose (○), or control diet only (□). Each point represents the mean ± standard deviation of counts from six to nine animals.

ically the effects of ETOH on the immune system using as many parameters of immunocompetency as possible. Using this model, in which ETOH is administered by gastric intubation, we have shown that ETOH administration to rats has profound effects on the immune system, including a loss of lymphocytes from the thymus, spleen, and peripheral blood, a dose-dependent loss of lymphocyte function as measured by reduced proliferation to mitogens, and an inability to respond to T-dependent antigens (9). In these studies, we have examined the effects of intubation of 8 to 11 g ETOH/kg body weight as well as one-half of this dose. As can be seen from the data resulting from these experiments, the loss of cells from the thymus and spleen (Figs. 1 and 2) was profound with the full dose of ETOH and occurred in these studies after 2 days of treatment. Cell loss seemed dependent on the dose of ETOH as evidenced by the lesser cell loss in animals treated with the half dose of ETOH.

Interestingly, high doses of ETOH markedly depleted lymphocytes from the circulation of the rat (Fig. 3), but the total leukocyte count was relatively unchanged. Examination of stained blood films showed that an increase in circulating granulocytes occurred concomitant with the loss of lymphocytes (Fig. 4), resulting in the relatively unchanged leukocyte count. These changes were also evident in animals treated with the half dose of ETOH, although the changes were not as pronounced. These data suggest that administration of ETOH results in a loss of immunocompetent cells from lymphoid organs, and this loss is proportional to the amount of ETOH administered.

The ability of the remaining lymphocytes obtained from the spleen or peripheral

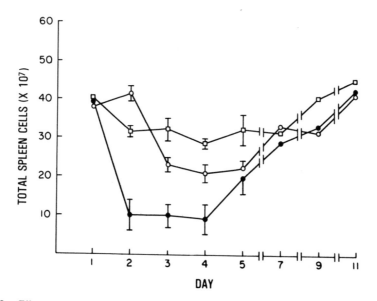

FIG. 2. Effects of ETOH administration on cell numbers in rat spleen. See legend for Fig. 1.

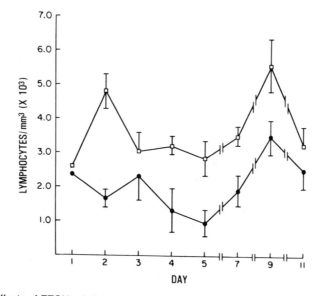

FIG. 3. Effects of ETOH administration on lymphocyte numbers in the peripheral blood of rats. Male Sprague–Dawley rats were intubated with either 8 to 11 g ETOH/kg body weight (●) or control diet only (□). Each point represents the mean ± standard deviation of duplicate counts from six animals.

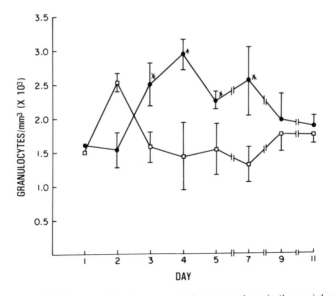

FIG. 4. Effects of ETOH administration on granulocyte numbers in the peripheral blood of rats. See legend for Fig. 3.

blood to proliferate to nonspecific mitogenic stimuli also was evaluated in these animals. The data from these experiments demonstrated a progressive loss of lymphocyte function throughout the course of ETOH administration; the most profound defect in lymphocyte proliferation, however, was seen at a time after ETOH administration was discontinued and physical signs characteristic of the withdrawal syndrome had become evident.

The data presented in Fig. 5 were obtained from animals treated with either a full or a half dose of ETOH at a time when withdrawal signs were evident. It is apparent that a defect in proliferation to Con A is present at all concentrations of Con A used, and the inability to respond to this mitogen was nearly as profound in the group treated with the half dose of ETOH. It could be argued from this finding that the inability to respond to Con A is not caused directly by the presence of ETOH but perhaps by secondary factors induced by ETOH. Lymphocyte proliferative defects were not associated with lymphocyte type in that the responses to both T-cell and B-cell mitogens were fairly equally affected.

The cell numbers in the various lymphoid organs recovered relatively quickly after ETOH administration was halted; the response to mitogenic stimulation, however, was impaired for somewhat longer periods and persisted even after cell numbers had returned to normal levels. This finding suggests that the inability to respond to mitogens resulted from more than a simple lack of cells in the spleen or peripheral blood.

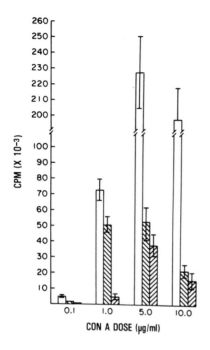

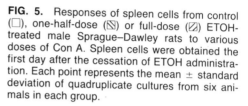

FIG. 5. Responses of spleen cells from control (□), one-half-dose (◨) or full-dose (▨) ETOH-treated male Sprague–Dawley rats to various doses of Con A. Spleen cells were obtained the first day after the cessation of ETOH administration. Each point represents the mean ± standard deviation of quadruplicate cultures from six animals in each group.

In further studies, the development of a primary immune response to a T-dependent antigen was evaluated by measuring the production of antibody-producing cells using a hemolytic plaque-forming cell assay after immunization of ETOH-treated and control rats with sheep erythrocytes (Fig. 6). The data from these studies showed that administration of ETOH for as little as 2 days after immunization markedly inhibited the immune response to this antigen relative to animals intubated with diet only. As before, suppression was dose dependent (not shown), and the most profound immune suppression was noted during the time of the withdrawal syndrome. Careful evaluation of the data revealed that the B-cell proliferative response to bacterial lipopolysaccharide was not impaired at a time after withdrawal when the production of antibody was still suppressed. This finding suggests that the inability to generate a primary immune response might be attributable to the effects of ETOH on T-helper cells and not directly on B cells.

This hypothesis is supported by data demonstrating that the antibody response to a T-independent antigen, TNP-Ficoll, is relatively unchanged in ETOH-treated animals (*unpublished data*). We have reported that most of the immune parameters were maximally depressed after the oral intubation of ETOH was halted and animals were showing signs of ETOH withdrawal, suggesting that the immunosuppression was not a result of the direct toxicity of ETOH in circulation. In related studies,

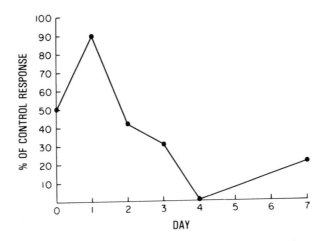

FIG. 6. Responses of ETOH-treated male Sprague–Dawley rats to sheep erythrocytes measured as plaque-forming cells. Each point represents the percentage of the mean of the group intubated with control diet only and was derived from duplicate determinations from six rats.

rats exposed to ETOH in an inhalation chamber for 14 days produced relatively consistent blood ETOH levels. This model avoids any stress associated with intubation as well as any effects of ETOH on the gastrointestinal tract. When these animals were evaluated for immunocompetency, similar changes in the immune system were observed as those found with oral intubation, including cell loss from spleen and thymus and lymphocyte loss from peripheral blood (C. A. Marietta et al., *unpublished data*). Preliminary data from this model indicated that lymphocyte proliferative responses were relatively unchanged, but only one time point was evaluated, and longer exposure by this route may be required.

In summary, it seems that exposure to ETOH, via various routes of administration, results in a reversible loss of lymphocytes from the thymus, spleen, and peripheral blood and a loss of lymphocyte function as measured by proliferation to mitogens and an inability to respond to T-dependent antigens in a primary antibody response. The rat model will now allow further studies to define the extent of the effect of ETOH on the immune system and, more importantly, to define the mechanisms of the noted immunosuppression.

EFFECTS OF ETOH ON RESPONSES TO RECALL ANTIGENS

Investigators studying guinea pigs given ETOH by intraperitoneal injections reported that the lymphocyte impairment resulting from ETOH was only in the response to mitogens and that the *in vitro* responses to recall antigens were not affected (14). The *in vitro* responses to antigens have been used as measures of the ability to sustain a previous immune response and have important implications for

TABLE 1. *Effects of ETOH administration on* in vitro *lymphocyte proliferative responses to mitogen or recall antigen*

In vitro stimulant (μg/ml)	Animal group[a]		
	Untreated	Treated control	ETOH treated
None	1,305[b]	779	918
KLH 500	4,181[c]	2,439[c]	807(33)[d]
KLH 250	2,714[c]	1,886[c]	525(28)
KLH 100	1,253	881	589
Con A 10	407,340	361,748	51,641(14)
Con A 5	420,127	377,096	62,953(17)
Con A 1	371,401	335,430	45,010(13)

[a]Adult male Lewis rats were immunized with keyhole limpet hemocyanin 14 days prior to treatment with 4 days of ETOH by gastric intubation (ETOH treated), treatment with diet only (treated control), or cage mates that were untreated. Microculture lymphocyte proliferation assay was set up using spleen cells obtained from animals on the day after ETOH administration was discontinued. Each group consisted of three to five rats.

[b]Mean counts per minute of tritiated thymidine uptake of quadruplicate cultures stimulated with the indicated material. Standard deviations were generally less than 15%.

[c]Positive response to recall antigen was defined as a stimulation that was at least twice the unstimulated value and significantly different ($p \le 0.01$) from the unstimulated value.

[d]Values in parentheses indicate the percentage of the treated control group's response attained by cells from the ETOH-treated group.

the ability of an animal to resist many infectious diseases. In many laboratories, the response to mitogens has been used as a model for studying the proliferation of T lymphocytes in a clonal manner after exposure to the specific antigen used for immunization. Conceptually, the proliferation in response to mitogens should mimic the response to an antigen, only at a higher magnitude, since more cells are stimulated. Because of this apparent dissociation in responses to mitogens and antigens in the guinea pig treated with ETOH and the obvious importance of secondary recall responses in host defense mechanisms, we have studied this question in our model system.

Rats were immunized with keyhole limpet hemocyanin (KLH) in adjuvant, administered ETOH mixed in a nutritionally adequate liquid diet, and then evaluated for *in vitro* responsiveness to KLH using lymphocyte proliferation. Data from a representative experiment are presented in Table 1, and it can be seen that the response to KLH in the ETOH-treated group was significantly less than the response of cells from animals treated with control diet only. In fact, the responses of the cells from the ETOH-treated animals did not differ from the responses of animals that received only adjuvant and must therefore be considered unresponsive to this antigen. The animals that were intubated with diet only did respond somewhat less than the untreated immunized group, but this difference was not significant.

The responses of cells from the three groups of rats to the T-lymphocyte mitogen

Con A were also suppressed in the ETOH group but not in the control groups. The mitogen responses of both control groups were not significantly different from the responses of age-, number-, and sex-matched animals that were untreated (data not shown). These data, although not conclusive, suggest that the lymphocyte impairment noted in our previous studies extends to antigen-induced responses. The implication of this finding is at least twofold. First, these data suggest that the mechanism of ETOH-induced immunosuppression in the rat is nonspecific and suppresses lymphocyte proliferation regardless of the stimuli. Second, the suppression of T-lymphocyte proliferation in response to recall antigens may be occurring *in vivo* and may in part explain the increased susceptibility to infection reported for alcoholics.

INFLUENCE OF ADRENOCORTICOSTEROIDS ON ETOH-INDUCED IMMUNOSUPPRESSION

Many of the effects of ETOH noted in our studies, most notably the thymic involution and granulocytosis, have also been associated with the administration of adrenocorticosteroids. This, along with previous studies showing elevated levels of corticosteroids in humans during ETOH intake or withdrawal (8,10) and in mice administered ETOH (18), prompted us to study the influence of corticosteroids on ETOH-associated immunosuppression in the rat model.

In initial studies, serum corticosterone levels were determined using RIA methodology in sera obtained from ETOH-treated and control-diet-treated rats at various times during treatment or after treatment was halted. At all times after ETOH administration, animals treated with ETOH showed elevated levels of corticosterone over control intubated rats (T. R. Jerrells et al., *unpublished data*). In both groups, an early (1 to 2 days after initiation of ETOH intubation) peak of corticosterone was noted that was likely caused by the stress of intubation; this peak was higher in animals treated with ETOH. Serum levels of corticosterone in animals intubated with the control diet rapidly declined to base-line levels. In contrast, steroid levels in ETOH-treated animals declined somewhat after the initial peak, but a relatively high serum level was maintained until the withdrawal period, after which a second peak was noted in this group only.

Since the production of corticosteroids was roughly associated with the extent of immunosuppression, we evaluated the effects of ETOH on immune parameters in animals depleted of the ability to make large amounts of corticosteroids by surgical adrenalectomy (ADX). The study of ADX rats was carried out with a lower dose of ETOH because ADX animals were found to be more susceptible to the effects of ETOH, and many did not survive the 8 to 11 g ETOH/kg body weight dose regimen. Even with the reduced dose of ETOH, many of the effects on the immune system that previously were described for rats with functional adrenal glands treated with similar doses of ETOH were observed. In contrast to the data with adrenal-bearing animals, the ADX group did not show as marked a loss of thymocytes or

TABLE 2. Effects of adrenalectomy on lymphoid cell numbers in rats administered ETOH by gastric intubation

Days of treatment[c]	Cell source	Percentage of control[a]	
		Normal[b]	ADX[b]
4	Spleen	100	49*
	Thymus	69*	48*
	Blood[d]	109	154
5	Spleen	63*	80
	Thymus	63*	51*
	Blood	78*	102
9	Spleen	107	103
	Thymus	103	88
	Blood	134	77

[a]Data expressed as a percentage of the cell count values obtained from animals intubated with diet only.
[b]Adrenalectomized or sham-operated rats were administered identical doses of ETOH by gastric intubation.
[c]Animals were given ETOH for 4 days. Withdrawal was on day 5.
[d]Lymphocyte numbers in peripheral blood determined by calculation using the total leukocyte count × percentage of lymphocytes from differentials.
*Significantly different from control at $p < 0.05$.

spleen cells (Table 2). In the majority of experiments, the animals in the ADX group demonstrated some loss of spleen and thymus cells, but the loss was in general significantly less than that observed in the paired group of adrenal-gland-bearing rats administered ETOH. The loss of peripheral blood lymphocytes associated with ETOH administration in this model was essentially reversed by adrenalectomy. In preliminary studies, the proliferative response to mitogens also was not suppressed in the ADX group compared with the treated adrenal-bearing animals (Fig. 7). If this finding is verified in further studies, an important mediating role of corticosteroids in the immunosuppression induced by ETOH can be established. It is also important to establish the role of steroids in the suppression of primary immune responses.

From the present data, it is concluded that many, but perhaps not all, of the effects of ETOH on the immune system are associated with changes in corticosteroid levels that accompany the pharmacologic effects of ETOH and its administration as well as with the corticosteroid changes accompanying ETOH withdrawal. The influence of other pharmacologic mediators in this system is unknown.

HUMAN STUDIES

Many immunological abnormalities have been described in humans in association with abusive ETOH ingestion (1,6,11,12,16,20), a large number of which are also

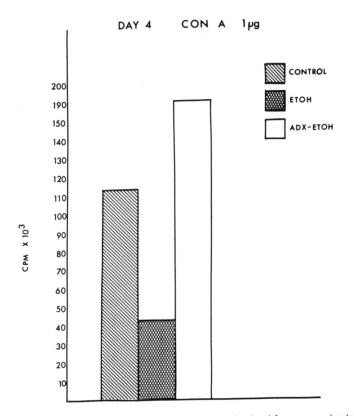

FIG. 7. Proliferative responses of spleen lymphocytes obtained from normal rats treated with control diet or ETOH and adrenalectomized rats treated with ETOH. Each point is the mean ± standard deviation of triplicate cultures. Each group consisted of six to nine animals.

observed in the animal model. In preliminary human studies, peripheral blood mononuclear cells were tested for *in vitro* proliferative responses at the time of hospital admission and at various times during the subsequent abstinence period. All alcoholic patients had detectable ETOH levels at the time of admission. Cells from control subjects were tested at the same time to establish a reference point. The data from one representative alcoholic patient are presented in Fig. 8. It can be seen from these data that the responses of cells from this male alcoholic were somewhat lower at the time of admission than the responses of the male control. A more marked depression of proliferative responses was noted in this patient at the next time cells were obtained, and this was during the period that the concomitants of ETOH withdrawal would be expected. With continued abstinence, the proliferative responses to mitogens were significantly increased over the patient's base-line level and the values obtained during the withdrawal period. The responses of the control subject remained relatively unchanged over this time period and are omitted for clarity.

This pattern, with minor variations, has been seen in several alcoholic patients,

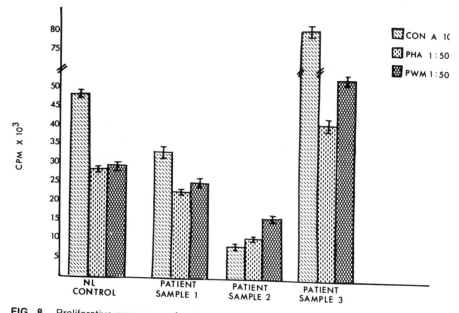

FIG. 8. Proliferative responses of peripheral blood mononuclear cells obtained from a patient at admission and after 3 and 10 days of abstinence. Each point is the mean ± standard deviation of quadruplicate cultures stimulated with concanavalin A, phytohemagglutinin, or poke weed mitogen.

and in our experience, the immunosuppression associated with ETOH withdrawal also is associated with elevated levels of serum cortisol. These data support the validity of the rat model and suggest the possibility that steroids mediate at least *in vitro* immunosuppressive events in human ETOH abuse. In these preliminary studies, we have not been able to document the relatively large cell losses in the human comparable to the cell losses seen in the rat. Using flow cytometry, however, we have noted some indication of shifts in T-lymphocyte subpopulations. It also is suggested by the human studies that adaptation may be a factor in the magnitude of the observable impairments in immune responses.

CONCLUSIONS

The studies we have performed in experimental animal model systems and in humans have established that the administration or consumption of large amounts of ETOH causes measurable changes in immune system functioning. Administration of large amounts of ETOH to rats by intubation is followed by a marked loss of lymphocytes from peripheral lymphoid organs and a depression of immune function, including an inability to respond to a T-dependent antigen with a primary immune response. This inability to produce a primary immune response is relevant to the long-known association of ETOH abuse and decreased resistance to infectious agents and opportunistic pathogens. The inability or deficiency of the primary immune response, along with other documented defects in nonspecific host defense mechanisms (5,7,12,17), are probably major factors involved in the increased susceptibility to infectious agents associated with ETOH abuse.

In contrast to other studies, our data show that the *in vitro* lymphocyte defect noted in ETOH-related animals extends to proliferative responses to recall antigens as well as to mitogens. This defect is the *in vitro* correlate of the skin test or delayed-type hypersensitivity anergy that has been observed in human subjects. The inability of lymphocytes from ETOH-treated animals to respond to a recall antigen suggests that another effect of ETOH abuse is a diminished ability to respond to agents to which the individual has been exposed previously. It is therefore possible that the impaired host defenses would include not only agents to which the individual has not been exposed previously and organisms such as the pneumococcus that do not induce a long-term memory-type immune response but also agents to which the individual may have been exposed or vaccinated against in the past.

It is important to note that the impairments noted in the rat are in the absence of overt liver pathology and in a system in which a large weight loss is not obvious, thus minimizing the influence of hepatic disease and nutritional deficiencies in the immunosuppression noted. It also is interesting to note that many of the findings occurred regardless of how ETOH was administered to the animal, suggesting that the effects observed are caused by ETOH and are not artifacts of how the ETOH is given to the animal.

REFERENCES

1. Berenyi, M. R., Straus, B., and Cruz, D. (1974): *In vitro* and *in vivo* studies of cellular immunity in alcoholic cirrhosis. *Am. J. Dig. Dis.*, 19:199–205.
2. Brayton, R. G., et al. (1970): Effect of alcohol and various diseases on leukocyte mobilization, phagocytosis and intracellular bacterial killing. *N. Engl. J. Med.*, 282:123–128.
3. Caizza, S. S., and Ovary, Z. (1976): Effects of ethanol intake on the immune system of the guinea pig. *J. Stud. Alcohol.*, 37:959–964.
4. Ericsson, C. D., et al. (1980): Mechanisms of host defense in well nourished patients with chronic alcoholism. *Alcoholism Clin. Exp. Res.*, 4:261–265.
5. Galante, D., et al. (1982) Decreased phagocytic and bactericidal activity of the hepatic reticuloendothelial system during chronic ethanol treatment and its restoration by levamisole. *J. Reticuloendothel. Soc.*, 32:179–187.
6. Gluckman, S. J., Dvorak, V. C., and MacGregor, R. R. (1977): Host defenses during prolonged alcohol consumption in a controlled environment. *Arch. Intern. Med.*, 136:1539–1543.
7. Gluckman, S. J., and MacGregor, R. R. (1978): Effect of acute alcohol intoxication on granulocyte mobilization and kinetics. *Blood*, 52:551–559.
8. Jenkins, J. S., and Connolly, J. (1968): Adrenocortical response to ethanol in man. *Br. Med. J.*, 2:804–805.
9. Jerrells, T. R., et al. (1986): Effects of ethanol administration on parameters of immunocompetency in rats. *J. Leukocyte Biol.*, 39:499–510.
10. Kissin, B., Schenker, V., and Schenker, A. C. (1960): The acute effect of ethanol ingestion on plasma and urinary 17-hydroxycorticoids in alcoholic subjects. *Am. J. Med. Sci.*, 239:690–705.
11. Lauria, D. B. (1963): Susceptibility to infection during experimental alcohol intoxication. *Trans. Assoc. Am. Physicians*, 76:102–112.
12. MacGregor, R. R., Gluckman, S. J., and Senior, J. R. (1978): Granulocyte function and levels

of immunoglobulins and complement in patients admitted for withdrawal from alcohol. *J. Infect. Dis.*, 138:747–753.

13. Majchrowicz, E. (1975): Induction of physical dependence upon ethanol and the associated behavioral changes in rats. *Psychopharmacologia*, 43:245–254.
14. Roselle, G. A., and Mendenhall, C. L. (1984): Ethanol-induced alterations in lymphocyte function in the guinea pig. *Alcoholism Clin. Exp. Res.*, 8:62–67.
15. Slone, F. L., Smith, W. I., and VanThiel, D. H. (1977): The effects of alcohol and partial portal ligation on the immune system of the rat. *Gastroenterology*, 72:1133.
16. Smith, W. I., et al. (1980): Altered immunity in male patients with alcoholic liver disease: Evidence for defective immune regulation. *Alcoholism Clin. Exp. Res.*, 4:199–206.
17. Spagnuolo, P. J., and MacGregor, R. R. (1975): Acute ethanol effect on chemotaxis and other components of host defense. *J. Lab. Clin. Med.*, 86:24–31.
18. Tabakoff, B., Jaffe, R. C., and Ritzmann, R. F. (1978): Corticosterone concentrations in mice during ethanol drinking and withdrawal. *J. Pharm. Pharmacol.*, 30:371–374.
19. Tennenbaum, J. I., et al. (1969): The effect of chronic alcohol administration on the immune responsiveness of rats. *J. Allergy*, 44:272–281.
20. Young, G. P., et al. (1970): Lymphopenia and lymphocyte transformation in alcoholics. *Experientia*, 35:268–269.

*Psychological, Neuropsychiatric, and
Substance Abuse Aspects of AIDS,*
edited by T. Peter Bridge et al.
Raven Press, New York © 1988.

Psychoimmunology and AIDS

Lydia Temoshok

*Department of Psychiatry, Langley Porter Psychiatric Institute, University of California at
San Francisco School of Medicine, San Francisco, California 94143*

A BIOPSYCHOSOCIAL APPROACH TO AIDS

The acquired immune deficiency syndrome (AIDS) and AIDS spectrum disorders have emerged as perhaps the most critical public health problem of the 1980s. Although a great deal of effort has been devoted to biomedical research on AIDS etiology and treatment, there is to date no known cure and no known vaccine for AIDS. This situation has led to a search for "cofactors" in AIDS onset and progression.

The complexity of interacting variables in the pathogenesis of immune deficiency and consequent vulnerability to a variety of infections and to cancer led the distinguished immunologist Norman Talal (37) to state, "AIDS teaches us that immunoregulatory diseases are truly multifactorial" (p. 183). The biopsychosocial model of disease, credited to Engel (9), is multifactorial, taking into account the interaction of genetic, biological (specific and nonspecific), emotional (state and trait), behavioral, situational ("stress"), and cultural factors in pathogenesis of all disease, not just those classically considered "psychosomatic." Given a particular genetic composition and/or physical exposure to a disease agent, a number of environmental factors can modify the host's basic immunocompetence to produce a temporarily enhanced immunity or acquired immunodeficiency. Perhaps the most prevalent but least understood of the environmental modulators of human immunocompetence are behavioral or psychosocial factors.

Since AIDS is under an epidemiologic, clinical, and psychosocial cloud of such uncertainty and bleakness, it is difficult to see a silver lining. One pinpoint of light, however, is that because of the increasingly well-documented immunologic relationships as well as the relatively rapid disease progression involving infection and/ or neoplasia, AIDS may be an ideal laboratory to investigate psychoimmunologic relationships. The term psychoimmunology, coined by Solomon in 1964 (34), refers to psychological influences (experience, stress, emotions, traits, and coping) on immune function and on the onset and course of immunologically resisted or mediated diseases (32). The larger field of psychoneuroimmunology deals with the complex bidirectional interactions of the central nervous system and the immune system (1). It is the conviction of our research team, the University of California Biopsychosocial AIDS Project (UCSF-BAP), that a biopsychosocial approach to AIDS research is necessary and that research questions emanating from the fields of health psychology, behavioral medicine, and psychoimmunology/psychoneuroimmunology may provide critical information for understanding and treating AIDS (5).

In this chapter, we consider areas of research that provide appropriate points of departure for psychoimmunologic investigations of AIDS. (The neurology and neuropsychology of AIDS form a complex area of intense recent investigation; a consideration of this work and of psychoneuroimmunologic approaches to AIDS research goes beyond the scope of this chapter.) Evidence from our own investigations in UCSF-BAP is presented for each of these areas.

STRESS, BEHAVIOR, AND IMMUNOLOGY

A number of recent studies in animals and humans have linked stress and/or behavior factors with immune response (e.g., 3,14,28,30) and with disease outcome (e.g., 26,41,42). There are only a handful of studies, however, that examine psychologic and immunologic variables in human patients with immunologically implicated diseases (10,12,20,25,38).

Can Psychosocial Variables Be Correlated with Specific Alterations in Immune Function Associated with HIV Infection?

Psychoneuroimmunologic studies of AIDS spectrum disorders with adequate funding to obtain sufficient laboratory data on a variety of immunologic measures are just underway. Up to this point, the longitudinal psychosocial study of persons with AIDS and ARC conducted by UCSF-BAP has been dependent, unfortunately, on laboratory tests conducted for clinical purposes within 2 weeks of the psychological assessments. Although the timing and the choice of tests are not ideal (i.e., helper/suppressor ratios were not conducted on most subjects), we were able to obtain data on an adequate number of AIDS/ARC subjects ($n = 43$–55 for any given analysis) for numbers of lymphocytes and polymorphonuclear leukocytes (PMNs).

Preliminary results (Table 1) indicate that overall dysphoric affect (as assessed by standard self-report measures of anxiety, mood state, and hopelessness) reflective of relative failure of psychological defenses and/or coping was positively correlated with total white blood cell count as well as with both numbers of polymorphonuclear leukocytes and lymphocytes on differential counts (eight out of 18 significant correlations; two near-significant correlations). The higher number of PMNs in persons psychologically more distressed seems consistent with the greater likelihood of clinical and subclinical infection in those with distress-induced incre-

TABLE 1. *Correlations of PMNs and lymphocytes with psychological self-report scales*

Scales	PMNs	p	Lymphocytes	p	n
Total dysphoria	0.26	<0.10	0.32	0.03	44
Taylor anxiety	0.31	0.02	0.37	0.006	55
Beck hopelessness	0.18	NS	0.27	<0.10	50
POMS confusion	0.08	NS	0.28	0.04	54
POMS dep–dej	0.10	NS	0.30	0.03	54
POMS fat–inr	0.33	0.01	0.29	0.03	53
POMS ten–anx	0.01	NS	0.38	0.004	54
POMS vig–act	−0.36	0.008	−0.23	<0.10	55
POMS ang–host	0.08	NS	0.18	NS	52
"Hardiness"	−0.09	NS	−0.32	0.04	43

mental immune impairment. Because HIV attacks lymphocytes and ultimately results in lymphopenia, the relative lymphocytosis in more distressed individuals is difficult to interpret. Higher lymphocyte and PMN counts also were associated (at near-significant and significant levels, respectively) with lower vigor–activity on the Profile of Mood States scale, whereas only higher lymphocyte counts were associated significantly with lower scores on Kobasa's Hardiness Scale. Perhaps early secondary infection, particularly bacterial, might be an explanation.

As we continue our longitudinal follow-up of these subjects and begin to study new cohorts of HIV antibody-positive, HIV antibody-negative, and ARC subjects, we hope to have the capacity for more meaningful laboratory correlations, including helper–inducer/suppressor–cytotoxic T-cell ratios. However, one of the many difficulties inherent in this area of investigation is that AIDS is such a relatively new phenomenon that the immunologic meaning of some of these laboratory measures is often unclear. For example, although John Fahey at UCLA has documented the importance of absolute number of helper (CD4) T cells in both progression of the disease and survival curves, the decreased number of helper T cells may be merely an indicator of the overall poor health status of the individual and not in itself the cause of that state. Another problem is that many individuals with AIDS and even those with ARC or positive HIV antibody tests are engaged in biological and/or psychosocial interventions that may affect their immunologic and psychologic status. For these reasons, we must be extremely cautious in making any causal interpretations of the findings in Table 1.

PSYCHOSOCIAL FACTORS IN THE PROGRESSION AND OUTCOME OF CANCER

Although one recent prospective study (4) found no relationship between psychosocial factors and the length of time to cancer relapse, there are several reports of positive results (6,7,11,24,27,38). It is difficult to compare the results of these studies because different types of cancer, different levels of severity, different measures, and different follow-up periods were used. However, there appears to be a thread running through all these studies concerning expression or report of emotion or distress, particularly as it relates to adjustment to cancer. Congruencies across studies, both prospective and retrospective, have prompted a number of investigators to posit the existence of a cancer-prone personality style that at least two authors have labeled "type C" (22,39).

Findings by Temoshok et al. (40) suggest that certain psychosocial factors reflecting a theoretical "type C" coping style are associated with unfavorable prognostic indicators for cutaneous malignant melanoma. "Type C" characteristics (e.g., being passive, appeasing, helpless, other-focused, and unexpressive of emotion, particularly anger) were theorized to be the opposite of "type A" characteristics (e.g., being aggressive, impatient, self-involved, and hostile). Temoshok et al. have hypothesized that lack of emotional expression is the pathological core of the type C style. A recent study found that measures of more emotional expression were positively correlated with a prognostically favorable host immune factor and negatively correlated with prognostically unfavorable tumor factors (38).

Solomon's (33) notions of an "autoimmune" pattern (31) and an "immunosuppression-prone" personality share common features with the "type C" coping pattern. Related concepts include McClelland's (21) "inhibited power motivation" and "alexithymia," which is thought to be related to somatic rather than psychological manifestations of emotional conflict (2). Common to all these proposed patterns are compliance, conformity, self-sacrifice, denial of hostility or anger, and nonexpression of emotion.

Is Length of Survival Related to Psychosocial Factors Assessed at an Earlier Time?

A corollary question is whether long survival with AIDS and any psychosocial correlates of long survival are related, in turn, to specific aspects of immune function. UCSF-BAP has begun to explore the possible relationship between psychosocial measures assessed within 2 to 8 weeks of an AIDS or ARC diagnosis and subsequent health outcomes.

Scores on self-report scales obtained at the time of the initial interview were compared for men who were alive as of March, 1986 and those who were deceased. Because most of the variance in outcome is most likely explainable by biological factors, particularly the type of AIDS-associated disorder, we conducted separate analyses for three groups: AIDS subjects with *Pneumocystis carinii* pneumonia (PCP) ($n = 21$), AIDS subjects with Kaposi's sarcoma ($n = 28$), and ARC subjects ($n = 53$). The results of this analysis that bear on the current topic are those for the subjects with ARC. (The results for subjects with AIDS-PCP will be discussed in the two subsequent sections. There were no significant differences between outcome groups on psychosocial scales for AIDS subjects with Kaposi's sarcoma.)

For ARC subjects, three psychosocial variables were significantly different between the deceased and alive groups: (a) the Marlowe–Crowne Social Desirability Scale ($M = 12.9$ in the deceased group, $M = 8.9$ in the alive group; $p < 0.009$, two-tailed); (b) and anger–hostility subscale on the Profile of Mood States scale ($M = 4.2$ for the deceased group, $M = 7.1$ for the alive group; $p = 0.05$, two-tailed); and (c) Kobasa's "commitment" subscale ($M = 56.4$ for the deceased group, $M = 53.3$ for the alive group; $p < 0.03$, two-tailed).

Because of the small sample sizes, group differences in average length of time in the study at follow-up, and the fact that numerous univariate tests for differences were conducted in this analysis, extreme caution is warranted in interpreting these results. Further, the variables cited above as significant may be only incidentally related to outcome because they are associated with another variable that is causally related to outcome. Thus, these preliminary results are presented more to engage other researchers in posing hypotheses about the possible relationships of psychosocial variables to outcome in AIDS.

Finding higher social desirability scores in the unfavorable-outcome group for men with ARC is consistent with some reports in the cancer literature about the negative effects of the so-called "type C" coping style (40) and the "autoimmune personality" pattern (31). Other investigators in psychosocial oncology (11,24) have provided evidence for the beneficial effects on cancer outcome of "fighting spirit" as an adjustment style. Such work supports the finding that the favorable ARC outcome group was initially significantly higher on the Profile of Mood States anger–hostility subscale than the unfavorable-outcome group. The finding about Kobasa's "commitment" subscale (explained below) was unexpected. Although a sense of meaning is an important variable in times of stress and coping with disease, it may be particularly critical for individuals who may be further along on the disease trajectory. Thus, it may be that we tapped this higher level of commitment (as more of a state than a trait) in the group of individuals who may have felt that their death was nearer at hand and who did indeed die.

"HARDINESS" AND HEALTH

Kobasa and her colleagues have produced an impressive array of studies providing evidence for a buffering effect of a personality style they call "hardiness" and exercise on stress and consequent stress-related illness (16). According to these authors, hardiness has three components: control, commitment, and challenge. People low in control tend to feel powerless in the face of overwhelming forces. They have the "helpless–hopeless" attitude associated in an increasing number of studies in both humans and animals (19) with poor health outcomes. Commitment is the opposite of alienation, according to Kobasa et al.; people high on this dimension find meaning in their work, values, and personal relationships. People high on the challenge dimension interpret potentially stressful events as challenges to be met with expected success rather than as threats.

Preliminary Outcome Data on Men with AIDS-PCP

In our longitudinal psychosocial study of men with AIDS and ARC described above, we compared self-report measures obtained 2 to 8 weeks after the diagnosis of AIDS-PCP (*Pneumocystis carinii* pneumonia) for men who had died ($n = 10$) by follow-up and those who were still alive ($n = 11$). The men in the favorable-outcome group had scored significantly ($p < 0.05$) higher than those in the unfavorable-outcome group on Kobasa's control measure (mean $= 65.0 \pm 5.6$ versus 60.0 ± 5.3). As above, however, caution must be used in interpreting these results because of the small sample sizes and the number of univariate tests conducted. Further, causation cannot be assumed from this correlation. The two outcome groups are significantly different in terms of time from initial interview to follow-up, the favorable-outcome group having a shorter period of time in the study (378.3 days) than the unfavorable-outcome group (481.5 days). Moreover, Kobasa's control measure is positively correlated ($r = 0.56$; $p = 0.01$) with time of the initial interview, which means that subjects with a longer time in the study score lower on the control measure. Again, this may be a state rather than a trait influence: subjects with a longer time in the study have been diagnosed longer (initial interviews were conducted for all subjects within 2 to 8 weeks of diagnosis), and it may well be that the longer one has AIDS, the less in control one feels as a succession of treatments fail to work and one gets progressively weaker and more ill.

With these caveats in mind, we will speculate briefly on the possible meaning of these preliminary findings. We view the significant differences between AIDS-PCP outcome groups on Kobasa's "control" subscale as consistent with the literature on helplessness–hopelessness (11,18,19,24,29). According to Kobasa (16), people low in control (as a "trait") tend to feel powerless in the face of overwhelming forces. When stressful events occur, such persons have little basis for optimistic cognitive appraisals or decisive actions that could transform events or concerns. As their coping styles provide little or no buffer, stressful events are given free rein to have a debilitating effect on health (18).

SOCIAL SUPPORT

For over a decade, social support has been posited to play a significant role in health and illness. In recent years, however, several critical reviews have tempered the enthusiasm among social scientists for social support as either a causal agent or a powerful buffering mechanism in disease morbidity and mortality (13,36). Nonetheless, there remains a general consensus among reviewers that social support has both theoretical and practical importance as a health-related resource. Further, there are several recent studies (e.g., 14) in which aspects of social support have been related to immunologic measures.

Preliminary Outcome Data on Men with AIDS-PCP

In our longitudinal psychosocial study of AIDS and ARC, we examined differences between ratings of emotionally sustaining forms of help (i.e., someone to talk to; someone who understands your problems; someone who expresses confidence in you) and problem-solving help (i.e., someone who gives you suggestions or advice about how to solve a problem; someone who explains or shows you how he/she has dealt with problems similar to your own) for subjects with AIDS-PCP (*Pneumocystis carinii* pneumonia) who had died or who were alive by follow-up. (This was the same comparison made in the section above discussing Kobasa's Hardiness construct.)

The only social support measure that distinguished the group of AIDS-PCP subjects still alive ($n = 11$) from those who had died ($n = 10$) was the rating of Problem-Solving Help Used ($t = 2.56$, $df = 19$, $p < 0.05$). The favorable-outcome group seems to have utilized significantly more problem-solving help than the unfavorable-outcome group. Problem-Solving Help Used was not significantly related to time of the initial interview. As with the other AIDS outcome result reported above, however, this finding should be regarded as preliminary and interpreted with caution. The finding that the favorable-outcome group seems to have utilized significantly more problem-solving help is consistent with research at UCLA on the benefits to mental health, at least, of active–behavioral coping (in comparison to active–cognitive and avoidance coping methods) in men with AIDS (23). Professionally led group interventions with AIDS patients aimed to enhance problem solving and coping or relaxation led to less depression and anxiety and to more active and less avoidant coping. An unstructured "emotional support group" seemed to engender greater anxiety and had many drop-outs.

LINKING PSYCHOLOGIC AND IMMUNOLOGIC FACTORS TO OUTCOME

There are no published studies of which we are aware that relate psychologic and immunologic variables to disease outcome variables (although many have been proposed and some are currently underway). Possible reasons for this include (a) the expense of conducting adequate immunologic tests, (b) the unknown temporal relationship between an external stressor, behavior, or intrapsychic event and immunologic reaction, (c) the usually unclear causal relationship between immunologic events and disease outcome, and (d) the typically long delays in prospective or longitudinal studies between psychologic testing and outcome—disease initiation, progression, or death.

The University of California Biopsychosocial AIDS Project has almost completed an intensive psychoimmunologic study of survival and AIDS (35). Although the prevalent belief among the general public, persons with AIDS, and even the professional community is that AIDS is invariably fatal, there are a growing number of individuals who are alive and well 3, 4, and even 5 years after an AIDS diagnosis. Our aim in the current study is to look intensively at the exceptional AIDS "survivors" in order to understand how they are different from others who have a more expected course of disease.

An important aspect of the present study is to understand the complex interactions among emotional expression, autonomic activity, and immune measures in persons with AIDS. Our interest in psychophysiological variables was prompted by a previous study (15) that defined "repressive coping style" as the interactive combination of certain psychological and psychophysiological measures and found that malignant melanoma patients were significantly more "repressive" in style, whereas matched cardiac patients were the most "sensitized." We based our methods in the current study on another relevant report (8), which found a robust differentiation in autonomic nervous system activity among six basic emotions. To the extent that behavior, including emotional expression or suppression/repression, has psychophysiological concomitants, it will affect immunologic state and, consequently, immunologically mediated diseases such as AIDS. In the "AIDS survivors" study, we will be able not only to compare psychological, emotional, psychophysiological, and immunologic variables in the exceptional AIDS survivor and the AIDS patient who is doing as expected, but we will be able to assess the prospective relationship of these variables to length of survival for all our subjects, who will have medical follow-ups until death (or interim follow-up data analysis). Such a study may provide important clues to why some AIDS patients survive longer, even when biological and treatment variables are equivalent. These clues can then form the basis of a biopsychosocial intervention study. Such a study may also provide a step in the understanding of mediators of relationships among cognitive, emotional, autonomic, and immunologic phenomena.

COMMENT

We believe that AIDS as a multifactorial disease offers a unique opportunity to explore the relationships among psychological, immunologic, and health outcome variables. Certain underlying uncertainties affect all research that attempts to explore relationships between psychosocial and immune variables. Problems are compounded by effects of disease processes themselves on the immune system, particularly in the case of a disease whose agent is "lympholethal." Certain diseases, including cancer and infections (particularly viral), are both immunosuppressive and psychologically distressing. How can one sort out "direct" from indirect psychologically mediated effects?

Other problems are of particular relevance to psychoimmunologic studies of AIDS. Such studies need to take into account sexual and drug use histories (semen and many recreational drugs are immunosuppressive) as well as medical and other interventions that may also affect the immune system. In the current state of knowledge about immunology and AIDS, it is unclear whether a certain level of a parameter is "good" or "bad" in terms of a person's current state of health and/or AIDS prognosis.

We need to apply what is known in the field of immunity to some basic issues in order to understand the psychosocial correlates of immunopathology and disease and to be convinced that these associations are meaningful. A major problem is timing of assessment of immune variables in relationship to the psychosocial variables. What is the "lag" between the presence of a psychological state and its influence on an immune function; or conversely, what is the "lag" between a particular immunologic aberration and the psychological state? Does it not seem likely that such "lags" vary among specific aspects of immune function? What specific aspects of immune function are most relevant to health? What homeostatic adjustments may compensate for insults or defects? At this point in psychoimmunologic research on AIDS or, indeed, any disease, there are many questions and virtually no answers. We believe, however, that by posing some of these questions in the context of previous work in psychoimmunology and our own preliminary findings, other researchers may be stimulated to approach this research frontier.

ACKNOWLEDGMENTS

Some of the concepts in this chapter have appeared, in another context, in a paper by G. F. Solomon and L. Temoshok, A psychoneuroimmunologic perspective on AIDS research: Questions, preliminary findings, and suggestions (*Journal of Applied Social Psychology,* 17:286–308, 1987). All the psychosocial AIDS research reported in this chapter was supported by NIMH grant No. MH39344 (principal investigator: L. Temoshok). The intensive psychoimmunologic study of long-surviving persons with AIDS is being supported by a grant from the Kroc Foundation in Los Angeles (co-principal investigators: L. Temoshok and G. F. Solomon). The immunologic component of that study was developed by Daniel P. Stites at the University of California San Francisco School of Medicine. I wish to thank the following members of the UCSF Biopsychosocial AIDS Project who have contributed to the work presented in this chapter: Mildred Dubzinsky, Susan Engleman, Robert Gorter, Phillip Hull, Ulrich Ledermann, Jeffrey S. Mandel, Jeffrey M. Moulton, Ann O'Leary, George F. Solomon, Kristy Straits, David M. Sweet, William Woods, and Jane Zich. I am particularly indebted to Dr. Solomon for many of the ideas presented in this chapter.

REFERENCES

1. Ader, R., editor (1981): *Psychoneuroimmunology.* Academic Press, New York.
2. Apfel, R., and Sifneos, P. (1979): Alexithymia: Concept and measurement. *Psychother. Psychosom.,* 32:180–190.

3. Bartrop, R. W., et al. (1977): Depressed lymphocyte function after bereavement. *Lancet,* 1:834–836.
4. Cassileth, B. E., et al. (1985): Psychosocial correlates of survival in advanced malignant disease? *N. Engl. J. Med.,* 312:1551–1555.
5. Coates, T. J., Temoshok, L., and Mandel, J. S. (1984): Biopsychosocial research is essential to understanding and treating AIDS. *Am. Psychol.,* 39:1309–1314.
6. Derogatis, L. R., Abeloff, M. D., and Melisaratos, N. (1979): Psychological coping mechanisms and survival time in metastatic breast cancer. *J.A.M.A.,* 242:1504–1508.
7. DiClemente, R. J., and Temoshok, L. (1985): Psychological adjustment to having cutaneous malignant melanoma as a predictor of follow-up clinical status. *Psychosom. Med.,* 47:81.
8. Ekman, P., Levenson, R. W., and Friesen, W. V. (1983): Autonomic nervous system activity distinguishes among emotions. *Science,* 221:1208–1210.
9. Engel, G. (1960): A unified concept of health and disease. *Perspect. Med. Biol.,* 3:459–485.
10. Glaser, R. J., et al. (1985): Stress, loneliness and changes in herpes virus latency. *J. Behav. Med.,* 8:249–260.
11. Greer, S., Morris, T., and Pettingale, K. W. (1979): Psychological response to breast cancer: Effect on outcome. *Lancet,* 13:785–787.
12. Kemeny, M., Zegans, L. S., and Cohen, F. (1987): Stress, mood, immunity and recurrence of genital herpes. *Ann. N.Y. Acad. Sci.,* 496:735–736.
13. Kessler, R. C., and McLeod, J. (1984): Social support and psychological distress in community surveys. In: *Social Support and Health,* edited by S. Coehn and L. Syme, pp. 219–240. Academic Press, New York.
14. Kiecolt-Glaser, J. K., et al. (1984): Urinary cortisol levels, cellular immunocompetency, and loneliness in psychiatric inpatients. *Psychosom. Med.,* 46:15–23.
15. Kneier, A. W., and Temoshok, L. (1984): Repressive coping reactions in patients with malignant melanoma as compared to cardiovascular disease patients. *J. Psychosom. Res.,* 28:145–155.
16. Kobasa, S. C. (1979): Stressful life events, personality and health: An inquiry into hardiness. *J. Pers. Soc. Psychol.,* 37:1–11.
17. Kobasa, S. C., Maddi, S. R., and Courington, S. (1980): Personality and constitution as mediators in the stress-illness relationship. *J. Health Soc. Behav.,* 22:368–378.
18. Laudenslager, M. D., et al. (1983): Coping and immunosuppression: Inescapable but not escapable shock suppresses lymphocytes proliferation. *Science,* 221:568–580.
19. Levy, S. M. (1985): Behavior as a biological response modifier: The psychoimmunoendocrine network and tumor immunology. *Behav. Med. Abstr.,* 6:1–4.
20. Levy, S. M., et al. (1985): Prognostic risk assessment in primary breast cancer by behavioral and immunological parameters. *Health Psychol.,* 4:99–113.
21. McClelland, D., et al. (1980): Stressed power motivation, sympathetic activation, immune function, and illness. *J. Hum. Stress,* 6:11–19.
22. Morris, T. (1980): A 'type C' for cancer? Low trait anxiety in the pathogenesis of breast cancer. *Cancer Detect. Prev.,* 3: Abstract no. 102.
23. Namir, S., Fawzy, D., and Wolcott, D. (1988): Group interventions in people with AIDS: Results of three interventions. *Psychiatric Med., (in press).*
24. Pettingale, K. W. (1984): Coping and cancer prognosis. *J. Psychosom. Res.,* 28:363–364.
25. Pettingale, K. W., Greer, S., and Tee, D. E. H. (1977): Serum IgA and emotional expression in breast cancer patients. *J. Psychosom. Res.,* 21:395–399.
26. Riley, V. (1981): Psychoneuroendocrine influences on immunocompetence and neoplasia. *Science,* 212:1100–1109.
27. Rogentine, S., et al. (1979): Psychological factors in the prognosis of malignant melanoma. *Psychosom. Med.,* 41:647–658.
28. Schleifer, S. J., et al. (1983): Suppression of lymphocyte stimulation following bereavement. *J.A.M.A.,* 250:374–377.
29. Schmale, A. H., and Iker, H. P. (1966): The affect of hopelessness and the development of cancer. *Psychosom. Med.,* 28:714–721.
30. Sklar, L., and Anisman, H. (1979): Stress and coping factors influence tumor growth. *Science,* 205:513–515.
31. Solomon, G. F. (1981): Emotional and personality factors in the onset and course of autoimmune disease, particularly rheumatoid arthritis. In: *Psychoneuroimmunology,* edited by R. Ader, pp. 159–182. Academic Press, New York.

32. Solomon, G. F. (1987): Psychoneuroimmunologic approaches to research on AIDS. *Ann. N.Y. Acad. Sci.*, 496:628–636.
33. Solomon, G. F. (1987): Psychoneuroimmunology. In: *The Encyclopedia of Neuroscience*, edited by G. Adelman, pp. 1001–1004. Birkhauser, Cambridge, MA.
34. Solomon, G. F., and Moos, R. H. (1964): Emotions, immunity, and disease: A speculative theoretical integration. *Arch. Gen. Psychiatry*, 11:657–764.
35. Solomon, G. F., Temoshok, L., O'Leary, A., and Zich, J. (1987): An intensive psychoimmunologic study of long-surviving persons with AIDS: Pilot work, background studies, hypotheses, and methods. *Ann. N.Y. Acad. Sci.*, 496:647–655.
36. Starker, J. (1986): Methodological and conceptual issues in research on social support. *Hosp. Commun. Psychiatry*, 37:485–490.
37. Talal, N. (1983): A clinician and a scientist looks at acquired immune deficiency syndrome, AIDS: A validation of immunology's theoretical foundation. *Immun. Today*, 4(Suppl.):180–183.
38. Temoshok, L. (1985): Biopsychosocial studies on cutaneous malignant melanoma: Psychosocial factors associated with prognostic indicators, progression, psychophysiology, and tumor-host response. *Soc. Sci. Med.*, 20:833–840.
39. Temoshok, L., and Fox, B. H. (1984): Coping styles and other psychosocial factors related to medical status and to prognosis in patients with cutaneous malignant melanoma. In: *Impact of Psychoendocrine Systems in Cancer and Immunity*, edited by B. H. Fox and B. H. Newberry, pp. 258–287. C. J. Hogrefe, Inc., Toronto.
40. Temoshok, L., et al. (1985): The relationship of psychosocial factors to prognostic indicators in cutaneous malignant melanoma. *J. Psychosom. Res.*, 29:139–153.
41. Temoshok, L., et al. (1987): Stress-behavior interactions in hamster tumor growth. *Ann. N.Y. Acad. Sci.*, 496:501–509.
42. Visintainer, M. A., Volpicelli, J. R., and Seligman, M. E. (1982): Tumor rejection in rats after inescapable or escapable shock. *Science*, 216:1100–1109.

*Psychological, Neuropsychiatric, and
Substance Abuse Aspects of AIDS,*
edited by T. Peter Bridge et al.
Raven Press, New York © 1988.

Immunomodulation by Classical Conditioning

*Nicholas Cohen and †Robert Ader

*Departments of *Microbiology and Immunology and †Psychiatry, University of Rochester
School of Medicine and Dentistry, Rochester, New York 14642*

Application of the principles and techniques of behavioral conditioning represents one of the more dramatic lines of evidence that underscores the importance of behavioral (and therefore central nervous system) processes in the modulation of immunity. Since we recently reviewed conditioning and immunomodulation elsewhere in great detail (4), this contribution will only highlight facets of this area of active research.

Our hypothesis that immunological reactivity could be conditioned derived from the serendipitous observation of mortality in an experiment on taste aversion learning (1). Following consumption of different volumes of a novel, saccharin-flavored drinking solution (the conditioned stimulus or CS), rats were injected with the immunosuppressive drug cyclophosphamide (the unconditioned stimulus or US). After the single conditioning trial, animals were reexposed to the saccharin solution every 3 days without being injected with the drug. An unexpected mortality rate was found to vary directly with the volume of the saccharin solution consumed on the conditioning trial (i.e., with the magnitude of the conditioned aversion to saccharin).

In our initial experiment designed to test the hypothesis that the immunopharmacological effects of cyclophosphamide (CY) had been conditioned (2), similarly conditioned animals were immunized with sheep red blood cells (SRBC). Conditioned animals that were reexposed to the CS at the time of antigenic stimulation (and/or 3 days later) had lower antibody titers than control groups that were comprised of (a) conditioned animals that were not reexposed to the CS, (b) unconditioned animals that were presented with saccharin, and (c) placebo-treated animals. These data were taken as evidence of a conditioned immunosuppressive response.

Despite the initial reaction to these observations, our early findings were rapidly verified by other investigators (20,24). Conditioned immunosuppressive antibody responses have now been observed in mice (as well as rats) in response to a T-cell-independent antigen (11) and in experiments involving different conditioned stimuli (4). Conditioned suppression of antibody responses has also been observed in studies measuring splenic plaque-forming cells (PFCs) (15,18). Also, the phenomenon has been confirmed in the use of conditioning to attenuate arthritic inflammation in rats (16) and in depression of the PFC response in mice to a CS previously paired with "stressful" stimulation (22).

The generality of the phenomenon has been further documented by studies indicating that conditioning with CY as an US can influence cell-mediated as well as antibody-mediated immunity. In one study (9), a graft-versus-host (GvH) response was induced in rats 7 weeks after they had been conditioned by pairing saccharin with CY. Conditioned animals reexposed to the CS showed an attenuated GvH response, and when unreinforced CS reexposures were introduced during the interval between conditioning and immunogenic stimulation, extinction of the conditioned immunosuppressive response proved to be a function of the number of unreinforced CS presentations (10). In another more recent study (19), the natural killer cell response of rats was suppressed following CS exposure.

The acquisition and extinction of a conditioned increase in the precursor frequency of cytotoxic T lymphocytes has also been demonstrated (14). This experiment involved neither an immunosuppressive regimen nor taste aversion learning; the CS consisted of the procedures and stimulation associated with skin allotransplantation in mice. Other observations of conditioned alterations of immunity have involved: the conditioned release of histamine (21); the use of antilymphocyte serum (a biological rather than a pharmacological immunosuppressant) as the US (17); a conditioned impairment of antitumor immunity that could be reversed by cimetidine, an antagonist of type-II histamine receptors found on suppressor T cells (13); and a conditioned enhancement of a delayed hypersensitivity (DH) reaction to SRBC (12). Other preliminary data suggest that conditioning can also modify DH reactions in humans (23).

Conditioned immunosuppression does not appear to be antigen dependent (i.e., the antigen does not need to interact with the CS to effect immunosuppression). This statement is based on experiments in which conditioned rats were presented with the CS and then, at varying times afterward, injected with antigen. In one protocol (5), when animals were immunized with SRBC 4 weeks after conditioning (2 weeks after the CS was presented), a significantly depressed response was still noted in the conditioned group relative to the nonconditioned controls or conditioned animals that were never exposed to the CS. This experiment underscores the idea that the conditioned immunosuppression is not antigenically specific. In other words, antigen is but one of several possible probes that can be used to reveal that conditioning effects an alteration in the immune system.

These conditioned immunopharmacological effects cannot be attributed to a stress-induced or conditioned elevation in adrenocortical steroids (6). Lithium chloride, for example, is effective in inducing a conditioned taste aversion and in elevating steroid levels, but it is not immunosuppressive under these conditions and does not result in an attenuated antibody response when conditioned animals are reexposed to the CS (2). Also, in animals conditioned with CY, injections of LiCl or corticosterone instead of reexposure to the CS does not depress the antibody response (6).

To assess the biological impact of conditioned immunosuppressive responses, conditioning techniques were applied in the chemotherapy of autoimmune disease in New Zealand mice (3). These animals develop systemic lupus erythematosus and die within 8 to 14 months of age, a process that can be delayed by weekly treatments with CY. Based on conditioning principles, we paired saccharin consumption with CY and, in experimental animals, presented only saccharin plus intraperitoneal injections of saline on half of the chemotherapy trials. As hypothesized, the development of disease and mortality were delayed in conditioned mice relative to non-conditioned animals treated with the same amount of saccharin and CY. Preliminary studies of extinction indicated that when chemotherapy was discontinued, the mortality rate in conditioned mice that continued to be exposed to the CS on a weekly basis approximated that of mice that continued to receive active drug.

Although no one has yet fully delineated the mechanisms involved in the behavioral modulation of immunity, those data that we and others have collected on conditioned alterations of immunological reactivity provide compelling evidence of a fundamental integration of behavioral, neuroendocrine, and immune processes of adaptation. Our experiments with autoimmune mice dramatically point out that even if conditioned modulation reveals only fine tuning of the immune system, fine tuning can have profound effects on the health of an animal. It appears that, like all other biological systems functioning in the interests of homeostasis, the immune system is integrated with other psychophysiological processes and, as such, is subject to regulation or modulation by the brain. It is reasonable to hypothesize that such regulation is involved in mediating at least some of the effects of psychosocial factors on the susceptibility to and/or progression of some disease processes. Since there is increasing evidence that the interactions between CNS and the immune system are reciprocal (4), it is also reasonable to expect that the immune status of an animal may, in fact, modify that animal's behavior. Recent studies with another strain of autoimmune-prone mouse suggest that this expectation may indeed be a reality (8).

ACKNOWLEDGMENTS

Support for research from the authors' laboratory has been provided by grant MH-42051 from the U.S.P.H.S.; R.A. is the recipient of Research Scientist Award MH-06318 from the U.S.P.H.S.

REFERENCES

1. Ader, R. (1974): Letter to the editor. *Psychosom. Med.*, 36:183–184.
2. Ader, R., and Cohen, N. (1975): Behaviorally conditioned immunosuppression. *Psychosom. Med.*, 37:333–340.
3. Ader, R., and Cohen, N. (1982): Behaviorally conditioned immunosuppression and murine systemic lupus erythematosus. *Science*, 215:1534–1536.

4. Ader, R., and Cohen, N. (1985): CNS–immune system interactions: Conditioning phenomena. *Behav. Brain Sci.*, 8:379–426.
5. Ader, R., Cohen, N., and Bovbjerg, D. (1982): Conditioned suppression of humoral immunity in the rat. *J. Comp. Physiol. Psychol.*, 96:517–521.
6. Ader, R., Cohen, N., and Grota, L. F. (1979): Adrenal involvement in conditioned immuno-suppression. *Int. J. Immunopharmacol.*, 1:141–146.
7. Ader, R., Cohen, N., and Grota, L. J. (1987): Adrenocortical steroids in the conditioned suppression and enhancement of immune responses. In: *Hormones and Immunity*, edited by I. Berczei, pp. 231–246. MTP Press, Lancaster, England.
8. Ader, R., Grota, L. J., and Cohen, N. (1987): Conditioning phenomena and immune function. *Ann. N.Y. Acad. Sci.*, 496:532–544.
9. Bovbjerg, D., Ader, R., and Cohen, N. (1982): Behaviorally conditioned suppression of graft-vs-host responses. *Proc. Natl. Acad. Sci. U.S.A.*, 79:583–585.
10. Bovbjerg, D., Ader, R., and Cohen, N. (1984): Acquisition and extinction of a graft-vs-host response in the rat. *J. Immunol.*, 132:111–113.
11. Cohen, N., Ader, R., Green, N., and Bovbjerg, D. (1979): Conditioned suppression of a thy-mus-independent antibody response. *Psychosom. Med.*, 41:487–491.
12. Bovbjerg, D., Cohen, N., and Ader, R. (1987): Behaviorally conditioned enhancement of de-layed type hypersensitivity in the mouse. *Brain Behav. Immunity*, 1:64–71.
13. Gorczynski, R., Kennedy, M., and Ciampi, A. (1985): Cimetidine reverses tumor growth en-hancement of plasmacytoma tumors in mice demonstrating conditioned immunosuppression. *J. Immunol.*, 134:4261–4266.
14. Gorczynski, R. M., Macrae, S., and Kennedy, J. (1982): Conditioned immune response asso-ciated with allogeneic skin grafts in mice. *J. Immunol.*, 129:704–709.
15. Gorczynski, R. M., Macrae, S., and Kennedy, M. (1984): Factors involved in the classical conditioning of antibody responses in mice. In: *Breakdown in Human Adaptation to Stress: Towards a Multidisciplinary Approach*, Vol. 2, edited by R. Ballieux, J. Fielding, and A. L'Ab-bate, pp. 704–712. Martinus Nijhoff, The Hague.
16. Klosterhalfen, W., and Klosterhalfen, S. (1983): Pavlovian conditioning of immunosuppression modifies adjuvant arthritis in rats. *Behav. Neurosci.*, 97:663–666.
17. Kusnecov, A. W., Sivyer, M., King, M. G., Husband, A. J., Cripps, A. W., and Clancy, R. L. (1983): Behaviorally conditioned suppression of the immune response by antilymphocyte serum. *J. Immunol.*, 130:2117–2120.
18. McCoy, D. F., Roszman, T. L., Miller, J. S., Kelly, K. S., and Titus, J. J. (1986): Some parameters of conditioned immunosuppression. Species differences and CS-US delay. *Physiol. Behav.*, 36:731–736.
19. O'Reilly, C. A., and Exon, J. H. (1986): Cyclophosphamide-conditioned suppression of the natural killer cell response in rats. *Physiol. Behav.*, 17:759–764.
20. Rogers, M. P., Reich, P., Strom, T., and Carpenter, C. B. (1976): Behaviorally conditioned immunosuppression: Replication of a recent study. *Psychosom. Med.*, 38:447–451.
21. Russell, M., Dark, K. A., Cummins, R. W., Ellman, G., Callaway, E., and Peeke, H. V. S. (1984): Learned histamine release. *Science*, 225:733–734.
22. Sato, K., Flood, J. G., and Makinodan, T. (1984): Influence of conditioned psychological stress on immunological recovery in mice exposed to low-dose X-irradiation. *Radiat. Res.*, 98:381–388.
23. Smith, G. R., and McDaniels, S. M. (1983): Psychologically mediated effect on the delayed hypersensitivity reaction to tuberculin in humans. *Psychosom. Med.*, 45:65–70.
24. Wayner, E. A., Flannery, G. R., and Singer, G. (1978): Effects of taste aversion conditioning on the primary antibody response to sheep red blood cells and *Brucella abortus* in the albino rat. *Physiol. Behav.*, 21:995–1000.

Psychological, Neuropsychiatric, and
Substance Abuse Aspects of AIDS,
edited by T. Peter Bridge et al.
Raven Press, New York © 1988.

Stress-Associated Immune Suppression and Acquired Immune Deficiency Syndrome (AIDS)

*Ronald Glaser and †Janice Kiecolt-Glaser

*Department of Medical Microbiology and Immunology, *Comprehensive Cancer Center,
and †Department of Psychiatry, The Ohio State University College of Medicine,
Columbus, Ohio 43210

Studies from several laboratories have shown that a variety of stressors down-regulate the immune response in animals as well as humans. Several components of the cellular immune response have been shown to be involved in this association, including the ability to control and maintain latent herpesviruses. It has now been shown that the oncogenic retrovirus (HTLV-III/LAV) associated with acquired immune deficiency syndrome (AIDS) can latently infect human T lymphocytes. The data obtained from studies on neuroimmunodulation may have implications for the clinical course of immune suppression associated with AIDS.

It has now been established that there are multiple mechanisms whereby the central nervous system (CNS) and the immune system interact with each other. For example, it has been shown that there are nerve endings in different lymphoid organs, such as the spleen and lymph nodes. The endocrine system has also been implicated as a mediator between the CNS and the immune systems; certain hormones such as cortisol can regulate certain aspects of cellular immunity (9,25). In addition, it has been possible to demonstrate receptors on the surface of lymphocytes to hormones such as ACTH, and lymphocytes may be able to produce certain hormones as well (32). Thus, the demonstration of neuroimmunomodulation in animals and humans may partially explain anecdotal data suggesting that certain kinds of stressors may increase risk for a variety of infectious diseases, and perhaps even cancer, providing some legitimate scientific evidence. The study of "psychoneuroimmunology" has included the examination of the immune response in association with severe stressors such as depression and bereavement, and decrements in cellular immunity have been demonstrated (1,35,54).

It has now been shown by several laboratories that a variety of stressors can modulate cellular immunity. It has been hypothesized that stress-related alterations in immune function may be associated with increased susceptibility to infectious disease and perhaps to cancer. Previous work from our laboratory has been concerned with studying the effect of commonplace stressors on cellular immune function. For example, we have found reproducible significant decrements in natural killer (NK) cell activity using two different target cells in three different medical student studies in which we examined the impact of academic stress on immunity. We have also found a decrease in the percentage of NK cells using two independent measures. Similar reliable immunological changes found associated with examinations were also found in the total number of T lymphocytes as well as in changes in the percentages of subpopulations of T lymphocytes, mitogen responsiveness, interferon (IFN) production by peripheral blood lymphocytes (PBLs) stimulated with concanavalin A (Con A), and the ability of the cellular immune response to be modulated in connection with the expression of three latent herpesviruses (17,23,36,37).

CHANGES IN CELLULAR IMMUNITY ASSOCIATED WITH PSYCHOLOGICAL STRESS

Over the past several years, our laboratory has been involved in studying different aspects of cellular immunity and the impact of a variety of psychological stressors on the maintenance of the cellular immune response, including percentages of subpopulations of lymphocytes. Blood samples were obtained at a base-line period approximately 1 month prior to a block of examinations at The Ohio State University College of Medicine in the first 2 years of the curriculum. The examinations in different specialties are given all together over a 1- to 3-day period throughout the academic year; thus, the medical class in this program cycles together as a group through examination periods. We have taken advantage of this arrangement to study the effects of academic stress on immunity and health. The cellular immune response was studied by testing for quantitative and qualitative changes in lymphocytes obtained from base-line blood samples as well as from blood samples obtained on the day of examinations. In addition, self-report data were also obtained in order to determine if there were changes in psychological stress associated with taking examinations. The results obtained from multiple studies with first-year and second-year medical students are reproducible and have demonstrated that there is a decrease in the mitogenic response to both Con A and phytohemagglutinin (PHA) by lymphocytes obtained on the day of examinations. We have also found that there was a decrease in NK lysis and in the percentages of OKT-4$^+$ (helper) T lymphocytes and OKT-8$^+$ (suppressor) lymphocytes under these circumstances as well as changes in total T lymphocytes (OKT-3$^+$). The reduction in NK cell lysis was not dependent on the target cell used in the assay (17,36,37).

In a separate study, we examined the mitogenic response of lymphocytes obtained from inpatient psychiatric patients (nonmedicated) as well as NK activity. The patient population was divided into high- and low-loneliness groups using the UCLA Loneliness Scale. We found that the patients in the high-loneliness group had a poorer mitogenic response to PHA as well as poorer NK lysis when compared to the patients in the lower-loneliness group (38). These data are consistent with data from our studies on academic stress.

EFFECT OF STRESS ON THE MAINTENANCE OF LATENT HERPESVIRUS

There has been speculation that links stress and the appearance, duration, and intensity of herpesvirus infections with the presumption that these changes reflect alterations in cellular immunity. For example, it was found that there was an increased risk for infection by Epstein–Barr virus (EBV) in West Point cadets associated with certain psychological risk factors: high levels of motivation, poorer academic performance, and having a father who was an overachiever (33). In another study, Luborsky et al. (41) found that unhappiness among nursing students was a predictor for herpes labialis lesions.

The role of immunity in controlling the recurrence of latent herpesvirus infections is not well understood. Normally, after an active herpesvirus infection, the virus is repressed in a latent state in certain host cells. It is common that in individuals who become immune suppressed, either naturally by infection with other viruses or, for example, after radiation therapy in cancer patients, there is often an increase in antibody titers to one or more of the herpesviruses, including herpes simplex virus type 1 (HSV-1), EBV, and cytomegalovirus (CMV). These antibody increases are presumably caused by the humoral immune response to the increase in virus-specific antigens after reactivation. It is thought that the cellular immune response is very important for the limitation of the primary infection and controlling the expression of latent EBV (26,39,51). Animal studies have shown that induced immune suppression can reactivate latent HSV (45,46).

We have attempted to assess possible stress-related changes in herpesvirus antibody titers using a prospective design. We have studied the effect of academic stress on the maintenance of EBV, HSV, and CMV. Any changes observed in antibody titers to any one or all of these herpesviruses would presumably reflect modulation of latent virus genomes by the cellular immune response. In one study, we examined a total of 49 EBV-seropositive medical students for changes in EBV antibody titers that could be related to academic stress. The average age of the 16 women and 33 men was 23 years. The first blood sample was obtained 1 month before final examinations, at the end of April. A second sample was obtained the first day of final examinations, at the end of May, and a third blood sample was collected during the first week of September, after the students had returned from vacation. As in all our studies, blood was obtained at the same time during the day (in the middle of the day) to avoid diurnal variations. Self-report data were also obtained at the time the blood was drawn.

The self-report measures used in this study included the Brief Symptom Inventory (BSI), a short form of the Symptom Checklist-90 (10). We also used the UCLA Loneliness Scale (52) to provide a brief subjective measure of the overall adequacy of interpersonal contacts. The EBV virus capsid antigen (VCA) mean antibody titers

(GMT) were obtained using the indirect immunofluorescence test. Antibody titers to HSV and CMV were obtained by ELISA. The results of the BSI for the three sample points confirmed that the examination sample was associated with the most distress, followed by the base-line sample, with the lowest self-ratings of distress occurring after the students' return from summer vacation. We found a significant change in EBV VCA antibody titers across the three sample points. We also found that high-loneliness subjects had significantly higher VCA titers than low-loneliness subjects. The interaction between loneliness and change across sample points did not reach significance. Similar changes were also observed for antibody titers to the EBV early antigen (EA). When antibody titers were assayed for HSV and CMV from the same blood samples, similar fluctuations were observed (16).

In order to evaluate the possibility that there were fluctuations in IgG antibody titers to other antigens as well, rather than specifically to the three latent herpesviruses, we measured antibody titers to poliovirus type 2 as a recall antigen. The widespread use in school vaccination programs provided some assurance that most students would have antibody to this virus. We did not find any significant change in antibody titers to poliovirus type 2 in the same samples in which we found changes to the three herpesviruses, supporting the hypothesis that the herpesvirus data reflect stress-related changes in virus latency. In addition, in order to evaluate the possibility that there was a subclinical epidemic of EBV infections in our medical students at the time the study was taking place, we measured antibody titers to EBV VCA IgM. All plasma specimens were found to be negative for EBV VCA IgM antibody, suggesting that the results that we obtained were not caused by an epidemic of EBV infections in this group (16).

It has been shown, both in humans and in laboratory animals, that the immune function generally declines with age. For example, it is known that T-lymphocyte-mediated immune function for the production of certain autoantibodies, such as antinuclear antibodies, tends to increase with aging (2,49,50,58). There are also data that suggest that although there are no changes in levels of IgM in plasma, there is an increase in IgG and IgA in older individuals (49). In order to examine another aspect of cellular immunity and its control of the latent EBV genome under natural conditions in otherwise normally healthy individuals, we examined EBV antibody titers in a geriatric population (24). We assayed levels of VCA IgG and IgA as well as EA IgG in a geriatric population in order to determine if there were any differences in the antibody patterns to these antigens when compared to a younger population, i.e., our medical students. We found that 89% of the geriatric blood samples were positive for EA IgG, and 83% of the medical students were positive for EA IgG. One hundred percent of the geriatric blood samples were positive for VCA IgG, and 87% of the medical students had antibodies to VCA IgG. We found that approximately 7% of the plasma samples obtained from the medical students were positive for VCA IgA antibody; however, 36% of the samples obtained from the geriatric population were found to be positive for this antibody. Statistical analyses of these data show that the EA GMT in the medical students is significantly lower than the EA GMT of the geriatric group, as determined using analysis of variance. A similar statistically significant difference was found between VCA IgG GMTs in the two populations as well. A statistically significant difference was found in VCA IgA levels.

At no time during the course of the study did any one of the geriatric participants complain of symptoms compatible with infectious mononucleosis or present with persistent EBV infection, and the higher levels of antibody in the geriatric group were not associated with clinical disease. The data suggest that there may be some loss of control over the latent EBV genome in geriatric individuals, presumably because of a less efficient cellular immune response. This could be related, for example, to a depression in T-lymphocyte-mediated immune function, already discussed. These data are consistent with the data obtained with the medical students, suggesting that negative modulation of the cellular immune response, either with aging or because of psychological factors such as academic stress, can allow at least some reactivation of latent herpesviruses.

DEPRESSION IN THE SYNTHESIS OF INTERFERON ASSOCIATED WITH ACADEMIC STRESS

There is good evidence that NK cell activity has an important role in the immune response to viral infections and perhaps cancer (27,28). Interferon is a major regulator of NK cell activity. It can activate the lytic activity of target binding cells, enhance cytolysis of target cells, and increase the number of target cells that then can be killed by an effector cell. In addition, there is also evidence that NK cells themselves can produce IFN (27,28).

In studies with rodents, it was suggested that there may be CNS mediation of IFN synthesis. Stress-associated changes in IFN production were found in virus-infected mice after the mice were exposed to physical stress such as shock (7,31). In addition, various stressors might also reduce responsiveness of certain immune functions to IFN stimulation. It was found that from 52 to 75% reduction in macrophage tumoricidal function in interferon-treated mice was observed following restraint (47).

As discussed earlier, in two studies from our laboratory we found a significant decrease in NK cell activity using both K562 cells and MOLT-4 cells (23,36). In the same studies, we measured changes in total IFN production by Con-A-stimulated PBLs taken at base line and at the time of examinations. We also determined the number of NK cells using two different protocols: the Leu-7 monoclonal antibody that recognizes a surface marker on NK cells and the number of large granular lymphocytes (LGLs), the phenotype of NK cells. As in previous studies, self-report data were obtained along with the immunological data. Again, we were able to document significantly increased distress associated with examinations, in comparison to base line. We found that the production of IFNs by Con-A-stimulated lymphocytes declined sharply from the first (base-line) to the second (examination) samples (23). We also measured IFN levels in plasma from both blood samples and found that no measurable levels could be detected in either sample point, as expected. These data have been confirmed in a second study in which medical students were followed over an entire academic year (three base-line and three examination periods). The ability of Con-A-stimulated PBLs to synthesize γ IFN was markedly inhibited during the examination periods as compared to base-line controls (22). We found that the percentage of anti-Leu-7$^+$ NK cells declined significantly in the PBL samples obtained during examinations as compared to the baseline sample. Similar results were obtained in the percentage of LGLs; NK cell lysis also decreased significantly, confirming previous studies.

The data obtained in these studies demonstrate a very large and significant decrease in the amount of γ IFN produced by Con-A-stimulated PBLs obtained from medical students during examinations in contrast to the base-line values obtained 6 weeks earlier (23). There was also a significant decrement in the activity of NK cells as represented by lysis of MOLT-4 target cells, and a decrease in the number of NK cells (percentage Leu-7$^+$ cells and percentage LGLs) was also found. Similar results were obtained when the absolute number of Leu-7$^+$ NK cells for each person and for each effector-to-target-cell ratio were calculated. These data suggest that the decrease in NK cell lysis reported earlier in animals and in studies from our laboratory may be caused at least in part by a decrease in the total number of NK cells (22). These data may have important health implications, particularly in regard to AIDS, and are discussed below.

CONTROLLING FOR OTHER FACTORS THAT COULD IMPACT ON CELLULAR IMMUNITY

In all of our studies, we have determined if other factors could have been implicated in the decrease in the cellular immune response. For example, we have determined that sex, age, loss of sleep, change in weight, smoking, alcohol, and caffeine intake in the medical student studies were not associated with any of the immunological changes we observed. Since poor nutrition has been shown to impact in a negative way on the immune response, in several of our studies we examined this possibility by using protein assays to obtain general nutritional status, for example, serum albumin and transferrin levels. These two protein markers have half-lives of approximately 20 days and 8 days, respectively, giving us a range of nutritional data. Serum proteins tend to decrease in protein malnutrition, and it has been shown that the serum transferrin levels can be used to assess the effectiveness of total parenteral nutrition (34). In all studies in which we measured these protein markers thus far, all participants were within normal ranges for albumin and transferrin.

LABORATORY STUDIES ON THE REACTIVATION OF LATENT EBV

The EBV is a human oncogenic herpesvirus that infects and becomes latently associated with human and certain nonhuman B lymphocytes and has also been detected in the epithelial cells of nasopharyngeal carcinoma (NPC) tumors. We have been interested in studying the expression and regulation of the EBV genome in nonlymphoblastoid cell lines, for example, epithelial/lymphoblastoid and NPC/epithelial hybrid cells, as a model for studying NPC, since there are no EBV-genome-positive NPC tumor cell lines. Thus far, it has been possible to obtain several EBV-genome-positive epithelial/lymphoblastoid and epithelial/epithelial hybrid cells (18–21,56,57). The latent EBV genome in these cells is generally in a repressed state; i.e., only the nuclear antigen (EBNA) is expressed, and EA and VCA are not synthesized. However, several years ago we found that by using iododeoxyuridine (IUdR), hybrid cells such as D98/HR-1, which contain a repressed EBV genome, can be induced to synthesize EA, VCA, and virus particles (15,19,21). It was of interest to us to determine whether the EBV genome latently associated with NPC epithelial tumor cells could also be induced to replicate in a similar way. Explant cell cultures were prepared from NPC biopsies and treated with IUdR and examined for the reactivation of the latent virus genome. We were able to demonstrate that, similar to the D98/HR-1 hybrid cells, the EBV genome in NPC tumor cells could be induced to synthesize at least EA after treatment with IUdR, suggesting that the association between the EBV genome and cell genomes in both the hybrid cells and NPC tumor epithelial cells may be the same and that the mechanisms whereby IUdR induces the endogenous genome may also be similar (14).

THE NEUROENDOCRINE AXIS AS A LINK BETWEEN THE CNS AND THE IMMUNE SYSTEM

It is not within the purview of this report to define stress. Suffice it to say that if the distress associated with taking examinations (academic stress) is sufficient to affect cell-mediated immunity, then the stress associated with the social interactions of the gay community could have immunological consequences. It has been shown in many studies that physiological stress results in changes in blood levels of a variety of hormones. It is thought that response to emotional stress is initiated in the hypothalamus, which ultimately modulates the release of pituitary hormones, as reviewed by Borysenko and Borysenko (5). Catecholamines are released and initiate a secondary cascade of hormonal effects. As demonstrated, corticosteroids and catecholamines are associated with stress; however, additional hormones such as growth hormone, somatotropin (6), adrenocorticotropin (43), melanocyte-stimulating hormone (29), prolactin (44), thyrotropin (11), vasopressin, aldosterone, calcitonin, parathyroid hormone, thyroxin, glucagon, renin, erythropoietin, and gastrin also have been found to be associated with stress (8). The impact of changes in blood levels of these hormones on the immune response in animals is reviewed by Landsberg (40). These changes include progressive atrophy of lymphoid organs, depression in the blastogenic response of lymphocytes, and changes in the percentage of lymphocytes and subpopulations of lymphocytes. Of interest is the fact that many of these inhibitory effects can occur even in the presence of low concentrations of hormones (3). What is not yet clearly understood is what the impact is of the release of endocrines *vis-à-vis* different kinds of stressors, for example, chronic stress versus acute stress, and what impact these changes have on the immune response, short term and long term.

As already discussed, physiological changes associated with stress include increases in blood levels of certain endocrines such as cortisol. Of interest and relevant to this discussion is a report by Markham et al. (42), who found that the ability to infect fresh normal human PBLs with HTLV-III productively was improved by supplementing cell culture medium with either the gonadal steroid chorionic gonadotropin or insulin, and even more substantially with the adrenal cortical steroid hydrocortisone. The data suggest a role for corticosteroids in the modulation of HTLV-III expression and/or replication and, put together with the data from our laboratory and others showing similar changes associated with stress, imply that there may be a connection. The high-risk populations for acquired immune deficiency syndrome (AIDS) and AIDS-related complex (ARC), such as homosexual men, may be a more psychologically stressed group because of societal and sociological pressures. Furthermore, this population, which is aware of the AIDS association with homosexuality, is under additional psychological stress because of the knowledge of the association of this devastating illness with their sexual practices.

THE ACQUIRED IMMUNE DEFICIENCY SYNDROME

Over the past several years, a severe disease syndrome involving opportunistic infections and Kaposi sarcoma has become a major health concern in the United States and several other countries. The AIDS has been linked to a human T-lymphotropic retrovirus, referred to as HTLV-III, lymphadenopathy-associated virus (LAV) (HTLV-III/LAV) (13). Associated with this immunosuppressive illness are opportunistic infections, for example, *Pneumocystis carinii, Toxoplasma gondii,* bacterial infections, and viral infections such as HSV. A common denominator for these clinical entities is abnormalities in cellular immunity, particularly demonstrated by a reduction in helper (inducer) T lymphocytes and abnormalities in the helper T-cell to suppressor T-cell ratio, as well as other immune dysfunctions. In addition, complications involving the CNS have also been described (55). The isolation of HTLV-III/LAV has been accomplished from lymphocytes from both AIDS and ARC patients. It is not known what controls the clinical course of ARC patients to frank AIDS patients. As discussed in this chapter, it is possible that stress-associated immune depression may be one component that affects the clinical course of both ARC and AIDS.

IMPLICATIONS OF NEUROIMMUNOMODULATION FOR ARC AND AIDS PATIENTS

As already discussed, there is evidence that supports the theory that the etiological agent for immune dysfunctions culminating in clinically defined ARC and AIDS is related to the HTLV-III/LAV virus (4,13). Evidence for this association is based primarily on a high correlation between the presence of antibody to viral structural proteins in the serum from a high proportion of patients as well as clinically healthy individuals with an elevated risk of being exposed, such as promiscuous homosexual males, heterosexual contacts of AIDS and ARC patients, and hemophiliacs (30,53). In addition, the isolation of HTLV-III/LAV from cultured lymphocytes from both ARC and AIDS patients as well as donors at risk for AIDS also supports the etiology of this virus(es) with the disease. It has also been shown that HTLV-III/LAV is cytopathic for T lymphocytes with the helper-inducer phenotype OKT-4/Leu-3$^+$ (13). It is of interest and relevant to this discussion that HTLV-III/LAV virus was isolated from lymphocytes of nearly 80% of ARC patients but initially only from 35% of patients with AIDS (13,48). Therefore, simply having the virus and carrying the virus in T lymphocytes does not necessarily imply that a person will have clinical disease. For reasons that are not clear, only a certain percentage of ARC patients potentially become AIDS patients. What determines the clinical course of the disease is not yet known. However, it is possible that any negative modulation of the immune response could result in an impact on the relationship between the virus and the lymphocytes such that virus could be reactivated from "latently infected" T lymphocytes. This reactivated virus could then be available for infecting other T lymphocytes, and so on. If this happens concomitantly in an individual whose immune system is less efficient than normal, then enhancement of virus replication could take place.

IMPLICATIONS FOR HTLV-III/LAV LATENCY AND PSYCHOLOGICAL STRESS

The data obtained in studies from our laboratory, already discussed in this chapter, show that at least for three latent herpesviruses, psychological stress can impact on the ability of the cellular immune response to control the maintenance of the virus genomes in the cells in which the virus is latent. Are there circumstances that provide a similar situation for HTLV-III/LAV, and, if so, can we extrapolate from the data on herpesvirus latency to AIDS? We have shown not only that the EBV genome can be induced from cell lines in which the virus is latently associated with drugs such as IUdR but, more importantly, that a similar phenomenon actually takes place using NPC tumor biopsies.

In a recent study, Folks and co-workers (12) infected a human T-cell line, A3.01, with HTLV-III/LAV. The virus lytically replicated in these cells and killed a high percentage of the cells. However, a small number of cells that lacked the Leu-3 surface marker survived infection. After growing out these remaining viable cells and reestablishing the cell culture, they found that the cells did not produce virus and that they could not be infected by the virus as well. What is of interest, however, is that HTLV-III/LAV could be induced to replicate and produce infectious virus from the A3.01 cells after treatment with IUdR, even after long-term culture up to 3 months. It is possible that individuals who harbor the virus in the latent form may do so for significant periods of time in the absence of expression of virus proteins or infectious viral particles, similar to cells latently infected with EBV. Under certain conditions, such as found for herpesviruses, it is possible that modulation of the cellular immune response and other factors involved in the reactivation of herpesviruses, such as stress, could result in the reactivation of the HTLV-III/LAV, perhaps as a consequence of the combination of down-regulation of cellular immunity and increases in stress-associated hormone levels. It is possible that this sequence of events could take place in clinically normal or ARC patients, resulting in a more acute form of immunosuppression, i.e., AIDS.

CONCLUSION

In this chapter, we have attempted to evaluate the data obtained in our laboratory and others on the psychological mediation of the immune response, sometimes called "psychoneuroimmunology" or "neuroimmunomodulation." We have demonstrated significant changes in several aspects of cellular immunity, many of which have potential significance for AIDS, such as NK cell activity and numbers and γ IFN production. We have also shown that reactivation of latent herpesvirus genomes may also be affected by psychological stress, presumably through the mediation of cellular immunity and its control over virus expression. The mechanisms whereby the nervous system and immune system react with each other are still not clear, but it is thought in part at least to be associated with certain endocrines. We have tried to speculate on how these phenomena may be related to AIDS or ARC. The data obtained in other studies on the expression of HTLV-III/LAV and hormones, and on the possibility that this virus can latently infect certain T lymphocytes and be reactivated with certain drugs such as IUdR, may have implications in regard to the data obtained in our laboratory on herpesviruses. Whether psychological stress in some way can modulate the expression of HTLV-III/LAV and whether factors such as stress can have implications for whether an ARC patient progresses to AIDS and the rate of appearance and severity of clinical symptoms remain speculative, and further studies will be necessary to determine whether this is so.

REFERENCES

1. Ader, R., editor (1981): *Psychoneuroimmunology.* Academic Press, New York.
2. Adler, W. H., and Nagel, J. E. (1981): Studies of immune function in a human population. In: *Immunological Aspects of Aging,* edited by D. Segre and L. Smith, pp. 295–320. Marcel Dekker, New York, Basel.
3. Bach, J. F., Duval, D., Dardenne, M., et al. (1975): The effects of steroids on T-cells. *Transplant. Proc.,* 7:25–30.
4. Barre-Sinoussi, F., Chermann, J. C., Rey, F., Nugeyre, M. T., Chamaret, S., Gruest, J., Dauguet, C., Axler-Blin, C., Vezinet-Brun, F., Rouzioux, C., Rozenbaum, W., and Montagnier, L. (1983): Isolation of a T-lymphotropic retrovirus from a patient at risk for acquired immune deficiency syndrome (AIDS). *Science,* 220:868–871.
5. Borysenko, M., and Borysenko, J. (1982): Stress, behavior, and immunity: Animal models and mediating mechanisms. *Gen. Hosp. Psychiatry,* 4:59–67.

6. Brown, G. M., and Reichlin, S. (1972): Psychologic and neural regulation of growth hormone secretion. *Psychosom. Med.*, 34:45–61.
7. Chang, S., and Rasmussen, A. F. (1965): Stress-induced suppression of interferon production in virus-infected mice. *Nature*, 205:623–624.
8. Claman, H. N. (1977): Corticosteroids and lymphoid cells. *N. Engl. J. Med.*, 287:388–397.
9. Claman, H. N., Moorhead, J. W., and Benner, W. H. (1971): Corticosteroids and lymphoid cells *in vitro*. *J. Lab. Clin. Med.*, 78:499–507.
10. Derogatis, L. R., and Spencer, P. M. (1982): *The Brief Symptom Inventory (BSI): Administration, Scoring, and Procedures Manual—I.* Clinical Psychometrics Research, Baltimore.
11. Dewhurst, K. E., El Kabir, D. J., Harris, G. W., et al. (1968): A review of the effect of stress on the activity of the central nervous–pituitary–thyroid axis in animals and man. *Confin. Neurol.*, 30:161–174.
12. Folks, T., Powell, D., Lightfoote, M. M., Benn, S., Martin, M. A., and Fauci, A. S. (1986): Induction of HTLV-III/LAV from a nonvirus-producing T-cell line: Implications for latency. *Science*, 231:600–602.
13. Gallo, R. C., Salahuddin, S. Z., Popovic, M., Shearer, G. M., Kaplan, M., Haynes, B. F., Palker, T. J., Redfield, R., Oleske, J., Safai, B., White, F., Foster, R., and Markham, P. D. (1984): Frequent detection and isolation of cytopathic retroviruses (HTLV-III) from patients with AIDS and at risk for AIDS. *Science*, 224:500–503.
14. Glaser, R., de-The, G., Lenoir, G., and Ho, J. H. C. (1976): Superinfection of epithelial nasopharyngeal carcinoma cells with Epstein–Barr virus. *Proc. Natl. Acad. Sci. U.S.A.*, 73:960–963.
15. Glaser, R., Farrugia, R., and Brown, N. (1976): Effect of the host cell on the maintenance and replication of Epstein–Barr virus. *Virology*, 69:132–142.
16. Glaser, R., Kiecolt-Glaser, J. K., Speicher, C. E., and Holliday, J. E. (1985): Stress, loneliness, and changes in herpesvirus latency. *J. Behav. Med.*, 8:249–260.
17. Glaser, R., Kiecolt-Glaser, J. K., Stout, J. C., Tarr, K. L., Speicher, C. E., and Holliday, J. E. (1985): Stress-related impairments in cellular immunity. *Psychiatry Res.*, 16:233–239.
18. Glaser, R., and Nonoyama, M. (1974): Host cell regulation of induction of Epstein–Barr virus. *J. Virol.*, 14:174–176.
19. Glaser, R., Nonoyama, M., Decker, B., and Rapp, F. (1973): Synthesis of Epstein–Barr virus antigens and DNA in activated Burkitt somatic cell hybrids. *Virology*, 55:62–69.
20. Glaser, R., and O'Neill, F. J. (1972): Hybridization of Burkitt–lymphoblastoid cells. *Science*, 176:1245–1247.
21. Glaser, R., and Rapp, F. (1972): Rescue of Epstein–Barr virus from somatic cell hybrids of Burkitt lymphoblastoid cells. *J. Virol.*, 10:288–296.
22. Glaser, R., Rice, J., Sheridan, J., Fertel, R., Stout, J., Speicher, C., Pinsky, D., Kotur, M., Post, A., Beck, M., and Kiecolt-Glaser, J. (1987): Stress-related immune suppression: Health implications. *Brain Behav. Immun.*, 1:7–20.
23. Glaser, R., Rice, J., Speicher, C. E., Stout, J. C., and Kiecolt-Glaser, J. K. (1986): Stress depresses interferon production by leukocytes concomitant with a decrease in natural killer cell activity. *Behav. Neurosci.*, 100:675–678.
24. Glaser, R., Strain, E. C., Tarr, K. L., Holliday, J. E., Donnerberg, R. L., and Kiecolt-Glaser, J. K. (1985): Changes in Epstein–Barr virus antibody titers associated with aging. *Proc. Soc. Exp. Biol. Med.*, 179:352–355.
25. Guyre, P. M., Bodwell, J. E., and Monck, A. (1981): Glucocorticoid actions on the immune system: Inhibition of production of an Fc-receptor augmenting factor. *J. Steroid Biochem.*, 15:35–39.
26. Harada, S., Bechtold, T., Seeley, J. K., and Purtilo, J. T. (1982): Cell-mediated immunity to Epstein–Barr virus (EBV) and natural killer (NK) cell activity in the X-linked lymphoproliferative syndrome. *Int. J. Cancer*, 30:734–744.
27. Herberman, R. B. (1982): Possible effects of central nervous system on natural killer (NK) cell activity. In: *Biological Mediators of Health and Disease: Neoplasia*, edited by S. M. Levy, pp. 235–248. Elsevier, New York.
28. Herberman, R. B., Ortaldo, J. R., Riccardi, C., Timonen, T., Schmidt, A., Maluish, A., and Djeu, J. (1982): Interferon and NK cells. In: *Interferons*, edited by T. C. Merigan and R. F. Freedman, pp. 287–294. Academic Press, London.
29. Hirata, Y., Sakamoto, N., Matsukura, S., et al. (1975): Plasma levels of β-MSH and ACTH during acute stresses and metapyrone administration in man. *J. Clin. Endocrinol. Metab.*, 41:1092–1097.

30. Jaffe, H. W., Sarngadharan, M. G., DeVico, A., Bruch, L., Getchell, J. P., Kalyanaraman, V. S., Haverkos, H. W., Stoneburner, R. L., Gallo, R. C., and Curran, J. W. (1987): Serologic evidence of an etiologic role for a human T-lymphotropic retrovirus (HTLV-III/LAV) in transfusion-associated AIDS. *J.A.M.A.* (*in press*).
31. Jensen, M. M. (1968): Transitory impairment of interferon production in stressed mice. *Proc. Soc. Exp. Biol. Med.*, 128:230–234.
32. Johnson, H. M., Smith, E. M., Torres, B. A., and Blalock, J. E. (1982): Neuroendocrine hormone regulation of *in vitro* antibody production. *Proc. Natl. Acad. Sci. U.S.A.*, 79:4171–4174.
33. Kasl, S. V., Evans, A. S., and Neiderman, J. C. (1979): Psychosocial risk factors in the development of infectious mononucleosis. *Psychosom. Med.*, 41:445–466.
34. Keyser, J. W. (1979): *Human Plasma Proteins*. John Wiley & Sons, New York.
35. Kiecolt-Glaser, J. K., Fisher, L. D., Ogrocki, P., Stout, J. C., Speicher, C. E., and Glaser, R. (1987): Marital quality, marital disruption, and immune function. *Psychosom. Med.* (*in press*).
36. Kiecolt-Glaser, J. K., Garner, W., Speicher, C. E., Penn, G. M., Holliday, J., and Glaser, R. (1984): Psychosocial modifiers of immunocompetence in medical students. *Psychosom. Med.*, 46:7–14.
37. Kiecolt-Glaser, J. K., Glaser, R., Strain, E., Stout, J., Tarr, K., Holliday, J., and Speicher, C. (1986): Modulation of cellular immunity in medical students. *J. Behav. Med.*, 9:5–21.
38. Keicolt-Glaser, J. K., Ricker, D., George, J., Messick, G., Speicher, C. E., Garner, W., and Glaser, R. (1984): Urinary cortisol levels, cellular immunocompetency and loneliness in psychiatric patients. *Psychosom. Med.*, 46:15–23.
39. Klein, E., Ernberg, I., Masucci, M. G., Szigeti, R., Wu, Y. T., Masucci, G., and Svedmyre, E. (1981): T-cell response to B-cells and Epstein–Barr virus antigens in infectious mononucleosis. *Cancer Res.*, 41:4210–4215.
40. Landsberg, L. (1977): The sympathoadrenal system. In: *The Year in Endocrinology, 1977*, edited by S. H. Ingbar, pp. 355–358. Plenum Press, New York.
41. Luborsky, L., Mintz, J., Brightman, V. J., and Katcher, A. H. (1976): Herpes simplex and moods: A longitudinal study. *J. Psychosom. Res.*, 20:543–548.
42. Markham, P. L., Salahuddin, S. Z., Veren, K., Orndorff, S., and Gallo, R. C. (1986): Hydrocortisone and some other hormones enhance the expression of HTLV-III. *Int. J. Cancer*, 37:67–72.
43. Mason, J. W. (1968): A review of psychoendocrine research on the pituitary–adrenal cortical system. *Psychosom. Med.*, 30:576–607.
44. Noel, G. L., Suh, H. K., Stone, G., et al. (1972): Human prolactin and growth hormone release during surgery and other conditions of stress. *J. Clin. Endocrinol. Metab.*, 35:840–851.
45. Oakes, J. E., Davis, W. B., Taylor, J. A., and Weppner, W. A. (1980): Lymphocyte reactivity contributes to protection conferred by specific antibody passively transferred to herpes simplex virus-infected mice. *Infect. Immun.*, 29:642–649.
46. Openshaw, H., Sekizawa, T., Wohlenberg, C., and Notkins, A. L. (1981): The role of immunity in latency and reactivation of herpes simplex viruses. In: *The Human Herpesviruses: An Interdisciplinary Perspective*, edited by A. J. Nahmias, W. R. Dowdle, and R. F. Schlanazi, Elsevier/North-Holland, New York.
47. Pavilidis, N., and Chirigos, M. (1980): Stress-induced impairment of macrophage tumoricidal function. *Psychosom. Med.*, 42:47–52.
48. Popovic, M., Read-Connole, E., and Gallo, R. C. (1984): T4 positive human neoplastic cell lines susceptible to and permissive for HTLV-III. *Lancet*, 2:1472–1473.
49. Radl, J. (1981): Immunoglobulin levels and abnormalities in aging humans and mice. In: *Immunological Techniques Applied to Aging Research*, edited by W. H. Adler and A. A. Nordin, pp. 121–136. CRC Press, Boca Raton, FL.
50. Radl, J., Sepers, J. M., Skvaril, F., et al. (1975): Immunoglobulin patterns in humans over 95 years of age. *Clin. Exp. Immunol.*, 22:84–90.
51. Rickinson, A. B., Moss, D. J., Wallace, L. E., Rowe, M., Misko, I. S., Epstein, M. A., and Pope, J. H. (1981): Long-term T-cell mediated immunity to Epstein–Barr virus. *Cancer Res.*, 41:4216–4221.
52. Russell, D., Peplau, L. A., and Cutrona, C. E. (1980): The Revised UCLA Loneliness Scale: Concurrent and discriminant validity evidence. *J. Pers. Soc. Psychol.*, 39:479–480.
53. Sarngadharan, M. G., Popovic, M., Bruch, L., Schupbach, J., and Gallo, R. C. (1984): Antibodies reactive with a human T-lymphotropic retrovirus (HTLV-III) in the sera of patients with acquired immune deficiency syndrome. *Science*, 224:506–508.

54. Schleifer, S. J., Keller, S. E., Camerino, M., Thornton, J. C., and Stein, M. (1983): Suppression of lymphocyte stimulation following bereavement. *J.A.M.A.*, 250:374–377.
55. Spivak, J. L., Selonick, S. E., and Quinn, T. C. (1983): Acquired immune deficiency syndrome and pancytopenia. *J.A.M.A.*, 250:3084–3087.
56. Takimoto, T., Sato, H., Ogura, H., and Glaser, R. (1986): Rescue of a biologically active Epstein–Barr virus (EBV) from nonproducer cells. *Cancer Res.*, 46:2085–2027.
57. Takimoto, T., Sato, H., Ogura, H., Miyawaki, T., and Glaser, R. (1986): Superinfection of epithelial hybrid cells (D98/HR-1, NPC-KT, and A2L/AH) with Epstein–Barr virus and the relationship to the C3d receptor. *Cancer Res.*, 46:2541–2544.
58. Toh, B. H., Roberts-Thomson, I. C., Mathews, J. D., et al. (1973): Depression of cell-mediated immunity in old age and the immunopathic diseases, lupus erythematosus, chronic hepatitis and rheumatoid arthritis. *Clin. Exp. Immunol.*, 14:193–202.

*Psychological, Neuropsychiatric, and
Substance Abuse Aspects of AIDS,*
edited by T. Peter Bridge et al.
Raven Press, New York © 1988.

Major Life Changes, Chronic Stress, and Immunity

*Janice Kiecolt-Glaser and †Ronald Glaser

*Departments of *Psychiatry and †Medical Microbiology and Immunology and
†Comprehensive Cancer Center, The Ohio State University College of Medicine,
Columbus, Ohio 43210*

Data from human studies suggest that (a) psychiatric patients with a major depression diagnosis have poorer immune function than nondepressed comparison subjects; (b) poorer marital quality is associated with poorer performance on qualitative indices of immune function; (c) length of separation and degree of continued attachment to the (ex-)husband are significantly associated with immune function and distress in separated and divorced women; and (d) family caregivers of AD victims have poorer immune function than well-matched comparison subjects. Taken together, these data provide good evidence of more chronic distress-related alterations in immune function. Thus, in contrast to data obtained from studies with rodents, it appears that chronic stress in humans does not lead to immunological adaptation to the level of sociodemographically-matched peers.

A number of studies have shown a relationship between an accumulation of stressful life changes and subsequent health impairments (24). Unfortunately, the effect has generally been small, and correlations between life change scores and self-reported health are typically in the 0.30s or lower (31). In addition, the great majority of life events studies find organic disease in only a minority of subjects when objective assessment procedures are used, and the mechanisms whereby such effects might be produced have not been well understood.

We suggest that the increased distress that normally accompanies major life changes (or more enduring chronic stressors) also has adverse effects on immunity. Distress-related changes in immunity would theoretically have their greatest impact in individuals whose immune system functioning is already compromised to some extent, either by an immunosuppressive disease like AIDS or by a natural process such as aging. For these individuals, smaller decrements in immune function could have larger biological consequences, because they would exacerbate existing immunological deficits at the onset. Within this framework, we argue that psychosocial resources such as supportive interpersonal relationships that buffer or moderate

217

the distress associated with stressful life changes may also concurrently attenuate adverse immunological changes.

We are unaware of any relevant evidence from studies with AIDS patients linking greater distress with more rapid disease progression or mortality. However, there is some epidemiological evidence from the aging literature that is consistent with this framework. Within the first year after psychiatric admission, there are 50 times more deaths from pneumonia among elderly psychiatric patients than among their age-matched general-population contemporaries; the ratio drops to 20 times that of their age peers by the second year of hospitalization, suggesting that the transition may be a more important factor than the hospital environment (6). Although it is reasonable to assume that psychiatric patients are more distressed than the general population, it should also be noted that depression is the modal reason for psychiatric hospitalization in the elderly (29).

The immunological consequences of relatively commonplace stressful events such as academic examinations are reviewed elsewhere (see R. Glaser and J. K. Kiecolt-Glaser, *this volume*); in this chapter we focus on immunological and health-related consequences associated with major stressful life events as well as more chronic and enduring stressors.

CHRONIC STRESS AND IMMUNE FUNCTION IN RODENTS AND MONKEYS

Data from several studies with rodents suggest that the chronicity of a stressor may mediate tumor growth and certain immunological responses. For example, a single session of inescapable shock had adverse consequences for tumor size and survival in mice injected with a transplantable tumor (28). In contrast, mice that experienced 10 daily shock sessions had tumors that were significantly smaller than those of controls; survival times were quite similar to those of controls.

In related work, Monjan and Collector (19) operationalized the results of "chronic stress" in mice as the changes occurring over a 45-day period of exposure to daily high-intensity intermittent noise. The acute or short-term consequences of the stressor appeared to be immunosuppressive, with mitogen responsiveness falling below base-line levels. However, data from blastogenic assays began to show an increase above base-line levels between days 10 and 20 and were returning to base-line levels by the end of the study.

There are a number of problems in drawing parallels between the outcome of research with rodents and the expectation of similar processes in humans. Although both rodents and humans are mammals, the immune system in rodents is more sensitive to steroids, and there is evidence that both tumor induction and growth are mediated through somewhat different pathways (e.g., ref. 9). Moreover, the stressors that are used in research with rodents are normally physical stressors such as shock, noise, restraint, or rotation (1). It is not clear if adaptation to these physical stressors follows the same course as adaptation to the psychological stressors that are of primary interest in research with humans.

There is evidence from work with nonhuman primates that adaptation does not easily occur to a repeated psychosocial stressor. Research with unweaned squirrel monkeys showed that the characteristic behavioral response to repeated 1-hr separations from their mothers adapted over time. However, the monkeys still showed reliable elevations in plasma cortisol in response to repeated separations, even after 20 such separations had occurred. A related form of separation distress has also been associated with significant immunological alterations. Completely weaned squirrel monkeys that were separated from their mothers showed decrements in several indices of humoral immunity at 7 and 14 days after the separation compared to preseparation samples (5); those monkeys who were caged with others showed less immunosuppression than those who were caged alone.

In the remainder of this chapter we discuss related evidence from human studies that suggests that longer-term psychosocial stressors do not eventuate in immunological adaptation to the level of matched comparison subjects. We also briefly review evidence that suggests an association between distress and morbidity and mortality for infectious and malignant disease.

DEPRESSION AS A LONGER-TERM STRESSOR

If there were indeed simple parallelism between the observed enhancement of immunity in rodents following a stressor prolonged over several weeks (19), then one might expect that individuals who had been quite distressed for several weeks would show enhanced immune function or would not differ from their well-matched, nondistressed community counterparts. However, data from human studies stand in contrast to the results obtained with rodents. For example, the DSM-III diagnostic classification of major depression, the psychiatric patient subpopulation most closely studied to date, specifies that the essential symptoms must have been present for a period of at least 2 weeks; in fact, most of the patients with a major depression diagnosis in our psychiatric hospital retrospectively report that the salient depressive symptoms had been present for periods of several weeks to several months before they decided to seek treatment.

Work from several laboratories has suggested that patients with a major depression diagnosis have poorer immune function than nondepressed comparison subjects. Depressed patients have poorer blastogenic responsiveness (26) and lower percentages of helper T lymphocytes (16) than their nondepressed counterparts. Other data suggest that depressed patients may have lower percentages of peripheral T lymphocytes (27).

MARITAL DISRUPTION: SHORTER- AND LONGER-TERM EFFECTS

The disruption of a marriage, through either divorce of death, appears to be one of the most stressful of life experiences (4,12,22). Both bereavement and divorce are associated with high rates of physical and emotional disorders; marital disrup-

tion is the single most powerful sociodemographic predictor of physical and emotional illness (30). Separated adults have about 30% more acute illnesses and physician visits than married adults, and divorced people have six times more deaths
from pneumonia than their married counterparts (18). Both bereaved and separated/
divorced adults have a higher incidence of cancer than similar married individuals (7).

Research in behavioral immunology has shown an association between bereavement and impaired mitogen responsiveness in both cross-sectional and prospective
work. Bartrop et al. (2) found that 26 bereaved spouses had an impaired proliferative response 2 to 6 weeks after their spouse's death. In a prospective study of 15
men whose wives were dying of breast cancer, Schleifer et al. (25) collected blood
samples before and after the wife's death. The men showed poorer lymphocyte
proliferation after the death than before.

Separation and divorce are consistently associated with greater morbidity and
mortality than bereavement; in studies that provide separate data for separation and
divorce, separation is reliably associated with greater health impairments than divorce (4,32). Summarizing the differences for separated and divorced women, Verbrugge (32) concluded:

> Separated women are strongly disadvantaged, compared to married ones, for acute
> incidence, all short-term disability measures, major activity limitations, and partial
> work disability. . . . Divorced women are also strongly disfavored. . . (p. 283).

Based on these epidemiological data, we designed a cross-sectional study to address
the possibility that there were distress-related immunological differences between
married and separated/divorced individuals.

We recruited 38 separated or divorced women and 38 sociodemographically
matched married comparison women (13). The two groups were matched for age,
education, number of years married, and socioeconomic status of the (ex-)husband.
The shorter-term consequences of marital disruption were striking: the 16 women
in the sample who had been separated 1 year or less had significantly poorer immune function on five of the six immunological assays than their 16 sociodemographically matched married counterparts. There were also longer-term differences
as well; comparisons of the entire cohort of 38 separated/divorced women with the
38 married women showed significant differences on three of the six immunological
assays, even though the women in the separated/divorced cohort had been separated
from 1 month to 6 years, with an average separation time of about 2 years. Moreover, within the separated/divorced cohort, shorter separation periods and/or greater
continued attachment to the (ex-)husband were associated with poorer immune
function and greater depression.

It has been suggested that the differences in health between married and nonmarried individuals may largely be a function of differences in lifestyle, with nonmarried individuals engaging in behaviors that pose greater health risks. For example, nonmarried adults might have poorer nutrition or poorer sleep, and/or they
might drink, smoke, or use drugs more than comparable married individuals (32).

Both our married and our separated/divorced samples were selected in part based on criteria that included limited alcohol intake and an absence of drug use; although we did not select subjects on the basis of nutritional or sleep criteria, we found no evidence of systematic differences of a magnitude that would account for the observed differences in immune function. Therefore, although it is certainly possible that lifestyle factors may contribute to the reliable differences in morbidity and mortality found in epidemiological studies, it is also possible that there are persistent stress-related changes in physiological functions such as immunity that might have some cumulative impact on health.

POORER MARITAL QUALITY AS A CHRONIC STRESSOR

In addition to the possible differences between separated and divorced individuals, we were interested in the possibility that there might also be a relationship between immune function and marital quality. On the average, unmarried individuals are less distressed than those in troubled marriages (10,21). Data from Renne (23) also suggested a relationship between marital quality and health: unhappily married people reported poorer health than either divorced or happily married individuals of the same age, sex, and race.

Using the data from the 38 married women described above, we found that marital quality was a significant predictor of depression and loneliness in hierarchical multiple-regression equations even after subject's education, the husband's socioeconomic status, and the number of negative life events were entered on previous steps. In addition, poorer marital quality was associated with a poorer response on the three qualitative measures of immune function.

Longitudinal data from Levinson and Gottman (17) provide evidence of one physiological pathway through which chronically abrasive relationships might mediate immune function. They found that greater autonomic arousal in interacting married couples was strongly predictive of subsequent declines in marital satisfaction 3 years later. In addition, poorer health ratings at follow-up were strongly correlated with greater declines in marital satisfaction. If the presence of a spouse in a disturbed relationship is associated with persistent physiological arousal, then there may be concurrent alterations in endocrine function (20) that could contribute to the observed relationship between marital quality and immunity.

IMMUNOLOGICAL CORRELATES OF CHRONIC STRESS IN FAMILY CAREGIVERS FOR ALZHEIMER'S DISEASE VICTIMS

Alzheimer's disease (AD) is thought to affect two million older adults in this country. The characteristic progressive cognitive impairments associated with AD lead to increasing needs for supportive care of the victims. Although mild memory impairments may be the only obvious symptom in the early stages, the irreversible deterioration of brain tissue eventually results in profound behavioral and cognitive changes including disorientation, incontinence, and an inability to provide any self-care (11). Since 8 years is the modal time for survival after onset, the long-term care of these patients by family members is conceptualized as a chronic stressor (8). Alzheimer's disease family caregivers appear to be at high risk for depression (8).

In order to study health-related consequences of caregiving for a demented relative, we obtained psychological and immunological data from 34 AD family caregivers and 34 sociodemographically matched (age, sex, and education) comparison subjects (14). Family caregivers for AD victims were significantly more depressed than comparison subjects and had poorer immune function on most of the cellular immunological assays (i.e., percentages of total T lymphocytes and helper T cells, the helper/suppressor ratio, and antibody to Epstein–Barr virus). These data suggest that chronically stressed AD family caregivers do not show immunological or psychological adaptation to the level of their well-matched age peers.

IMPLICATIONS

We have presented data from human studies that suggest that (a) psychiatric patients with a major depression diagnosis have poorer immune function than non-depressed comparison subjects; (b) poorer marital quality is associated with poorer performance on qualitative indices of immune function; (c) length of separation and degree of continued attachment to the (ex-)husband are significantly associated with immune function and distress in separated and divorced women; and (d) family caregivers of AD victims have poorer immune function than well-matched comparison subjects. Taken together, these data provide good evidence of more chronic distress-related alterations in immune function. Thus, in contrast to data obtained from studies with rodents (19,28), it appears that chronic stress in humans does not lead to immunological adaptation to the level of sociodemographically matched peers.

At present little is known about the importance of psychological factors in the progression of AIDS, especially in terms of possible changes related to HTLV-III/LAV latency (see R. Glaser and J. K. Kiecolt-Glaser, *this volume*). The well-publicized growth in the incidence of AIDS and its fatal consequences have led to creased depression and fear in groups at greater risk for the disease (3). Learning that one has AIDS is often followed by social ostracism at the very time when increased interpersonal support is needed and desired (3). Further research is needed to understand better the possible consequences of these and other acute and chronic psychosocial stressors for health and well-being in AIDS patients and those individuals who are at risk for AIDS.

ACKNOWLEDGMENTS

Work on this chapter was supported in part by grant No. 1 RO1 MH40787 from the National Institute of Mental Health.

REFERENCES

1. Ader, R., editor (1981): *Psychoneuroimmunology.* Academic Press, New York.
2. Bartrop, R. W., Luckhurst, E., Lazarus, L., Kiloh, L. G., and Penny, R. (1977): Depressed lymphocyte function after bereavement. *Lancet,* 1:834–836.
3. Batchelor, W. F. (1984): AIDS: A public health and psychological emergency. *Am. Psychol.,* 39:1279–1284.
4. Bloom, B. L., Asher, S. J., and White, S. W. (1978): Marital disruption as a stressor: A review and analysis. *Psychol. Bull.,* 85:867–894.
5. Coe, C. L., and Levine, S. (1987): Psychoimmunology: An old idea whose time has come. In: *Biological and Behavioral Correlates of Psychopathology,* edited by T. Perez, J. Chido, and J. H. Harvey. Texas Tech University, Lubbock (*in press*).
6. Craig, T. J., and Lin, S. P. (1981): Mortality among elderly psychiatric patients: Basis for preventive intervention. *J. Am. Geriatr. Soc.,* 29:181–185.
7. Ernster, V. L., Sacks, S. T., Selvin, S., and Petrakis, N. L. (1979): Cancer incidence by marital status: U.S. Third National Cancer Survey. *J. Natl. Cancer Inst.,* 63:587–589.
8. Fiore, J., Becker, J., and Coppel, D. B. (1983): Social network interactions: A buffer or a stress. *Am. J. Commun. Psychol.,* 11:423–429.
9. Fox, B. H. (1981): Psychosocial factors and the immune system in human cancer. In: *Psychoneuroimmunology,* edited by R. Ader, pp. 103–158. Academic Press, New York.
10. Glenn, N. D., and Weaver, C. N. (1981): The contribution of marital happiness to global happiness. *J. Marriage Family,* 43:161–168.
11. Heckler, M. M. (1985): The fight against Alzheimer's disease. *Am. Psychol.,* 40:1240–1244.
12. Jacobs, S., and Ostfeld, A. (1977): An epidemiological review of bereavement. *Psychosom. Med.,* 4:4–13.
13. Kiecolt-Glaser, J. K., Fisher, L., Ogrocki, P., Stout, J. C., Speicher, C. E., and Glaser, R. (1987): Marital quality, marital disruption, and immune function. *Psychosom. Med.,* 49:13–35.
14. Kiecolt-Glaser, J. K., Glaser, R., Dyer, C., Shuttleworth, E. C., Ogrocki, P., and Speicher, C. E. (1987): Chronic stress and immune function in family caregivers of Alzheimer's disease victims. *Psychosom. Med.,* 49:523–535.
15. Kiecolt-Glaser, J. K., Glaser, R., Williger, D., Stout, J., Messick, G., Sheppard, S., Ricker, D., Romisher, S. C., Briner, W., Bonnell, G., and Donnerberg, R. (1985): Psychosocial enhancement of immunocompetence in a geriatric population. *Health Psychol.,* 4:25–41.
16. Krueger, R. B., Levy, E. M., Cathcart, E. S., Fox, B. H., and Black, P. H. (1984): Lymphocyte subsets in patients with major depression: Preliminary findings. *Advances,* 4:5–9.
17. Levenson, R. W., and Gottman, J. M. (1985): Physiological and affective predictors of change in relationship satisfaction. *J. Pers. Soc. Psychol.,* 49:85–94.
18. Lynch, J. (1977): *The Broken Heart.* Basic Books, New York.
19. Monjan, A. A., and Collector, M. I. (1977): Stress-induced modulation of the immune response. *Science,* 196:307–308.
20. O'Dorisio, M. S., Wood, C. L., and O'Dorisio, T. M. (1985): Vasoactive intestinal peptide and neuropeptide modulation of the immune response. *J. Immunol.,* 135:792s–796s.
21. Pearlin, L. I., and Lieberman, M. A. (1979): Social sources of emotional distress. In: *Research in Community and Mental Health,* edited by R. Simmons, pp. 217–248. JAI Press, Greenwich, CT.
22. Rees, W. D., and Lutkins, S. G. (1967): Mortality of bereavement. *Br. Med. J.,* 4:13–16.
23. Renne, K. S. (1971): Health and marital experience in an urban population. *J. Marriage Family,* 23:338–350.
24. Sarason, I. G., Sarason, B. R., Potter, E. H., and Antoni, M. H. (1985): Life events, social support, and illness. *Psychosom. Med.,* 47:156–163.
25. Schleifer, S. J., Keller, S. E., Camerino, M., Thornton, J. C., and Stein, M. (1983): Suppression of lymphocyte stimulation following bereavement. *J.A.M.A.,* 250:374–377.
26. Schleifer, S. J., Keller, S. E., Meyerson, A. T., Raskin, K. L., and Stein, M. (1984): Lymphocyte function in major depressive disorder. *Arch. Gen. Psychiatry,* 41:484–486.
27. Schleifer, S. J., Keller, S. E., Siris, S. G., Davis, K. L., and Stein, M. (1985): Depression and immunity. *Arch. Gen. Psychiatry,* 42:129–133.
28. Sklar, L. S., and Anisman, H. (1979): Stress and coping factors influence tumor growth. *Science,* 205:513–515.
29. Solomon, K. (1981): The depressed patient: Social antecedents of psychopathologic changes in the elderly. *J. Am. Geriatr. Soc.,* 29:14–18.

30. Somers, A. R. (1979): Marital status, health, and use of health services. *J.A.M.A.*, 241:1818–1822.
31. Thoits, P. A. (1983): Dimensions of life events that influence distress: An evaluation and synthesis of the literature. In: *Psychosocial Stress: Trends in Theory and Research,* edited by H. B. Kaplan, pp. 33–103. Academic Press, New York.
32. Verbrugge, L. M. (1979): Marital status and health. *J. Marriage Family,* 41:267–285.

Psychological, Neuropsychiatric, and Substance Abuse Aspects of AIDS, edited by T. Peter Bridge et al. Raven Press, New York © 1988.

Behavioral Risk Factors and Host Vulnerability

Sandra M. Levy

Pittsburgh Cancer Institute, University of Pittsburgh School of Medicine, Pittsburgh, Pennsylvania 15213

For decades, clinical anecdotes of mysterious cancer regression suggest that host characteristics do have some effect on the course of disease. For example, the following story is often told in various works concerned with belief and disease. In the 1950s, Krebiozen (a now debunked anticancer drug) was being tested. A particular patient with advanced lymphosarcoma was terminally ill and asked for Krebiozen treatment. Subsequently, he went into remission, returned to work, and resumed his normal activities. As published reports began to appear that Krebiozen was ineffective in the treatment of malignancy, the man immediately relapsed and again became terminally ill. His physician, feeling justified by his deteriorating condition, reportedly told him that a special, purified form of Krebiozen was in fact effective and instead gave his patient distilled water (believing that the earlier rally was a placebo effect). The patient subsequently made a remarkable recovery. Approximately 2 months later, an authoritative government report on Krebiozen was published; it concluded that the drug was absolutely worthless. The man died a few days later.

Stories such as this one provided the clinical and anecdotal background on which our research program, begun in 1979 at the National Cancer Institute, National Institutes of Health, was launched. In fact, it has only been in recent years that both the laboratory technology and the behavioral science technology have been available to allow careful examination of the links between behavior and cancer outcome.

In this chapter, I first review the biological evidence linking central nervous system, endocrine, and immune factors with disease outcome. I concentrate on malignancy because most of our own work has been carried out in this area. However, given the major focus of this volume on acquired immunodeficiency disorder, I also extrapolate where relevant to this disease end-point. I also concentrate on breast cancer and malignant melanoma, as these are the two tumor systems that have been most frequently studied by interdisciplinary teams examining mechanisms linking behavior with cancer progression. I then review findings from our program of studies over the last 7 years. In the last section of this chapter, I describe a psychosocial schema, extracted from findings in the literature, linking behavioral factors with cancer outcome.

BREAST CANCER AND MELANOMA: IMMUNOLOGICAL AND NEUROENDOCRINOLOGICAL MECHANISMS

Breast Cancer: Potential Endogenous Control Mechanisms

For breast cancer, both immunologic and hormonal factors have been implicated as mechanisms modulating tumor growth. Primary breast tumors have been reported to induce an immune response at least capable of modifying tumor growth by various mechanisms (25,38). Similarly, many studies have shown that hormone levels play an important part in contributing to breast cancer risk as well as in modifying the course of primary breast cancer, the growth of metastatic foci, and the maintenance of the disease-free interval (2,20,39,45). But here we focus on the role of the immune system in tumor control because of recently demonstrated links between the immune and central nervous systems.

Breast Cancer and Immunologic Responses

Many reports have been published on the clinical significance of lymphocytic infiltration of cancer tissues, including human malignancies (8,38,48). The study of tumor immunology has been marked by both failures and successes, and the history of this research field is not reviewed here. The weight of experimental and clinical evidence strongly suggests that cellular immune effector functions are involved in the host–tumor relationship and play a modifying role related to tumor growth within the host.

We are especially concerned here with the role of immunological responses in resistance to the growth of breast cancer and melanoma. There have been reports (41,44) of microscopic studies of *in situ* and invasive breast cancer revealing lymphoid cell infiltrations of the primary tumor. A recent study (51) showed that T-cell infiltration in breast tumors was scanty in scirrhous carcinoma but more ample in infiltrating papillotubular carcinoma, the latter known to have better prognosis. These investigators also found a significant inverse correlation between the intensity of the T-cell infiltration and clinical stage of disease (stage IV having practically no T-cell-relevant activity). The intensity of the T-cell infiltration was significantly higher in patients without spread of cancer cells to the regional lymph nodes. Although the authors noted that these correlational data do not prove causal effects, they cited animal experiments with autochthonous tumor systems (32) that have shown that some T-cell populations have a suppressive effect on cancer cell growth.

Malignant Melanoma

A disproportionate share of all cases of spontaneous regression have been reported for malignant melanoma, and such regressions have served to increase interest in melanoma as a model for host response and endogenous tumor control (6).

Melanoma is a malignant tumor originating from the melanocyte and has the capacity to invade and metastasize to vital host organs. Although still a relatively rare malignancy, both the incidence and the mortality rates from malignant melanoma are rising rapidly in all countries in which they have been studied. Mortality rates are rising by around 3% to 9% per year, so that the rates have doubled in about the last 15 years (7). In the United States and Canada, the rate of increase is greater than that for any other tumor except lung cancer, and such changes have been shown to be independent of improved diagnosis. There is some sign that incidence rates have risen more rapidly, showing that improved diagnosis and treatment have reduced case fatality, but not to a great extent (7). In addition, the rise in incidence and mortality has been much greater in young individuals than in those over the age of 65. Therefore, the average age of those who die from melanoma is decreasing, and the loss of productive years for the individual and the community is even greater than the rise in mortality alone would suggest. Moreover, malignant melanoma is virtually untreatable by radiation or chemotherapy, and survival for the most part depends on the excision of very early lesions. For advanced stage I and stages II and III, survival rates rapidly fall off.

Melanoma and Hormones

The melanocyte develops embryologically from the neural crest and has a common origin with other tissues that later secrete peptide hormones or hormone-like substances such as ACTH, gastrin, and glucagon. There have even been reports of malignant melanoma lesions producing serotonin (7). Melanocyte-stimulating hormone (MSH) also arises from the same pituitary precursor molecule—the pro-opiomelanocortin molecule—as do ACTH and β-endorphin. Therefore, central nervous system paths linking higher cortical function with hypothalamic–pituitary hormone secretion and melanocyte activity are plausible.

Melanoma and Immune Containment

Spontaneous regression of melanoma is sometimes associated with infectious episodes and may be characterized by the presence of lymphoid infiltrates within tumor tissues (47). It therefore appears that the rate of tumor progression is not only controlled by tumor cell kinetics but also modulated by the patient's immune response to his or her malignant cells. Space does not allow for a review of the extensive tumor immunology literature relevant to melanoma. Because of our earlier findings suggesting the relevance of natural killer (NK) cells to cancer prognosis, we concentrate on evidence linking NK activity with melanoma progression or containment.

The most common form of melanoma is the superficial spreading type, representing 60% of all melanomas. This malignancy has a biphasic evolution, characterized by a relatively slow horizontal growth phase followed by a rapid vertical growth pattern. Metastasis coincides with this second vertical phase. During the initial horizontal growth phase, there is commonly dense lymphocytic activity. The vertical growth phase is correlated with a much weaker lymphocyte reaction.

Recent *in vitro* studies with melanoma patients have shown reduced NK activity relevant to normal controls. This decrease was significantly associated with advancing stage of disease. Kadish et al. (35) showed that NK functional decrease seemed not to be secondary to suppressor cell activity, and response to interferon (normally an NK enhancer) was also impaired in patients with advanced disease. The number of effector-to-target bindings was normal, even in patients with reduced NK function. However, the number of active lytic effectors was decreased. These results suggested that the cells that bind tumor targets are present in patients with advanced cancer, but these cells are either functionally inactive or immature. Other recent investigators (24,53) have also shown defective NK activity in patients with advanced malignancy.

Recent work by Hanna and colleagues (18,19) has definitively demonstrated in an *in vivo* model that NK cells can inhibit tumor spread, including the metastatic spread of circulating tumor emboli from a transplanted melanoma cell line. Therefore, the weight of clinical and recent experimental evidence suggests that NK cells play an important role in controlling the growth of malignant melanoma.

Again, with progressing disease, such lymphocytic activity has been reported to decrease. Such decreasing functional activity result from lack of competent, sensitized cells, lack of tissue antigenicity, or both. One explanation for reduced containment of tumor cells is that those that "slip through" are antigenically altered and, thus, escape being killed by sensitized effector cells. It has also been suggested that migrating tumor cells actually lose their antigenic quality and are therefore no longer detected as foreign.

NATURALLY OCCURRING CYTOTOXICITY AND TUMOR CONTROL

As previously discussed, tumor cells are adaptive within an immunological environment, and subpopulations within heterogeneous tumors have been reported to escape specific T-cell cytolytic attack. In contrast, populations of cells within the natural immune system have been shown to be effective in killing such heterogeneous tumor masses, including circulating tumor emboli (19). Such natural effector cells include natural killer (NK) cells and a phagocytic cell, the macrophage. A major focus for our studies has been concerned with NK activity and its influence on progression of breast carcinoma or malignant melanoma, and this lymphocyte subset is further described here.

Natural killer cells comprise a defense system in which the effector cells appear to have an innate ability to recognize and kill neoplastic cells (21,23) as well as other targets. Unlike cytotoxic T cells, no antigen priming is required for NK cells to exert their toxic activities. Various *in vivo* models suggest that defects in NK activity can be correlated with increased susceptibility to malignancies, particularly lymphomas (20). A study of ours (35) demonstrated that there was a high correlation between reduced NK activity and spread of breast cancer to regional lymph nodes.

Other evidence for the importance of NK cell activity includes correlations between levels of this cell function and the growth of transplanted tumors in animal models (19,22). Similarly, susceptibility to spontaneous mammary tumors in C3H mice and spontaneous lymphomas in AKR mice correlates with low NK function (17). *In vitro*, NK cells have been shown to be cytolytic for a broad spectrum of neoplastic cells (leukemias, carcinomas, sarcomas, melanomas) (22).

Recent studies (54; D. Strayer, W. Carter, and I. Brodsky, *unpublished data*) of healthy women with a family history of breast cancer, and of individuals with high familial incidences of various cancers including melanoma, showed significantly lower NK cytotoxicity compared to individuals without such a family history. Clinical studies indicate that patients with a variety of advanced cancers (including breast cancer and melanoma) had lower NK activity against K562 cells, a human lymphocytic leukemia cell line, than those with localized malignancies (40). Of note, the number of NK cells, as determined by monoclonal antibody studies, was normal, but the functional target cell-killing capacity was depressed.

The Immune System and the Neuroendocrine System

Increasing evidence indicates that the nervous system can effect considerable control over the immune system (4) and that proteins produced by monocytes also moderate glucocorticoid blood levels and ACTH via the pituitary–adrenal axis (11) (see supplement to *The Journal of Immunology,* Vol. 135, 2, August, 1985). Among the possible mediators of the CNS immune activities are neuropeptides and hormones such as steroids and catecholamines.

In addition, lymphocytes have receptors for neuropeptides (e.g., Met-enkephalin) and produce hormone-like substances (e.g., lymphokines such as interferon). In fact, Blalock (5) has argued that because of common peptide signals between the immune system and CNS–endocrine system (e.g., ACTH produced by both lymphocytes and pituitary), common receptors (e.g., receptors for neuropeptides on both endocrine and immune tissues), and common function (e.g., products of lymphocytes such as interferon have hormone-like action), both the central nervous system and the immune system serve sensory functions within the organism. Pert and colleagues (46) discussed the functional implications of the findings that a network of cells in the brain, glands, and immune system probably communicate via the same chemicals and receptors. They suggest that this "psychoimmunoendocrine network" plays a major role in regulating vertebrate homeostasis.

THE NATIONAL CANCER INSTITUTE AND PITTSBURGH STUDIES (1979–1987)

As indicated earlier, for decades there have been case reports and clinical anecdotes that suggested that attitudes, behaviors, and beliefs of cancer patients played some role in their disease progression. In 1979, there was a report published in the *Journal of the American Medical Association* (13) that demonstrated an independent association between psychosocial factors and survival in advanced breast cancer patients. This article attracted wide public attention. At that point, I and my collaborators decided to begin to address the question.

Below, I briefly describe findings from a series of studies that began at that time. On the basis of these findings, as well as the findings from other studies that have also appeared in the meantime, we have developed a causal schema that is discussed in the final section of this chapter.

Study of Survival in Advanced Breast Cancer Patients

In 1979, a study of survival time in advanced breast cancer patients (NCI Protocol #80-C-49) was initiated at the National Cancer Institute (37). Thirty-four first-recurrent breast cancer patients having no previous chemotherapy (mean age 52 years) were administered a structured interview and were given a self-report psychiatric rating instrument, the Symptom Checklist-90 (SCL-90) (12), as well as a mood measure, the Affect Balance Scale (ABS). The patients were rated on a brief behavioral rating form, the Global Adjustment to Illness Scale (GAIS) (42), which has also been shown in previous research to be a valid measure of psychological function in cancer patients (43). Patients were also rated by observers on the Karnofsky Scale (31), a measure of physical disability status.

Biological prognostic factors that have been shown to be associated with length of survival were recorded from patients' charts. These factors included the disease-free interval (DFI), number and direness of metastatic site(s), numbers of nodes positive at primary diagnosis, and age. Patients were assessed at base line and again at 3 months and were followed until recurrence of disease. Twenty-four patients in the original sample have died.

When stratified by living longer than, versus shorter than, 2 years, long survivors had significantly more positive affect at base line ($t = 2.3$, $p < 0.03$), a longer physician's prognosis ($t = 2.0$, $p < 0.05$), significantly more joy ($t = 3.0$, $p < 0.009$), and less depression ($t = 1.8$, $p < 0.08$) than shorter survivors. Using a Cox's survival hazards model (30), disease-free interval (DFI), number of metastatic sites, age, and cell histology were always entered into the stepwise analysis.

We then also attempted to enter psychological factors significantly associated, by Pearson correlations or by simple t tests, with survival time. The most significant model predicting length of survival included the variables disease-free interval, joy, physician's prognosis, and number of metastatic sites ($\chi^2 = 23.0, p < 0.0001$). A long DFI, more joy expressed at base line (measured by the Affect Balance Scale), longer physician's prognosis, and fewer metastatic sites were significantly associated with longer survival.

In all likelihood, the affect variable labeled joy had overlapping variance with a number of biologically relevant factors—host resilience, vigor, stamina, etc. But the psychological expression associated with this undoubtedly complex phenomenon was joy. This finding is consistent with recent epidemiological data reported by Reynolds and Kaplan (49). Cancer mortality data from the Alameda County cohort showed that well-being and happiness predicted reduced cancer incidence and mortality from hormonally dependent tumors for women in that large population study.

Study of Prognosis in Early-Stage Breast Cancer Patients

In late 1981, we began gathering data on early-stage breast cancer patients who were being studied at the National Cancer Institute. Because this study has been published (35), the findings are briefly summarized.

This study investigated the predictive power of natural killer (NK) cell activity as well as selected psychological and demographic factors on breast cancer prognostic risk status. It was found that NK activity predicted the presence or absence of cancer spread to the axillary lymph nodes. Those patients with higher NK activity tended to have fewer nodes positive with cancer.

We then investigated the relative contribution of both clinically and theoretically derived behavioral, psychological, and demographic variables to NK activity at the time of primary treatment by step-wise multiple-regression analysis. After the observer rating (GAIS), a measure of perceived social support, and the POMS subscale Fatigue were entered into the equation, the other variables, including delay in diagnosis and age, accounted for only a very small amount of additional NK variance. With all of the variables entered into the equation ($F_{3,41} = 14.3, p < 0.0001$), we could account for 52% of the NK activity variance. However, 51% of the NK variance could be accounted for by the first three variables alone. Patients who were rated as well adjusted, who reported having less than desirable support in their environment, and who responded with fatigue-like symptoms (lack of vigor, listless, apathetic, etc.) tended to have lower NK activity. We have also replicated these findings at the 3-month follow-up period (36).

We are continuing to follow the NCI samples, tabulating instances of recurrence and deaths. Final analyses will be performed in the next year. In the meantime, an expansion of the NCI investigation has been initiated at the University of Pittsburgh School of Medicine. We have expanded the number of biological mediators that are being examined to include various hormones—urinary catecholamines, cortisol, and endogenous opioids—as well as measurements of lymphocyte phenotypes and functional assays of NK cells. We have also refined the psychological measures of coping and social support. To date, we have accrued approximately 80 patients to this study and intend to increase accrual to a total of 122 patients.

Pilot Study of Survival and Biological Vulnerability in Melanoma Patients and Healthy Normals

As an outgrowth of the breast cancer work, a pilot study of stress, coping, and biological outcome in melanoma patients and normal volunteers (NCI Protocol #84-C-09) was initiated at the NCI. We expanded the biological mediators measure to include not only NK activity but also urinary catecholamine excretion as a general distress index.

For the advanced melanoma patients (stage III), although the pilot sample was quite small ($N = 13$), we found significant correlations between natural immunity and distress indicators. Negative associations were found between NK activity and tension (-0.87), depression (-0.61), fatigue (-0.85), total Profile of Mood States (POMS) score (-0.64), and state anxiety (-0.69). Interestingly, positive correlations were found between NK activity and vigor ($+0.70$), state curiosity ($+0.55$), state anger ($+0.60$), and trait curiosity ($+0.74$). Given the size of this pilot sample, such clusters of strong correlations are somewhat surprising. But on the whole, these findings make clinical sense. These results also indicated to us that psychosocial factors may also play a role even in advanced disease. Because of these findings, we are also studying prospectively intermediate and advanced melanoma patients with the aim of identifying factors predicting differential outcome of disease in these samples.

For the healthy volunteer sample, the most interesting finding, based on recent work in Japan (T. Aoki, T. Usuda, H. Miyakoshi, K. Tamura, and R. Herberman, *unpublished data*), was the identification of a subgroup at particular risk for follow-up infectious illness severity. These individuals were characterized as having persistently lower levels of NK activity (LNK syndrome) at all three base-line times of measurement. Individuals with normal functional levels of natural immunity were much less likely to report serious follow-up illness than individuals with persistently suppressed NK activity. Such "low-NK" individuals also tended to be younger and to report more hassles and less vigor than those with more normal levels of NK activity. Low-NK individuals also tended to have higher levels of norepinephrine excretion across the three times of base-line measurement, potentially reflecting higher levels of emotional distress in this subsample.

We are currently pursuing this line of investigation at the University of Pittsburgh. We will be studying comparison samples of normal and psychiatric populations to identify and characterize such immunologically compromised hosts and to develop intervention strategies—both immunological and behavioral—that will enhance host status.

GENERAL CONCLUSIONS

One general conclusion that we have begun to draw from this program of studies is that if one is interested in disease outcome as a major end-point in clinical studies of behavior and immunity, then one needs to be sophisticated in identifying samples at risk for such biological effects. Clearly, it is not difficult to demonstrate "stress" effects on immune function in a variety of populations. Studies have been carried out showing at least short-term depressive effects on T-cell subsets and NK activity as a function of stressors such as examination stress and bereavement. But very rarely is the last link made among stress, immune function, and illness end-points. Perhaps in the healthy organism there are buffering factors, not well understood, that protect the organism from deleterious stress effects associated with environmental insults. Perhaps it is only as the organism begins to fail, to become more fragile and biologically vulnerable, that such buffering factors cease to be effective. Perhaps the "So what?" can only be answered in such populations—cancer patients, those immunosuppressed for some reason, including HIV-infected individuals, or other compromised hosts such as the elderly.

We believe that we have begun to identify in this series of studies:

1. A particularly biologically vulnerable subgroup within a presumably normal population, with a particular psychological profile.
2. A particular coping style within a biologically compromised population of cancer patients, within a context of low familial support.
3. An immunological marker of host risk, principally involving functional levels of natural immunity, as well as an identification of one endocrine distress marker (catecholamine excretion) associated with host risk.

PSYCHOSOCIAL RISK FACTORS: A SCHEMATIC FRAMEWORK

Table 1 lists the major recent studies in this area—two concerned with psychological factors associated with cancer initiation and nine concerned with factors associated with prognosis or progression of disease. The major psychosocial risk factors are listed, as well as the measures used to assess these factors.

It is apparent from Table 1 that most of these studies measured different constructs and used different methods of assessment. A detailed review of these projects is beyond the scope of this chapter. But in attempting to make sense of these findings, one may consider three possibly interrelated factors associated with increased risk that emerge from this body of work: inadequate social support, cognitively generated helplessness, and inadequate expression of negative emotion. I first discuss each factor independently and then speculate about interrelationships among the factors in the proposed schema.

First, the effects of social support have been studied in cancer patient samples, but few investigators have examined the biological advantage of such support (3,10,14). Even fewer researchers have evaluated the possible mediating mechanisms linking social support and host vulnerability. As discussed previously, in our

TABLE 1 - SUMMARY OF PSYCHOBIOLOGICAL STUDIES LINKING BEHAVIOR AND CANCER END-POINTS

Investigator	Patients and Clinical End-Point	Major Constructs	Direction of Association with Worse Outcome	Measures
1. Shekelle, et al. 1981	All cancer mortality	Depression Other Psychiatric Variables	← ↔	MMPI
2. Reynolds and Kaplan 1986	All cancer incidence and mortality	Social Isolation and Unhappiness	→	Social Network Index
3. Derogatis, et al. 1979	Advanced breast cancer survival	Hostility, Guilt, Negative Affect "Adjustment" Positive Attitudes toward Treatment	← ↔ ← ↔	SCL-90 ABS GAIS Structured Interview
4. Rogentine, et al. 1979	Melanoma progression	"Adjustment to Illness"	→	Adjustment to Illness Rating Scale (1-100)
5. Visintainer and Casey 1984	Melanoma progression	Problem Minimization Anxiety, Hostility NK Cell Activity	← ↔ →	Ways of Coping Checklist SCL-90
6. Levy, et al. 1985	Early stage breast cancer prognosis	"Adjustment" Listlessness, Apathy Social Support NK Cell Activity	← ↔ ← ↔	GAIS POMS Interview Subscale
7. Temoshok, et al. 1985	Melanoma prognosis	Type C, Younger Ss (Cooperative, Unassertive, Suppresses Negative Emotions, Complies with External Authority)	←	Content Analysis of Videotaped Interview Subscale: Non-verbal Type C - 17 Semantic Differential Scales
8. Greer, et al. 1985	Early stage breast cancer survival	Stoic Helpless	← ↔	Categorical Ratings of Baseline Interview Content
9. Levy, et al. 1986	Early stage breast cancer prognosis– Predictors of NK activity on follow-up	"Adjustment" Listlessness, Apathy Social Support	← ↔ ←	GAIS POMS Interview
10. Levy, et al. 1986	Advanced breast cancer survival	Disease-free Interval Joy Doctor's Prognosis Number of Metastatic Sites	→ → → ←	Affect Balance Scale

study of early-stage breast cancer patients (35), perceived social support from family members proved to be a significant predictor variable. Women who complained about a lack of social support in their environment—for example, decreased communication with spouse and general inadequacy of family social support system—tended also to be in the worst prognostic category. This variable accounted for nearly 15% of the NK variance in our sample. Recently, Reynolds and Kaplan (49) reported findings from a large population study that showed that women who were socially isolated, and who also felt isolated, were at significantly enhanced risk for both cancer incidence (relative hazard $= 1.7$, $p < 0.05$) and mortality (relative hazard $= 2.5$, $p < 0.005$) from all sites and for cancer mortality from hormonally dependent tumor sites (relative hazard $= 4.8$, $p < 0.01$) after controlling for other risk factors.

The area of social support research has been fraught with methodological difficulties. But based on the weight of evidence, the quality of perceived social support may play an important role in host vulnerability to stress and, hence, disease risk.

Second, we have included cognitively generated helplessness because of preliminary findings linking this factor to cancer outcome (16,37) and especially because of the parallel animal model linking helplessness with experimental tumor growth (28,50,52). This latter work has demonstrated not only plausible biological mediating mechanisms linking helplessness and tumor outcome but also a causal direction linking behavior of a certain kind—"depressive-like"—and tumor response. In the recent reformulation of the learned helplessness construct (1), depression is thought to be caused by a function of self-statements or causal explanations. Although depression per se has not emerged as an independent factor in most clinical studies of cancer progression, such lack of association may be because of the third factor in this proposed schema, namely, distorted or inadequate negative emotional expression.

In a recent review of this area, Cox and MacKay (10) concluded that the inability to express emotion was probably the most significant psychological risk factor related to cancer progression. Variously characterized as repressive/defensive coping (27), stoicism (16), and type C behavior (55), such lack of negative emotional expression has been repeatedly associated with worse cancer outcome.

It is likely important to distinguish lack of distress from lack of distress expression. Jensen (27) found that although breast cancer patients with the worst prognosis reported little in the way of distress symptoms, they nevertheless reported physical symptoms of chronic tension (e.g., trouble sleeping, trouble relaxing, and higher levels of stress-associated hormones). Primate studies have shown a dissociation between overt distress in separated infants and biological indices of distress response (9,34).

Therefore, "distress" is probably associated with worse outcome in these samples, but it is distress of a certain kind. Sklar and Anisman (52) suggested that when the organism cannot effect coping behavior outwardly on its stress-producing environment, all homeostatic resolution is forced within, taxing the organism. Perhaps there is a parallel clinical phenomenon. For historical, constitutional, and/or developmental reasons, the at-risk patient may not express a negative emotional disturbance that nevertheless takes its toll. Perhaps the only distress-produced negative affect that does get expressed may take the form of depressive/fatigue-like somatic symptoms. In fact, such an individual might be at double risk, suffering the ill effects of distress and its chronic suppression.

In the prospective schema proposed, there are a variety of possible interrelationships among the schematic elements. I am hypothesizing that a major social–environmental background factor is the patient's quality of social support. There is, in fact, evidence that social support, measured in a variety of ways, has survival advantage. In our schema, social support could operate through cognitive factors, with other persons providing cues and modeling and reinforcing active coping solutions during environmental stress. Successful coping could enhance self-esteem, making it more likely that the person will attribute the source of positive outcomes to his or her own ability. Such successful coping may facilitate more rapid stress reduction, with homeostatic, neuroendocrine, and immune function relatively buffered from severe chronic stress sequelae. Such optimal physiological regulation would then presumably play a buffering role relative to disease end-points.

Alternatively, social factors could act directly on emotional expressiveness, perhaps by others shaping the person habitually to inhibit negative emotional expression. The opposite, optimal social support, could facilitate expression of distress in response to crisis, promoting facilitating of distress reactions and allowing the safe expression of negative affect. In fact, Lehman et al. (33) found that positive social support during a severe crisis provided the opportunity, welcomed by the victim, to express disturbance.

Of course, social support could operate directly on disease outcome by some mechanism other than those we considered here. For example, an adequate support system could enhance medical compliance and thus affect recurrence of disease. Similarly, social and psychological factors could affect disease end-points through biological mechanisms other than the specific neuroendocrine and immune factors we propose to examine. There currently exist data analytic techniques that allow for the examination of both simple and compound paths in order to test the causal direction proposed here.

The above are possible paths linking these psychosocial variables to cancer outcome via neuroendocrine and immune factors. Clearly, there are potential bidirectional effects that could occur. For example, cognitive helplessness and emotional distortion could affect the individual's quality of social support. Further, host status, reflected in hormonal and/or immunological function, could affect mood and behavior. More simply, worsening of disease status could alter the structure of social support. Again, there are statistical tests available (27) to test such directionality of association.

CONCLUDING REMARKS

The basic question is this. We and others have found ample correlations linking behavior and disease outcome. If we change the behavior, does it make any difference in terms of progression of disease? Animal work in this area suggests that it would (29). But we need to answer the question in human studies. Ultimately, to answer the question "So what?" we must demonstrate a causal link in man.

It is important to stress at this point that the major determiner of disease outcome—whether HIV infection or cancer—is the biology of the disease process itself. In addition, at least for malignancy, the stage of disease at diagnosis and the biological therapeutics that are applied are also of major significance in terms of outcome. But for HIV infection as well as malignancy, if behavior matters (and at least for cancer, it is beginning to look as though it does), then this is important because behavior can be changed. Whether such behavior change will make any difference or not is the question that we and others are just beginning to address.

REFERENCES

1. Abramson, L., Seligman, M., and Teasdale, J. (1978): Learned helplessness in humans: Critique and reformulation. *J. Psychosom. Res.*, 27:177–183.
2. Beatson, G. (1896): On the treatment of inoperable cases of carcinoma of the mammary: Suggestions for a new method of treatment with illustrative cases. *Lancet*, 2:104–107.
3. Berkman, L., and Syme, L. (1979): Social networks, host resistance, and mortality: A nine-year follow-up study of Alameda County residents. *Am. J. Epidemiol.*, 2:186–204.
4. Besedovsky, H., Del Rey, A., Sorkin, E., and Dinarello, C. (1986): Immunoregulatory feedback between Interleukin-1 and glucocorticoid hormones. *Science*, 233:652–654.
5. Blalock, J. (1984): The immune system as a sensory organ. *J. Immunol.*, 132:1067–1070.
6. Bodurtha, A., Berkelhammer, J., Kim, Y., Laucius, J., and Mastrangelo, M. (1976): A clinical, histologic, and immunologic study of a case of metastatic malignant melanoma undergoing spontaneous remission. *Cancer*, 37:735–742.
7. Carey, T. (1982): Immunologic aspects of melanoma. *CRC Crit. Rev. Clin. Lab. Sci.*, 18:141–182.
8. Cochran, A. (1978): *Man, Cancer, and Immunity*. Academic Press, New York.
9. Coe, C., and Levine, S. (1981): Normal responses to mother–infant separation in nonhuman primates. In: *Anxiety: New Research and Changing Concepts*, edited by D. Klein and J. Rabkin, pp. 155–177. Raven Press, New York.
10. Cox, T., and MacKay, C. (1982): Psychosocial factors and psychophysiological mechanisms in the etiology and development of cancers. *Soc. Sci. Med.*, 16:381–396.
11. Del Rey, A., Besedovsky, H., and Sorkin, E. (1984): Endogenous blood levels of corticosterone control the immunologic cell mass and B cell activity in mice. *J. Immunol.*, 133:572–575.
12. Derogatis, L. (1977): *Administration, Scoring, and Procedures Manual for the SCL-90-R*. Clinical Psychometric Research, Baltimore.
13. Derogatis, L., Abeloff, M., and Melisaratos, N. (1979): Psychological coping mechanisms and survival time in metastatic breast cancer. *J.A.M.A.*, 242:1504–1509.
14. Funch, D., and Mettlin, C. (1982): The role of support in relation to recovery from breast surgery. *Soc. Sci. Med.*, 16:91.
15. Funch, D., and Marshall, J. (1983): The role of stress, social support and age in survival from breast cancer. *J. Psychosom. Res.*, 27:177–183.

16. Greer, S., Pettingale, K., Morris, T., and Haybiate, J. (1985): Mental attitudes to cancer: An additional prognostic factor. *Lancet*, 1:750.
17. Hanna, N. (1986): *In vivo* activities of NK cells against primary and metastatic tumors in experimental animals. In: *Immunobiology of Natural Killer Cells*, edited by E. Lotzova and R. Herberman. CRC Press, Boca Raton, FL.
18. Hanna, N., and Barton, R. (1981): Definitive evidence that natural killer (NK) cells inhibit experimental tumor metastasis *in vivo*. *J. Immunol.*, 127:1754–1758.
19. Hanna, N., and Fidler, I. (1980): Role of natural killer cells in the destruction of circulating tumor emboli. *J. Natl. Cancer Inst.*, 65:801–809.
20. Henderson, D., and Cannellos, G. (1980): Cancer of the breast: The past decade, Part I. *N. Engl. J. Med.*, 302:17–30,78–90.
21. Herberman, R., and Holden, H. (1978): Natural cell-mediated immunity. *Adv. Cancer Res.*, 27:305–377.
22. Herberman, R., and Ortaldo, J. (1981): Natural killer cells: Their role in defenses against disease. *Science*, 214:24–30.
23. Herberman, R., and Santono, A. (1984): Regulation of natural killer cell activity. In: *Biological Responses in Cancer*, Vol. 2, edited by E. Mihich. Plenum Press, New York.
24. Hersey, P., Edmond, J., and McCarthy, W. (1980): Tumor-related changes in natural killer cell activity in melanoma patients: Influence of stage of disease, tumor thickness, and age of patients. *Int. J. Cancer*, 25:187–194.
25. Humphrey, L., Singla, O., and Volence, F. (1980): Immunologic responsiveness of the breast cancer patient. *Cancer*, 86:893–898.
26. James, J., Mulaik, S., and Brett, J. (1982): *Causal Analysis: Assumptions, Models, and Data*. Sage Publications, Beverly Hills.
27. Jensen, M. (1984): *Psychobiological Factors in the Prognosis and Treatment of Neoplastic Disorders*. Ph.D. dissertation, Department of Psychology, Yale University, New Haven.
28. Justice, A. (1985): Review of the effects of stress on cancer in laboratory animals: Importance of time of stress application and type of tumor. *Psychol. Bull.*, 98:108–138.
29. Kadish, A., Doyle, A., Steinhauer, E., and Ghossein, N. (1981): Natural cytotoxicity and interferon production in human cancer: Deficient natural killer activity and normal interferon production in patients with advanced disease. *J. Immunol.*, 123:1817–1822.
30. Kalbfleisch, J., and Prentise, R. (1980): *The Statistical Analysis of Failure Time Data*. John Wiley & Sons, New York.
31. Karnofsky, D., and Burchenal, J. (1949): The clinical evaluation of chemotherapeutic agents in cancer. In: *Evaluation of Chemotherapeutic Agents*, edited by C. MacLead. Columbia University Press, New York.
32. Kikuchi, K., Ishii, Y., Veno, H., and Koshiba, H. (1976): Cell-mediated immunity involved in autochthorious tumor rejection in rats. *Ann. N.Y. Acad. Sci.*, 276:188–206.
33. Lehman, D., Wortman, C., and Williams, A. (1984): Long-term effects of losing a spouse or child in a motor vehicle crash. American Psychological Association, Washington.
34. Levine, G., Johnson, D., and Gonzales, C. (1985): Behavioral and hormonal responses to separation in infant Rhesus monkeys and mothers. *Behav. Neurosci.*, 99:399–410.
35. Levy, S., Herberman, R., Maluish, A., Schlien, B., and Lippman, M. (1985): Prognostic risk assessment in primary breast cancer by behavioral and immunological parameters. *Health Psychol.*, 4:99–113.
36. Levy, S., Herberman, R., Lippman, M., and d'Angelo, T. (1987): Correlation of stress factors with sustained depression of natural killer cell activity and predicted prognosis in patients with breast cancer.
37. Levy, S., Seligman, M., Morrow, L., Bagley, C., and Lippman, M. (1987): Survival hazards analysis in first recurrent breast cancer patients: Seven-year follow-up.
38. Lewison, E. (1976): Spontaneous regression of breast cancer. *Nat. Cancer Inst. Monogr.*, 44:23.
39. Lippman, M. (1985): Can psychic factors transduced through the endocrine system alter the progression of human neoplasia? In: *Behavior and Cancer*, edited by S. Levy. Jossey-Bass Publishers, San Francisco.
40. Lotzova, E., and Herberman, R. (1986): *Immunobiology of Natural Killer Cells*, Vol. I. CRC Press, Boca Raton, FL.

41. Moore, O., and Foote, F. (1949): The relatively favorable prognosis of medullary carcinoma. *Cancer,* 2:635–642.
42. Morrow, G., Chiarello, R., and Derogatis, L. (1978): A new scale for assessing patients' psychosocial adjustment to medical illness. *Psychol. Med.,* 8:605–610.
43. Morrow, G., Feldstein, M., Adler, L., Derogatis, L., Enelow, A., Gates, C., et al. (1981): Development of brief measures of psychosocial adjustment to medical illness applied to cancer patients. *Gen. Hosp. Psychiatry,* 3:79–88.
44. Nathanson, L. (1977): Immunology and immunotherapy of human breast cancer. *Cancer Immunother.,* 2:209–224.
45. Papatestas, A., Paneviliwalla, D., Pertsemlides, D., Mulvihill, M., and Aufses, A. (1980): Association between estrogen receptors and weight in women with breast cancer. *J. Surg. Oncol.,* 13:177–180.
46. Pert, C., Ruff, M., Weber, R., and Herkendam, M. (1985): Neuropeptides and their receptors: A psychosomatic network. *J. Immunol.,* 135:820s–826s.
47. Pross, H. (1986): The involvement of natural killer cells in human malignant disease. In: *Immunobiology of Natural Killer Cells,* edited by E. Lotzova and R. Herberman. CRC Press, Boca Raton, FL.
48. Pross, H., and Baines, M. (1976): Spontaneous human lymphocyte-mediated cytotoxicity against tumour target cells. I. The effect of malignant disease. *Int. J. Cancer,* 18:593–604.
49. Reynolds, P., and Kaplan, G. (1986): Serial connections and cancer: A prospective study of Alameda County residents. In: *Society of Behavioral Medicine Meeting.*
50. Shavit, J., Lewis, J., Terman, G., Gale, R., and Liebeskind, J. (1984): Opioid peptides mediate the suppressive effect of stress on natural killer cell cytotoxicity. *Science,* 223:188–190.
51. Shimakowara, I., Imamura, M. Yamanaka, N., Ishii, Y., and Kikuchi, K. (1982): Identification of lymphocyte subpopulations in human breast cancer tissue and its significance. *Cancer,* 49:1456–1464.
52. Sklar, L., and Anisman, H. (1981): Stress and cancer. *Psychol. Bull.,* 89:369–406.
53. Steinhauer, E., Doyle, A., Reed, J., and Kadish, A. (1982): Defective natural cytotoxicity in patients with cancer: Normal number of effector cells but decreased recycling capacity in patients with advanced disease. *J. Immunol.,* 129:2255–2259.
54. Strayer, D., Carter, W., Mayberry, S., Pequignot, E., and Brodsky, I. (1984): Low natural cytotoxicity of peripheral and mononuclear cells in individuals with high family incidences of cancer. *Cancer Res.,* 44:320–324.
55. Temoshok, L., and Fox, B. (1984): Coping styles and other psychosocial factors related to medical status and to prognosis in patients with cutaneous malignant melanoma. In: *Impact of Psychoendocrine Systems in Cancer and Immunity,* edited by B. Fox and B. Newberry. C. J. Hogrefe, New York.

Psychological, Neuropsychiatric, and
Substance Abuse Aspects of AIDS,
edited by T. Peter Bridge et al.
Raven Press, New York © 1988.

Legal and Ethical Issues in the Neuropsychiatric Research in AIDS

T. Peter Bridge

Alcohol, Drug Abuse, and Mental Health Administration, Intramural Research Program, National Institute of Mental Health, National Institutes of Health, Bethesda, Maryland 20892

Reviewed elsewhere, the epidemiologic, immunopathologic, and neuropsychiatric aspects of acquired immunodeficiency syndrome (AIDS) have been discussed in detail (1,4–6). Based on the demonstrated knowledge derived from these areas of medical research, legal and ethical issues focused on AIDS evolve. As these issues are examined, it can be anticipated that clinical research policy-related decisions will likely occur. Informed decisions must be based on the experience available from those fields most likely to be affected by those decisions.

Although AIDS is a relatively new illness (2,8,15), the clinical impact [cognitive, behavioral, and motor impairment (11–13)] of the illness and the development of means to address these special needs in a research context are not new to neuropsychiatric research. Critical questions to the development of clinical research policy relevant to the mental health and drug abuse aspects of AIDS are therefore identified and examined in this chapter. Although the clear aim of research policy is the development of an integrated plan across all aspects of AIDS, such a goal is beyond the scope of this chapter. Discussion is limited, therefore, to consideration of issues and questions relevant to the mental health and substance abuse aspects of AIDS. In an area of health research such as AIDS, the data base is rapidly changing. Thus, it must be emphasized that the information presented here is current as of May, 1987 and that further research findings can considerably affect the points discussed here.

Although discussed in detail elsewhere, a brief enumeration of the basic facts of AIDS as we currently understand them is useful here.

AIDS is a fatal infectious disease transmitted through sexual contact and through parenteral exposure to instruments or blood contaminated with the virus known to cause AIDS, human immunodeficiency virus (HIV) (1,2,4–6,8,15).

Groups known to be at high risk for development of HIV infection are gay/bisexual males, intravenous (i.v.) drug users, infants born to parents with HIV infection, hemophiliacs and others transfused with blood contaminated with HIV, and sexual partners of persons with HIV infection. Of the major risk groups, approximately 66% are gay/bisexual men, 9% are gay/bisexual males who are also i.v. drug users, and 17% are i.v. drug users. Approximately 6% of current AIDS cases cannot be ascribed to any high-risk group, and half of these are from Haitian or central African backgrounds (1).

Recent research findings in the fight against AIDS are the identification of the causative viral agent for AIDS (HIV) and the development of a screening test for the presence of antibodies to HIV. This screening test, designed to detect units of blood contaminated by previous exposure to HIV, is now being utilized to screen for the presence of the antibody in humans. It is estimated that approximately 1,000,000 persons in the United States would test positive to the antibody screen. The test detects the presence of antibody to HIV but is not capable of determining the continuing presence of the virus in the blood, nor does it predict who among those infected with HIV will develop AIDS (1,4,8,15).

Current estimates are that approximately 20% of all individuals seropositive for HIV antibody will progress to develop AIDS or AIDS-related conditions (ARC). Further, it is believed that within 3 years almost all individuals with ARC will develop AIDS. By the end of this decade, it is expected that 100,000 people will die from AIDS, and by 1991, that there will be 250,000 diagnosed cases of AIDS (1,10).

AIDS is an infectious disease currently without effective medical prevention or cure. The means of preventing the spread of AIDS at present are behavioral. Clearly, behavioral science is known to those in the mental health and substance abuse fields. Many of the issues raised by these behavioral approaches have been addressed previously by those working in the mental health and substance abuse fields. Confidentiality, assessment of risk potential to society, and involuntary restraint as well as capacity to consent, poor predictors of illness outcome, and use of the physician as an agent of society are topics familiar to those working with psychiatric and substance abuse patients. Even the concept of contagious illness is not foreign to these workers. Recall that in the early 1970s substance abuse was presented in the model of an infectious public health problem and resulted in the "War on Drugs." Such observations must not be converted to the easy assumption that the answers to the behavioral controversy with AIDS are readily at hand, requiring no further consideration. AIDS presents many unique challenges to the public health community, but previous experience with behavioral techniques in the mental health and substance abuse fields can profitably be used in addressing the needs of AIDS patients, seropositive individuals, and society.

CONFIDENTIALITY

Among the most difficult issues that workers in the mental health and substance abuse fields have faced has been confidentiality of patient records. Traditionally, information revealed between physician and patient has been privileged and treated as confidential. Any diagnosis, once made and later disclosed, can prove limiting to that patient. Experience has shown, however, that neuropsychiatric and addiction diagnoses are perhaps the most prejudicial of all. These diagnoses, reflective of the behaviors associated with them, not only potentially limit the occupational aspirations of the patient but also may have impact on the ability of the patient to maintain family and community support systems, a means of livelihood, housing, and even residence in the community.

Where has the pressure come from to divulge psychiatric and substance diagnoses, and of what relevance is that to the AIDS/ARC patient or seropositive individual? The pressures are multifocal, but examples include the patient's family, employer, insurance carrier, and agencies of the government, including the courts. Certainly these examples must come to mind for the AIDS-affected communities as they hear (a) discussion of mandatory reporting of AIDS patients by name to governmental registries, (b) of donor deferral registries by name at blood banks, (c) of insurance carriers threatening to cancel health coverage to AIDS patients, or (d) of the screening of applicants to and members of the Armed Forces for HIV antibody (9,14).

Although caregivers have dealt with the process to limit confidentiality in a variety of ways, the records for both research and drug abuse clients have been given specific protections from violations of confidentiality (16). Clinicians have become circumspect regarding the data they enter into the medical record, balancing the need to provide adequate information with the need to protect the interests of their patients. Nonetheless, breaches in confidentiality of data from medical records have occurred. Because of this history, Federal statutes protect the information entered into the medical records of drug abuse clients. These protections were perceived as necessary in order to be able to enroll drug abuse clients into treatment programs. The needs of society were served by enrolling greater numbers of drug abuse clients into treatment, this benefit offsetting the evident risk of denying the courts and others access to these records. Analogous reasoning leads to the provision of confidentiality protection to participants in research projects if investigators successfully obtain Certificates of Confidentiality from the Department of Health and Human Services. Although not as broadly defined as the protections for drug abuse treatment clients, it is nonetheless the perception that the needs of society are served by providing legal protection for research participants in "sensitive" research areas with assurances of confidentiality (9).

It would seem clear that breaches in confidentiality have resulted in some negative outcomes for patients and made both the physician and patient wary of what information is included in the medical record. Further, specific legislation to protect the identity of drug abuse clients in treatment programs was enacted in order to make it more likely to enlist patients in these programs. Such action was perceived necessary to assuage the realistic concerns of the drug abuse clients that treatment would result in their identity being revealed to government (particularly legal) agencies. It is not surprising that such proposals as mandatory reporting of AIDS cases by name to state registries and case-finding techniques used with sexually transmitted diseases have generated so much controversy. Because nearly one-half of the states make homosexuality and/or i.v. drug use felonious acts, it is easy to understand the concerns of these communities affected by AIDS (9). In contrast to this history, have breaches in confidentiality ever proved of benefit to the patient?

It is a common experience in the treatment of substance-abusing patients that they must confront their behavior before any progress will be made in their treatment. Such confrontations often involve family, friends, employers, and agents of the legal system. Consider the approaches used with drunk drivers, employee assistance programs, impaired physician programs, and the like. Keeping the problem closeted often results in continuing the substance-abusing behavior pattern. Both patient and caregiver alike acknowledge the importance of such confrontations, with their attendant breach of confidentiality, as necessary for behavioral change. Behavioral responsibility relevant to AIDS means recognizing one's infectiousness, recognizing that repeated exposures to the virus can potentially accelerate the course of the illness, and initiating behavioral change to accomplish these needed behavioral changes. Similar to the situation with the substance-abusing patient, accepting responsibility for one's behavior is more likely to produce meaningful results early in the course of the illness. Although there is no intent here to "blame the victim," it is clear now that certain behaviors vastly increase the likelihood of exposure to HIV once it has been introduced into a population. To minimize this point is to endanger those potentially at risk for HIV infection and society in general. Although confrontation can be stigmatizing and patronizing, it can also be, depending on the situation, responsible. In the face of compelling, compulsive behaviors such as substance abuse or highly eroticized behavior, reification of the patient's autonomy has failed. In contrast, confrontation has worked.

Evidence that these changes are possible at the macro level of analysis exists. Reported from both New York and San Francisco are dramatic decreases in the rates of certain diseases such as rectal gonorrhea associated with high-risk sexual behavior (7). Survey data from intravenous drug users indicate that there is widespread knowledge of the association of AIDS and needle sharing and that self-acknowledged needle sharing has decreased (3). The threat of AIDS appears to have a considerable impact for many individuals. Nonetheless, many individuals continue to ignore the advice from public education efforts, and it is with these individuals that the rights to confidentiality and the public health needs of the community are opposed.

These processes impacting on confidentiality reflect here, as is the case with many of the other questions to be examined in this chapter, the inherent tension between the rights of the individual and the needs of society. This tension must be acknowledged forthrightly with the patient (and their family or friends) by those who care for them. Similarly, policymakers must not minimize the long-established principle that society must protect itself from individuals who threaten the integrity or safety of the community. To do less is to erode their credibility. At issue, then, is the process by which the nature and extent of the threat are assessed.

RISK ASSESSMENT

Risk assessment as it applies to behavior usually means determining the extent to which a given individual is dangerous. Evaluating the danger of any given patient to himself or to others has long been the province of those in the mental health field. It has had, however, a checkered history. With each episode of public dangerousness (presumably secondary to mental illness), there has been an outcry for more stringent application of criteria for defining dangerousness. At the opposite pole has been the move to deinstitutionalize patients, propelled by civil rights advocates and legislative fiscal concerns. In the breach has been the notoriously poor predictive ability of even skilled clinicians to determine future dangerousness. That notwithstanding, psychiatrists have often taken polar positions in this situation, and their public controversy has devalued the impact of their statements.

Among the processes that reflect the tension between the rights of the individual and the rights of society that touches on risk assessment is the "duty to warn," which is part of the Tarasoff ruling (17). Established in the Tarasoff rule is the responsibility of a treating physician to warn a potential victim based on knowledge gained in the treatment of a potentially dangerous patient. Although this rule was developed in the context of psychiatric illness, it nonetheless provides a fairly straightforward analogy in HIV infection. What does the physician treating a seropositive patient do with the information that a given patient is failing to practice safe sex or is continuing to share needles with others? Although there have been no cases to date testing this point, one can expect that litigation may arise. Failing litigation-established precedence, it is most likely that the majority of physicians will not assume this responsibility on their own. Since state legislatures and courts continue to ponder the relevance of the Tarasoff case in non-AIDS cases, this choice seems not surprising.

What can be learned from this experience of the mental health field that is relevant to the AIDS situation? Asking such a question should not seem to imply that psychiatrists and other mental health professionals have training to determine the risk of patients with infectious disease to the general community—they do not. Rather, it is their chastened state from having attempted the prediction of dangerousness with nonspecific or inaccurate instruments that is relevant. For the greatest part, informed psychiatrists now avoid making these predictions but acknowledge the value of having the tools to do so and strive to develop them. In addition, the societal pressure to make these predictions seems lessened, perhaps secondary to the perception that such predictions are highly inaccurate or perhaps secondary to the activities of civil libertarians to demonstrate the limited utility of these predictions. The same elements are present in the AIDS controversy: tests and procedures of limited predictive value, a highly volatile demand by the public for protection, and civil libertarians likely to act in concert with politically organized groups most affected by the demand for protection. It would seem, therefore, that history may repeat itself unless those working with AIDS recognize what has already taken place in the mental health arena. The lesson to be learned seems to be to rely on scientifically reliable and replicable methods. Absent that, the effort should be directed toward developing those methods rather than attempting premature efforts at risk assessment.

INVOLUNTARY RESTRAINT/QUARANTINE

Another issue addressed by those working in the mental health and drug treatment fields relevant to AIDS is that of involuntary restraint. Such actions flow naturally from the consideration of risk assessment. Not surprisingly, as the value placed in the mental health/drug treatment professional's ability to assess risk has eroded, so also has the widespread application of involuntary restraint. It remains but is considerably more difficult to institute and maintain than previously.

As before, the applicability of the experience with involuntary restraint in the mental health/drug treatment setting to the situation with AIDS must be considered. Such treatment is justified on the basis of "quarantining" someone of repeated demonstrable danger to himself or others or giving care to someone no longer capable of informed consent. Dangerous behavior as a justification for involuntary treatment has come to rest on observed behavior so compelling, or predictable by its repetitious nature, that other treatment alternatives are not feasible. Further, it is invoked when persuasion, coercion, and similar efforts have failed. Failure to be able to give consent for medically warranted treatment is a special case of involuntary treatment and has of late often resulted in the appointment of a guardian to consent for treatment. Patient advocates within the treatment system have also been utilized as a means to provide an observer from the patient's point of view to balance those provided by the caregivers.

The relevance of the experience with involuntary treatment to development of policy for AIDS appears to rest on two principles: (a) dangerousness is based on demonstrable, repeated, or compelling behavior, and (b) failure to be able to provide informed consent may prove to be common when as many as 50% of AIDS patients in advanced stages of the disease demonstrate cognitive impairment. Evidence to date indicates that spread of the HIV is linked to specific high-risk behaviors. Involuntary restraint would have to be linked not to the infection per se but to the behavior that spreads the infection. Infected individuals who continue to engage in high-risk behavior—observable, repeated, and compelling—may warrant involuntary restraint. This is particularly so if they also show evidence of cognitive impairment serious enough to affect their judgment. As was stated in the section on risk assessment, the experience of those working in behavioral treatment fields needs to be utilized in the fight against AIDS.

CONCLUSION

AIDS represents one of the most important challenges to the medical research and health care systems in this century. Much has already been accomplished, but those accomplishments (identification of the causative agent and development of the antibody test) have added to the need to mobilize behavioral and social research experience. Recognizing the behavioral component of AIDS is imperative to moving forward in the fight to combat the spread of AIDS. Drawing on the experience of those fields that have addressed issues of behavioral management and treatment would appear to be essential for the forseeable future. The identification of effective vaccines for HIV and the development of treatments for AIDS, ARC, and HIV infection in both the immune system as well as the central nervous system will make such interventions unnecessary. At the moment, however, behavioral treatments are available and effective. Vaccines and biologic treatments for AIDS are not.

REFERENCES

1. Centers for Disease Control (1986): Update: Acquired immunodeficiency syndrome. *Morbid. Mortal. Week. Rep.*, 35:22–223.
2. Centers for Disease Control (1985): Revision of the case definition of acquired immunodeficiency syndrome for national reporting—United States. *Morbid. Mortal. Week. Rep.*, 34:373–375.
3. Des Jarlais, D. C., Friedman, S. R., and Hopkins, W. (1985): Risk reduction for AIDS among intravenous drug users. *Ann. Intern. Med.*, 103:755–785.
4. Fauci, A. S., Masur, H., and Gelmann, E. P. (1985): The acquired immunodeficiency syndrome: An update. *Ann. Intern. Med.*, 102:800–813.
5. Fauci, A. S., Macher, A. M., and Longo, D. L. (1984): Acquired immunodeficiency syndrome. *Ann. Intern. Med.*, 100:92–106.
6. Gallo, R. C., Salahuddin, S. Z., and Popovic, M. (1984): Frequent detection and isolation of cytopathic retroviruses (HTLV-III) from patients with AIDS. *Science*, 224:500–502.
7. Institute of Medicine (1986): *Mobilizing Against AIDS*. Harvard University Press, Cambridge, p. 90.
8. Levy, J. A., Hoffman, A. D., and Kramer, S. M. (1984): Isolation of lymphocytotrophic retroviruses from San Francisco patients with AIDS. *Science*, 225:840–842.
9. Matthews, G. W., and Neslund, V. S. (1987): The initial impact of AIDS on public health law in the United States—1986. *J.A.M.A.*, 257:344–352.
10. Morgan, W. M., and Curran, M. W. (1986): AIDS: Current and future trends. *Public Health Rep.*, 101:459–465.
11. Navia, B. A., Jordan, B. D., and Price, R. W. (1986): The AIDS dementia complex I. Clinical features. *Ann. Neurol.*, 19:517–524.
12. Navia, B. A., Cho, E., and Petito, C. K. (1986): The AIDS dementia complex II. Neuropathology. *Ann. Neurol.*, 19:525–535.
13. Navia, B., and Price, R. W. (1987): AIDS dementia complex and the presenting sole manifestation of HIV infection. *Ann. Neurol.*, 44:65–69.
14. Pascal, C. B. (1987): Selected legal issues about AIDS for drug abuse treatment programs. *J. Psychoact. Drugs*, 19:1–12.
15. Weiss, S. H., Goedert, J. J., and Sarngadharan, M. (1985): Screening test for HTLV-III antibodies. *J.A.M.A.*, 253:221–225.
16. 42 U.S.C. 290ee-3.
17. 131 Cal. Rpt. 14, 551 P2d 340 (1976).

Subject Index

A

Abortion, spontaneous, 18
Acetylcholine receptor, for rabies virus, 57–71,78
  AIDS treatment implications, 68
  neuromuscular junction localization, 58,61
  neurotoxin binding and, 59–60,62–68,69
    synthetic glycoprotein peptide-neurotoxin competition, 64–68,69
    viral disease implications, 68,69
    viral glycoprotein-neurotoxin sequence similarity, 62–63,69
  pathogenesis and, 58,61
  saturation of binding, 60–61
  structure, 59–60
Acquired immune deficiency syndrome (AIDS). *See also* Human immunodeficiency virus (HIV) infection
  affective response in, 2,10,117
  amygdala in, 117,119
  anxiety in, 89,111
  anxiety disorder in, 111,112
  attentional deficits in, 120–122
    event-related brain potentials and, 121–122
  behavioral changes related to, 8,9,86,87–89
  biopsychosocial approach, 100–102,104,187–188
    patient care implications, 107
  in bisexuals, 145,159
  brain lesions in, 119
  in children
    gender-related differences, 160
    intravenous drug abuse and, 145
    Kaposi's sarcoma and, 166
    neuropathologic findings, 3
  cognitive function deficits in, 112–113
    event-related brain potentials, 121–122
    incidence, 246
  confidentiality regarding, 242–245
  dementia in, 19
  denial in, 88
  depression in, 8,89,90–91,92,93,112,222
    brain lesion-related, 119
    neuropsychological deficits and, 119–120
    prior depression and, 8

drug abuse and. *See also* Intravenous drug abusers, AIDS in; names of individual drugs of abuse
  neuroimmomodulatory effects, 145–158
dysphoria in, 89,117,119
emotional expression and, 194
epidemic curve, 85,86
fear related to, 222
in Haitians, 1,96–97
helplessness in, 89,100,104
hex death and, 95–100
in homosexuals
  drug abuse cofactor, 145
  first observed, 1
  hex death, 99–100
  Kaposi's sarcoma and, 165,166–167,168–169,170
  nitrate inhalant use cofactor, 165,168–169
  as percentage of total cases, 159
hopelessness in, 104,188,189
immune function in
  drug abuse and, 145–158
  stress effects, 188–189,210,212
incidence, 85,86
  predicted, 242
in intravenous drug abusers
  children of, 145
  cytomegalovirus cofactor, 161
  gender-related differences, 159–162
  Kaposi's sarcoma and, 160,161,166
  as percentage of total AIDS cases, 145
involuntary restraint/quarantine, 86,89,242,246
Kaposi's sarcoma and
  case comparison study, 167
  in children, 166
  cytomegalovirus cofactor, 170
  incidence, 166–167,170
  in intravenous drug users, 160,161,166
  nitrite inhalant use cofactor, 165–171
  Pneumocystis carinii pneumonia and, 166,167
  surveillance, 166–167
major depressive disorder in, 111,112
memory impairment in, 120
mood changes in, 117

249